MEDICAL TERMINOLOGY

Building Blocks for Health Careers

Mary E. Kinn, CPS, CMA-A

Former Assistant Professor, Health Technologies
Long Beach City College,
Long Beach, California

Past President, American Association of Medical Assistants

Past President, California Association of Medical Assistants

Former Chairman, AAMA Certifying Board

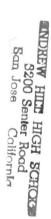
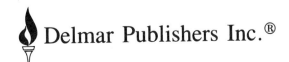

Delmar Publishers Inc.®

NOTICE TO THE READER

COVER ILLUSTRATION: Gabriel Molano

Delmar Staff

Executive Editor: Leslie F. Boyer
Associate Editor: Marjorie A. Bruce
Project Editor: Eleanor Isenhart
Production Supervisor: Karen Seebald
Design Coordinator: Susan C. Mathews

For information, address Delmar Publishers Inc.
3 Columbia Circle, PO Box 15015
Albany, New York 12212-5015

Printed in the United States of America
Published simultaneously in Canada
by Nelson Canada,
A division of The Thomson Corporation

10 9 8 7 6 5 4

Library of Congress Cataloging in Publication Data

Kinn, Mary E.
  Medical terminology.

    Includes index.
    1. Medicine—Terminology. I. Title. [DNLM: 1. Nomen-
clature. W 15 K55mb]
R123.K52   1990   610′.14   88-33415
ISBN 0-8273-3338-2 (pbk.)
ISBN 0-8273-3339-0 (instructor's guide)

CONTENTS

Part I
Introduction to Vocabulary Building

Chapter 1
The Elements of a Medical Vocabulary   **1**

Introduction   2
Commonly Used Terms   2
Learning and Remembering Medical Terms   3
Combining Vowels   5
Adjective Endings   6
A Guideline for Word Formation   7
Forming Plurals   7
Pronouncing Medical Terms   8
The Importance of Spelling Medical Terms Correctly   10
Reviews   11

Chapter 2
Frequently Used Building Blocks   **13**

Frequently Used Suffixes   15
Frequently Used Roots   18
Frequently Used Prefixes   21
Reviews   24

Chapter 3
General and Structural Terms   **31**

Using Your New Vocabulary   32
Points of Reference   33
Structural Units of the Human Body   33
Planes of the Body   34
Body Cavities   35
The Anatomic Position   36
Directional Terms   38
Body Motions   38
Anatomic Regions of the Abdomen   40
Clinical Divisions of the Abdomen   40
Anatomic Regions of the Back   41
Building Blocks   42
Vocabulary   44
Reviews   46

PART II
Body Systems

Chapter 4
Integumentary System 55

Overview 57
Structure of the Skin 57
Skin Appendages 59
Building Blocks 60
Vocabulary 62
Reviews 69

Chapter 5
Skeletal System 77

Structure and Function of the Skeletal System 78
Types of Bones, Structure, and Bone Markings 80
Divisions of the Skeleton 82
Joints 89
Fractures 89
Building Blocks 92
Vocabulary 93
Reviews 99

Chapter 6
Muscular System 109

Overview 110
Types of Muscle Tissue 110
Muscle Attachments 111
Muscle Parts 111
Muscle Functions 111
Building Blocks 115
Vocabulary 117
Reviews 123

Chapter 7
Circulatory, Lymphatic, and Immune Systems 133

Overview 136
The Heart 138
Blood Vessels 140
Blood 141
Lymphatics 142
Spleen 142
Thymus 142
Immune System 145
Building Blocks 147
Vocabulary 148
Reviews 158

Chapter 8
Respiratory System   169

Overview   170
Structure and Function   170
Building Blocks   176
Vocabulary   178
Reviews   185

Chapter 9
Digestive System   195

Overview   197
Primary Digestive Organs   197
Accessory Digestive Organs   201
Building Blocks   205
Vocabulary   206
Reviews   216

Chapter 10
Male Reproductive System   227

Overview   228
Male Gonads   229
Duct System   230
Glands   230
External Genitalia   231
Building Blocks   233
Vocabulary   234
Reviews   240

Chapter 11
Female Reproductive System   249

Overview   251
Female Gonads (Ovaries)   251
Internal Organs   252
External Structures   253
Mammary Glands (Breasts)   256
Hormones   256
Menstruation   257
Menopause   257
Building Blocks   257
Vocabulary   259
Reviews   272

Chapter 12
Urinary System   285

Overview   286
Kidneys   288

Ureters 290
Urinary Bladder 291
Urethra 291
Urine 291
Building Blocks 292
Vocabulary 293
Reviews 300

Chapter 13
Endocrine System

309

Overview 311
Structure and Function 311
Building Blocks 314
Vocabulary 315
Reviews 323

Chapter 14
Nervous System

331

Overview 332
Neurons and Nerves 332
Central Nervous System 335
Peripheral Nervous System 338
Medical Care and the Nervous System 338
Building Blocks 339
Vocabulary 340
Reviews 351

Chapter 15
Special Senses: Sight and Hearing

361

Overview 363
Structure and Function of the Eye 363
Visual Acuity 365
Refractive Disorders 366
Common Ophthalmic Diseases 366
Building Blocks 366
Vocabulary 367
Structure and Function of the Ear 374
Common Disorders of the Ear 377
Building Blocks 377
Vocabulary 378
Reviews 381

Chapter 16
Health Professions
395

Overview   396
Medicine   396
Nursing   400
Allied Health   401
Reviews   403

Appendix I
Additional Medical and Surgical Terms
406

Selected Terms Relating to Signs and Symptoms   406
Selected Terms Relating to Examination and Treatment   410
Selected Terms Relating to Diagnostic Procedures   415
Selected Terms Relating to a Disease or Condition   417

Appendix II
Commonly Used Abbreviations
421

Appendix III
Glossary of Building Blocks
435

Index
457

PREFACE

INTRODUCTION

Many of the available texts on medical terminology are too comprehensive to complete in the time allotted for the formal classroom, and too intimidating for self-study. *MEDICAL TERMINOLOGY—Building Blocks for Health Careers* is designed as a simplified approach to building a practical medical vocabulary. The text is appropriate for either self-paced home study or a short-term formal course.

The objectives in this study of medical terminology are to:

- correctly spell medical terms
- use accepted pronunciation for medical terms and
- precisely define medical terms.

To be useful, the medical terms must become a comfortable part of one's vocabulary. By completing the exercises throughout the text, learners can build a usable medical vocabulary. The sample readings in this text are representative of actual reports dictated by physicians in their practices. Working with these readings will give the learner a feel for the use of common terminology in context.

A grasp of medical terminology is a basic requirement for most career opportunities in the allied health occupations. Those who have a workable medical vocabulary will find positions in many settings, including physicians' offices, hospitals, laboratories, emergency care centers, medical and surgical equipment firms, insurance companies, medical associations, and federal, state and local medical administrations.

ORGANIZATION OF THE TEXT

Part I, Introduction to Vocabulary Building, consists of Chapters 1, 2 and 3. Chapter 1 relates medical terms to the learner's everyday vocabulary, illustrating that most medical terminology is based on combining easily learned word components, or *building blocks*. Chapter 2 provides an extensive list of frequently used *building blocks*. Chapter 3 follows with general and structural terms that apply to all parts of the body.

These three chapters are the foundation upon which the learner builds a medical vocabulary. If time is very limited, these introductory chapters can be the basis for a short course in medical terminology, with the learner following up with a self-paced study of the remaining chapters.

Part II, Body Systems, is presented in the generally accepted sequence of studies in anatomy and physiology. Therefore, the learner who is concurrently studying anatomy and physiology will find that one class reinforces learning in the other. However, each chapter is independent of the others and the instructor may use any preferred sequence.

Each chapter in Part II begins with objectives, followed by a brief list of key terms that assists the learner in understanding the synoptic review of the body system. The system review is followed by a listing of the *building blocks* for the chapter vocabulary. The vocabulary is subdivided into:

- general terms
- terms related to anatomy and physiology

- terms related to pathology
- terms associated with diagnostic devices and procedures
- terms related to surgery and treatment

Phonetic pronunciation is included for each term. Definitions are simplified as much as possible.

Every chapter includes review exercises to assist learners in their study, and then to reinforce and test the learning that has taken place. Each chapter in Part II includes actual medical records and reports that introduce the student to the world of health care. These reading comprehension exercises can be read aloud and discussed in the classroom if time permits. Reading aloud is important for gaining confidence in pronouncing medical terms. Learners can use them to test their own reading comprehension skills and add to their medical vocabulary. Some of the readings may be difficult for the learners to understand. They are not intended as testing materials, but they do illustrate how medical terms are used and they may serve as a springboard for further study. Chapter 16, Health Professions, briefly describes each medical specialty, the several levels of nursing, and allied health professions.

Appendix I provides an extensive vocabulary covering additional medical and surgical terms that do not relate specifically to one body system. These are divided into selected terms relating to:

- signs and symptoms
- examination and treatment
- diagnostic procedures
- disease or condition

Appendixes II and III include over 600 commonly used abbreviations and acronyms and a glossary of the *building blocks*. An index to the chapter vocabularies is also provided.

SUPPLEMENT

The text is accompanied by an Instructor's Guide which is designed to help the instructor implement a medical terminology course. The guide consists of the following content:

- General Plan of the Guide
- Organization of Text
- Planning the Course
- Study Methods
- Application of Learning
- Testing
- Reference Materials
- Instructional Objectives
- Answers to Text Reviews

- Chapter Tests
- Answers to Test Questions
- Application—Autopsy Report
- Transparency Masters

ACKNOWLEDGMENTS

The author acknowledges with grateful appreciation the contribution of material for this text from:

Kay Cox, RN   Joseph K. Cummings, MD
Hugh M. Firemark, MD   Stephen Goldberger, MD
Sondra Sue Hein, CMT   Edward W. Kim, MD
James A. Padova, MD   W. Allen Schade, MA
Arthur D. Silk, MD   Theodore Van Dam, MD

The following individuals provided extensive reviews of the manuscript and provided valuable guidance to the author. Their contributions are most appreciated.

Ann Frasier, Program Coordinator, Detroit College, Dearborn, MI 48126-3799

William J. Lorman, Director of Education, National Schools, Inc., Philadelphia, PA 19107

Lois H. Johnson, State Specialist, Health Occupations, State Department of Education, Montgomery, AL 36130

Helen R. Gemeinhardt, Medical Curriculum Specialist, National Education Centers, Inc. Irvine, CA 92714

Bernadette A. Bly, The Bryman School, Salt Lake City, UT 84111-3209

Ann Senisi, Coordinator of Nursing/Health Occupations, Nassau Tech Board of Cooperative Educational Services, Westbury, NY 11590

Janet Dancy, Central Piedmont Community College, Charlotte, NC 28210

PART I

INTRODUCTION TO VOCABULARY BUILDING

CHAPTER 1

The Elements of a Medical Vocabulary

OBJECTIVES

When you have successfully completed Chapter 1, you should be able to:
— Relate words in your everyday vocabulary to the building of medical terms.
— Understand the basic process of word building.
— Form plurals of most nouns.
— Correctly pronounce the terms you have learned.
— Understand the importance of spelling medical terms carefully.

adjective	A word used with a noun to modify its meaning
analyze	To separate into elements or parts
consonant	A letter of the alphabet other than *a, e, i, o, u*
diphthong	A blend of two vowel sounds in one syllable
interpret	To explain or tell the meaning of
noun	A word that is the name of something, such as a person, place, thing, or idea
plural	The form of a word denoting more than one
pronounce	To say words or syllables aloud
syllable	Several letters taken together to form one sound
vocabulary	A list or collection of words
vowel	One of the letters *a, e, i, o, u.* The letter *y* sometimes serves as a vowel.

INTRODUCTION

This text has two main purposes:

1. To help you build a medical vocabulary easily and quickly, and
2. To assist you in interpreting medical terms as they are used in medical practice.

In this first chapter, we will talk about the way that medical terms are built. We will analyze the terms, and you will have practice exercises to help you remember. In later chapters you will learn how to interpret medical terminology as it is used by physicians and other health professionals.

COMMONLY USED TERMS

You may not realize that many medical terms are already a part of your vocabulary. You've seen them in print—in advertisements, for instance; you've heard them in television programs; and you've used them in conversation. Let's analyze a few medical terms that you are likely to have heard. Like the new medical terms you'll be learning later on, they are formed from combinations of parts.

abnormal	*ab–* is a word beginning, or prefix, often used in medical terms. It means *away from.*

anemia	*an–* is a prefix meaning *not* or *without*. *–emia* is a word ending, or suffix, meaning *blood condition*.
appendectomy	*–ectomy* is a suffix used in surgical terms; it means *taking out* (excision) or *removing*; *append–* refers to the appendix.
arthritis	*arthr* is a word root meaning *joint*; *–itis* is a suffix meaning inflammation.
cardiogram	*cardio* is a combining form referring to the heart; *–gram* is a suffix meaning *a recording*.
diarrhea	*dia–* is a prefix meaning *through*; *–rhea* is a suffix meaning *flow*.
hydrophobia	*hydro–* is a root meaning *water*; *–phobia* means *fear*. It is the medical term for rabies, a disease in which the victim fears water because swallowing it leads to painful spasms.
hypodermic	The prefix *hypo–* means *beneath*; the suffix *–dermic* means *having to do with the skin*. A hypodermic syringe (needle) injects fluid beneath the skin.
neuralgia	*neur–* is the root for *nerve*; the word ending *–algia* means *pain* in the body part it follows.
tracheotomy	*trache* is the medical root for *trachea* (the windpipe); *–otomy* is a surgical suffix that means a *cutting* or *incision*.

These are only a few examples of words that you may already have heard and used. You may feel quite comfortable with them. As you work through this text, you'll find the new terms becoming just as comfortable.

LEARNING AND REMEMBERING MEDICAL TERMS

Let's begin by learning some word parts. Medical terms have three basic elements: (1) roots, (2) prefixes, and (3) suffixes (Figure 1.1).

- The *root* is that part of a word that can stand alone and have meaning.
- A *prefix* is a letter or group of letters placed *before* the root or roots to change (modify) their meaning.
- A *suffix* is a letter or group of letters placed after the root or roots to change (modify) their meaning.

Like the plastic blocks that children play with, these basics forms can be linked in hundreds of different ways to create different meanings. By thinking of them as *building blocks*, you can make building a medical vocabulary into a game.

Once you have learned a word and understand its meaning, you should be able to use it forever. Most medical terms do not change their meanings. Sometimes the logic of the way the word was formed no longer makes sense because of new discoveries. For example, the term *artery* comes from the Greek word *arteria*, which means windpipe yet we now know that arteries carry blood, not air. The ancient Greeks believed that the

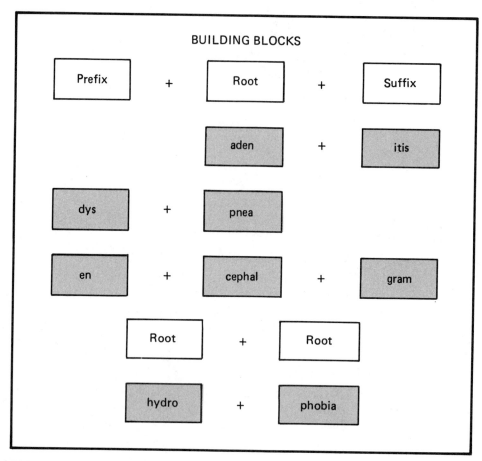

FIGURE 1.1 Constructing medical terms using building blocks

arteries carried only air because their physicians had never found blood in the arteries of a cadaver (a dead body). Even so, the word "artery" remains in the medical vocabulary today, as similar terms do.

This is not to say that a medical vocabulary never changes. As advances in medicine are made, new words are coined. Others are discarded. The new words are often formed from the very building blocks that you will be mastering. These basics will always be with you to help you build and interpret new terms.

Analyzing the Structure of Words

Now, let's explore some common building blocks (Figure 1.1). In the lists of examples, you will see the building block, then its meaning, then its use in the full word, where the building block is shown in *italics*.

ROOT. The *root* of a word can stand alone and have meaning. For example:

Root	Meaning	Example
aden	gland	*aden*itis
cardi	heart	*cardi*ology
cephal	head	en*cephal*ogram
derm	skin	*derm*atosis
flex	bending	ante*flex*ion
gastr	stomach	*gastr*oscopy
hydr	water	*hydr*ophobia
my	muscle	*my*algia
neur	nerve	*neur*itis
pnea	breath	dys*pnea*

PREFIX. Recall that a *prefix* is a letter or group of letters placed before a word to change (modify) its meaning. For example:

Prefix	Meaning	Example
a–	without, not	*a*pnea
ante–	before (in time or place)	*ante*flexion
dys–	bad, painful, difficult	*dys*function (**Note:** This is an example in which *y* serves as a vowel.)
endo–	within	*endo*crine
retro–	behind, backward	*retro*grade

SUFFIX. Recall that a *suffix* is a letter or group of letters placed after a word to change (modify) its meaning. For example:

Suffix	Meaning	Example
–algia	pain, painful condition	neur*algia*
–cele	herniation or bulging	hydro*cele*
–itis	inflammation	gastr*itis*
–ology	study or science of	cardi*ology*
–pathy	disease	myo*pathy*

COMBINING VOWELS

Sometimes in our word building we need a vowel to link the parts together. A vowel used this way is called a *combining vowel*. Often it is an *o*. It may link a root to another root or a root to a suffix. When a combining vowel is added to a root, we have what is called a *combining form*. For example, in the word *adenopathy*, the root is *aden*, and the suffix is *-pathy*. We join the root and the suffix with the combining vowel *o* to make a complete word that can be easily pronounced. *Adeno* is the combining form.

Now, try your hand at analyzing the following terms. Use a slash mark (/) to separate the building blocks: prefix (if any), root, combining vowel (if any), and suffix (if any). Then list the building blocks in the table below and write in the meaning as shown in the example.

	Prefix	Root	Suffix	Meaning
a/pnea	a	-pnea	—	lack of breathing
cephalalgia	_____	_____	_____	_____
dermatology	_____	_____	_____	_____
gastrocele	_____	_____	_____	_____
adenopathy	_____	_____	_____	_____
endocardium	_____	_____	_____	_____
retroflexion	_____	_____	_____	_____

How did you do? Check yourself against the explanations below.

cephal = root	–algia = suffix	cephal/algia—head pain
dermat = root	–ology = suffix	dermat/o/logy—study or science of the skin
gastr = root	–cele = suffix	gastr/o/cele—hernia of the stomach
aden = root	–pathy = suffix	aden/o/pathy—any glandular disease
endo = prefix	cardi = root	endo/cardium—within the heart
retro = prefix	flex = root	retro/flexion—bending backward

ADJECTIVE ENDINGS

Adjectives are words that describe *nouns* by specifying size, color, number, or some quality such as hard, soft, and so on. Several adjective endings occur over and over in medical terms. When you see them combined with a root, you know that the word means "having to do with" or "pertaining to" the root meaning. For example:

- *–ac* combined with *cardi* means pertaining to the heart: *cardiac arrest* means a stopping of the heartbeat.
- *–al* combined with *oro* means pertaining to the *mouth*; *oral hygiene* means cleansing of the mouth. (Note that the *o* is dropped in making the combination.)
- *–ary* combined with *pulmon* means pertaining to the lungs; *pulmonary obstruction* means blockage of the lungs.
- *–eal* combined with *corpus* (using *o* for the combining form) means pertaining to the physical body.

Similarly:

- Hypochondr*iac* refers to the region of the hypochondrium, from which obsession with one's health was once thought to originate. (**Note:** This is an example of a term that has outlived its logic.)
- Pept*ic* signifies that the word it modifies is related to digestion or the digestive organs: *peptic ulcer.*
- Morb*id* means pertaining to disease, as rab*id* means pertaining to rabies.
- Adip*ose* means pertaining to fat, as gluc*ose* means pertaining to a specific kind of sugar.
- Muc*ous* means pertaining to mucus: the *mucous membranes.*
- Opt*ic* means pertaining to sight or to the eye.

A GUIDELINE FOR WORD FORMATION

A guideline that may help you understand how terms are combined is this: When new medical terms are formed, usually, the ending of the medical term is the first word of its meaning.

    EXAMPLE: appendicitis
    appendix   appendic/
    inflammation   /itis
    Definition: Inflammation/of the appendix

    EXAMPLE: hysterectomy
    uterus   hyster/
    excision   /ectomy
    Definition: Excision/of the uterus

This guideline can be applied to about 90 percent of terms.

FORMING PLURALS

As you have seen, many medical words have Latin roots. The plural ending of a Latin noun is determined by its gender (masculine, feminine, or neuter). We are not accustomed to dealing with genders in the English language, and you do not need to concern yourself with whether medical terms have masculine, feminine, or neuter endings. It is enough to known the basic ways that plurals are formed. For example:

	Singular (one)	Plural (more than one)	Singular (one)	Plural (more than one)
Nouns ending in	a	ae	vertebr*a* macul*a*	vertebr*ae* macul*ae*
Nouns ending in	is	es	bas*is* diagnos*is*	bas*es* diagnos*es*
Nouns ending in	um	a	ov*um* dat*um*	ov*a* dat*a*

	Singular (one)	Plural (more than one)	Singular (one)	Plural (more than one)
Nouns ending in	us	i	bronch*us*	bronch*i*
			cocc*us*	cocc*i*
Nouns ending in	ix, ex	ces	ind*ex*	ind*ices*
			append*ix*	append*ices*

There are exceptions, but you can memorize them as you use them. When in doubt, consult a good medical dictionary.

PRONOUNCING MEDICAL TERMS

You may feel uncomfortable in your first attempts to pronounce unfamiliar medical terms. Following a few basic rules will make pronunciation easier for you.

Accenting Syllables

Here are some guidelines for where to place the accent as you pronounce the word.

- The last syllable is seldom accented in medical words.
- Most two-syllable and three-syllable words are accented on the first syllable (nexus, **NECK**-sus) (niacin, **NIGH**-ah-sin).
- Every vowel or diphthong (a blend of two vowel sounds in one syllable) makes a separate syllable.
- Medical terms, even those taken directly from Latin or Greek, are usually pronounced as though they were English, with each letter being pronounced.

Pronouncing Double Consonants

In English, a consonant is any letter other than *a, e, i, o,* or *u*. These five letters are called vowels. (As already mentioned, *y* is sometimes a vowel, sometimes a consonant.) In words with certain double consonants appearing at the beginning of a word, the first consonant is silent. If this pairing of consonants appears within a word, however, both are usually pronounced. For example:

Double Consonant at Beginning	Double Consonant Within Word
gn gnosis (**NOH**-sis)	prognosis (prog-**NOH**-sis)
mn mnemic (**NEE**-mick)	amnesia (am-**NEE**-zee-ah)
pn pneograph (**NEE**-oh-graf)	apnea (ap-**NEE**-ah)
ps pseudo (**SUE**-doh)	apsychia (ap-**SICK**-ee-ah)
pt ptosis (**TOH**-sis)	hemoptysis (hee-**MOP**-tih-sis)

Pronouncing Consonant Combinations

It is helpful to know how certain consonant combinations, such as the following, are usually pronounced.

ch	is often pronounced like *k*; for example:
	chlorine (**KLOH**-reen)
	chromosome (**KROH**-moh-sohm)
	technology (teck-**NOL**-oh-jee)

ph	has the sound of *f*; for example:
	phobia (**FOH**-bee-ah)
	ophthalmology (ahf-thal-**MOL**-oh-jee)
	encephalitis (en-**sef**-ah-**LIE**-tis)

rh	has the sound of *r*; for example:
	rheumatic (roo-**MAT**-ick)
	herniorrhaphy (**her**-nee-**OR**-ah-fee)

Pronouncing C and G

Before *e*, *i*, and *y*, *c* is often given the soft sound of *s*, and *g* the soft sound of *j*. For example:

cervical (**SER**-vih-kal)

cycle (**SIGH**-kl)

geriatrics (jer-ee-**AT**-ricks)

giant (**JYE**-ant)

Before other letters, *c* and *g* have a harsh sound, found in such words as

cardiac (**KAR**-dee-ack)

cocaine (koh-**KAYN**)

gauze (gawz)

gonorrhea (**gon**-oh-**REE**-ah)

When *cc* is followed by *e*, *i*, or *y*, the first *c* is pronounced as *k* and the second *c* as *s*. For example:

coccygeal (kock-**SIH**-jee-al)

streptococceae (**strep**-toh-**KOCK**-see-ee)

occipital (ock-**SIP**-ih-tal)

Pronouncing Combined Vowels

The combinations *ae* and *oe* are pronounced *ee*; for example:

fasciae (**FASH**-ee-ee)

coelom (**SEE**-lum)

Pronouncing Word Endings

When *i* is used at the end of a word to form a plural, it has a long sound like the sound in "eye." For example:

cocci (**KOCK**-sigh)

alveoli (al-**VEE**-oh-lie)

nevi (**NEE**-vie)

As the final letter or letters of a word, *e* or *es* may be pronounced as a separate syllable. For example:

rete (**REE**-tee)

nares (**NAY**-reez)

How Local Customs Affect Pronunciation

Many words have more than one acceptable pronunciation, so you may find members of the same medical community accenting different syllables and pronouncing words differently, depending on where they learned them. For example, you may hear the word *cerebrum* pronounced **SER**-*eh-brum* or *seh*-**REE**-*brum*. Local custom may determine which is the more common. You must learn to recognize the word either way it is pronounced.

Careless Pronunciations

Sometimes, careless pronunciations lead to misspelling. A notable example of this is

ophthalmology (**AHF**-thal-**mol**-oh-jee)

which is often mispronounced (**OP**-thal-**mol**-oh-jee). The mispronunciation leads to a common misspelling—omitting the first of the two *h*'s. Another example is the word

respiratory (**REH**-spih-rah-**toh**-ree)

often carelessly pronounced (**RES**-pih **toh**-ree), which again leads to misspelling.

Pronouncing Unfamiliar Terms

Unfamiliar medical words often seem long and difficult to pronounce. These long words are usually made up of several shorter ones. Look at the word carefully, and you will probably see word parts that are familiar. Look for a vowel that may tell you where a new syllable begins. Think about the rules for accenting syllables. With a little practice you will be able to arrive at an acceptable pronunciation.

THE IMPORTANCE OF SPELLING MEDICAL TERMS CORRECTLY

Misspelling a medical word, even by adding or leaving out one letter, can entirely change its meaning. For instance:

A*b*duction	carrying away from
A*d*duction	carrying toward
Arte*r*itis	inflammation of an artery
Arth*r*itis	inflammation of a joint

| Il*e*um | lower part of small intestine |
| Il*i*um | hip bone |

The spelling of medical terms is learned through (1) memorization, and (2) understanding the meaning of the term.

The person who understands the meaning of ileum and ilium would never misinterpret them when hearing them in context, but when they stand alone there is no way to determine which is meant except through correct spelling.

Some words have more than one correct spelling. For example, *disk* and *disc, leukocyte* and *leucocyte*. A medical dictionary will help you know which is currently preferred.

Chapter 2 will introduce more of the commonly used prefixes, roots, and suffixes. Before proceeding to the next chapter, review your understanding of the chapter you have just completed.

1.1 Review

DIRECTIONS: Complete the following statements by filling in the blanks.

1. The three basic elements of medical terms are:
   a. _____ , b. _____ , and c. _____ .

2. The element that can stand alone and have meaning is the _____ .

3. A letter or group of letters placed before a word to modify meaning is a _____ .

4. A letter or group of letters placed after a word to modify meaning is a _____ .

5. When we use a vowel to link two parts of a word, this vowel is called the _____ _____ .

6. How many adjective endings that mean "pertaining to" can you remember?
   _____
   _____

7. Write the plural form of the following words:

Singular	Plural
diagnosis	_____
basis	_____
vertebra	_____
datum	_____
coccus	_____
index	_____
macula	_____
bronchus	_____

8. Write the meanings of the following building blocks:

a. aden   _____

b. cardi   _____

c. cephal   _____

d. derm   _____

e. flex   _____

f. gastr   _____

g. hydr   _____

h. my   _____

i. neur   _____

j. pnea   _____

k. a–   _____

l. ante–   _____

m. dys–   _____

n. endo–   _____

o. retro–   _____

p. –algia   _____

q. –cele   _____

r. -itis   _____

s. –logy   _____

t. –pathy   _____

1.2   Review: Word Building

DIRECTIONS: Fill in the blanks with the appropriate building block or medical term.

1. The suffix for *inflammation* is _____ .

   The combining form for *stomach* is _____ .

   _____ is the term for inflammation of the stomach.

2. _____ is a prefix meaning *backward*.

   _____ is a root meaning *bending*.

   The term for bending backward is _____ .

3. _____ is the root for *muscle*.

   _____ is a suffix meaning *pain*.

   _____ is the term for muscle pain.

4. _____ is a suffix meaning *hernia*.

   _____ is the combining form for *stomach*.

   A _____ is a hernia of the stomach.

5. The prefix *a–* means _____ .

   The root *pnea* means _____ .

   Apnea means _____ .

CHAPTER 2

Frequently Used Building Blocks

OBJECTIVES

When you have successfully completed Chapter 2, you should be able to:
— Recognize and define frequently used suffixes, roots, and prefixes.
— Define medical terms using these word elements.
— Build new medical terms using the word elements introduced in this chapter.

anatomy	(ah-**NAT**-oh-mee)	The study of the structure of an organism
pathology	(pah-**THOL**-oh-jee)	The study of the basic nature of disease and the changes in the structure and function of cells, tissues, and organs that lead to disease
physiology	(**fiz**-ee-**OL**-oh-jee)	The study of how a living organism and its components function, and the physical and chemical processes involved in those functions
surgery	(**SER**-jer-ee)	The branch of medicine in which manual and operative procedures are used to correct deformities and defects, to repair injuries, to diagnose and treat certain diseases

On the following pages are prefixes, roots, and suffixes that you will use throughout this text in achieving your goal of developing a practical medical vocabulary. Some you will recognize from Chapter 1. Many of these building blocks will appear again and again in later chapters. They will soon seem like old friends as you become more comfortable with these basic word parts. In later chapters you will add new terms that relate to specific body systems.

The prefixes and roots are listed in alphabetic order. The suffixes are listed in three separate groups to help you remember how they are used (Figure 2.1). These groups are:

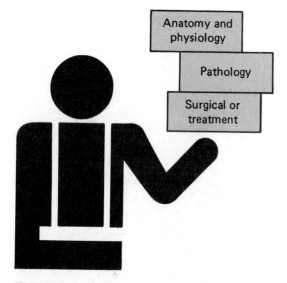

FIGURE 2.1 **Many word parts can be grouped by type of use**

- *Suffixes related to anatomy and physiology.* These word endings refer to a structure or function of the body in a normal state.
- *Suffixes related to pathology.* These word endings indicate the nature and cause of conditions that occur with a change from normal.
- *Suffixes related to surgery or treatment.* The surgical suffixes describe what was or will be done either manually or through a cutting procedure to change a body condition.

FREQUENTLY USED SUFFIXES

Anatomy and Physiology

Suffix	Meaning	Example Word and Definition
–blast	immature stage of cell	*myoblast* (**MY**-oh-blast): the immature stage of a muscle-forming cell
–cyte	mature cell	*leukocyte* (**LOO**-koh-sight): a white blood cell
–genesis	production, development	*myogenesis* (**my**-oh-**JEN**-eh-sis): development of muscle tissue
–genic	origination	*carcinogenic* (**kar**-sih-noh-**JEN**-ick): producing cancer
–phagia, phagy	eating, swallowing	*dysphagia* (dis-**FAY**-jee-ah): difficulty in swallowing
–phasia	speaking	*aphasia* (ah-**FAY**-zee-ah): loss or impairment of speech
–poiesis	formation	*hidropoiesis* (**high**-droh-poy-**EE**-sis): the formation of sweat

Pathology

Suffix	Meaning	Example Word and Definition
–algia	pain	*analgia* (an-**AL**-jee-ah): absence of pain
–cele	pouching, hernia	*enterocele* (**EN**-ter-oh-**seel**): hernia of the intestine
–dynia	pain	*gastrodynia* (**gas**-troh-**DIN**-ee-ah): pain in the stomach
–ectasis	dilatation, expansion	*angiectasis* (**an**-jee-**ECK**-tah-sis): dilatation of a blood or lymph vessel

–emia	blood	*glycemia* (glie-**SEE**-mee-ah): sugar in the blood. **Note:** In this form, the *h* is dropped from the root *heme,* which means *blood.*
–iasis	condition, presence of	*cholelithiasis* (**koh**-lee-lih-**THIGH**-ah-sis): presence of stones in the gallbladder
–itis	inflammation	*bronchitis* (brong-**KYE**-tis): inflammation of the breathing tubes
–lysis	dissolution, breaking down	*cytolysis* (sigh-**TOL**-ih-sis): dissolution or destruction of living cells
–malacia	softening	*splenomalacia* (**spleh**-no-mah-**LAY**-she-ah): softening of the spleen
–megaly	enlargement	*acromegaly* (**ack**-roh-**MEG**-ah-lee): enlargement of the extremities (arms and legs)
–oid	resembling, like	*fibroid* (**FIE**-broyd): containing or resembling fibers
–oma	tumor	*lipoma* (lih-POH-mah): a fatty tumor
–osis	abnormal condition	*dermatosis* (**der**-mah-**TOH**-sis): any skin disease
–pathy	disease	*uropathy* (you-**ROP**-ah-thee): any abnormality of the urinary tract
–penia	abnormal reduction	*cytopenia* (**sigh**-toh-**PEE**-nee-ah): deficient number of cells
–phobia	exaggerated fear	*agoraphobia*(**ag**-oh-rah-**FOH**-bee-ah): fear of being in a large open space
–plegia	paralysis	*hemiplegia* (**hem**-ee-**PLEE**-jee-ah): paralysis of half of the body
–ptosis	downward displacement	*blepharoptosis* (**blef**-ah-roh-**TOH**-sis): drooping of an upper eyelid
–rhage, –rhagia	excessive flow, hemorrhage	*rhinorrhagia* (**rye**-no-**RAY**-jee-ah): profuse bleeding from the nose

–rhea	discharge	*pyorrhea* (**pie**-oh-**REE**-ah): discharge of pus
–rhexis	rupture	*angiorrhexis* (**an**-jee-oh-**RECK**-sis): rupture of a vessel
–uria	urine	*hematuria* (**hem**-ah-**TOO**-ree-ah): blood in the urine

Surgery or Treatment

Suffix	Meaning	Example Word and Definition
–centesis	puncture for aspiration (draining)	*cephalocentesis* (**sef**-ah-loh-sen-**TEE**-sis): surgical puncture of skull
–desis	binding, fixation	*arthrodesis* (ar-throh-**DEE**-sis): surgical fixation of a joint
–ectomy	excision, cutting out	*appendectomy* (**ap**-en-**DECK**-toh-mee): excision of the appendix
–pexy	to fix in place	*orchiopexy* (or-kee-oh-**PECK**-see): suturing (stitching) of an undescended testis to fix it in the scrotum
–plasty	to mold or shape	*otoplasty* (**OH**-toh-**plas**-tee): plastic surgery of the ear
–rhaphy	suturing (stitching or closing)	*glossorrhaphy* (glaw-**SOR**-ah-fee): suturing of a wound of the tongue
–sclerosis	hardening	*arteriosclerosis* (ar-**tee**-ree-oh-skleh-**ROH**-sis). hardening of the arteries
–scope	examining instrument	*anoscope* (**AY**-noh-skohp): instrument for examining the lower rectum and anus
–scopy	internal examination	*cystoscopy* (sis-**TOS**-koh-pee): the process of examining the bladder with a cystoscope
–stomy	creation of opening	*enterostomy* (**en**-ter-**OS**-toh-mee): surgical creation of a permanent opening into an intestine through the abdominal wall

–tomy	incising or cutting	*nephrotomy* (neh-**FRAH**-toh-mee): cutting into the kidney
–tripsy	crushing, friction	*lithotripsy* (**LITH**-oh-**trip**-see): crushing of a stone. Used in referring to a stone in the bladder or urethra

FREQUENTLY USED ROOTS

The following list includes some commonly used roots. You may notice that two apparently different roots are used to refer to the same structure or organ. For example, the root *hyster* and the root *uter* are both used in words referring to the womb. The root *hyster* comes to us from the Greeks; the root *uter* is Latin. Today, the two roots are both used.

Root and Combining Vowel (if used)	Meaning	Example Word and Definition
aden/o	gland	*adenoid* (**ADD**-eh-noyd): resembling or having the appearance of a gland
angi/o	vessel	*angiotomy* (**an**-jee-**OT**-oh-mee): cutting of blood vessels
arter/i/o	artery	*arteriosclerosis* (ar-**tee**-ree-oh-skleh-**ROH**-sis): thickening ("hardening") of an artery
arthr/o	joint	*arthralgia* (ar-**THRAL**-jee-ah): pain in a joint
cardi/o	heart	*cardioptosis* (**kar**-dee-op-**TOH**-sis): prolapse of the heart
		cardioscope (**KAR**-dee-oh-skohp): An instrument for examining the inside of the heart
cephal/o	head	*cephalad* (**SEF**-ah-lad): toward the head
cerebr/o	brain	*cerebropathy* (**ser**-eh-**BROP**-ah-thee): any morbid condition of the brain
cheil/o	lip	*cheilosis* (**kye-LOH**-sis): abnormal condition of the lips

chondr/o	cartilage	*chondrocyte* (**KON**-droh-sight): a cartilage cell
cost/o	rib	*costectomy* (kos-**TECK**-toh-mee): surgical removal of a rib
crani/o	cranium, skull	*craniometer* (**kray**-nee-**AH**-meh-ter): instrument for measuring the skull
cyst/o	sac, bladder	*cystolith* (**SIS**-toh-lith): a bladder stone
cyt/o	cell	*cytoblast* (**SIGH**-toh-blast): a cell nucleus
derm/o, dermat/o	skin	*dermomycosis* (**der**-moh-my-**KOH**-sis): a skin disease caused by a fungus
encephal/o	brain	*encephalocele* (en-**SEF**-ah-loh-seel): herniation of the brain through a crack or fissure of the skull
enter/o	intestine	*enterospasm* (**EN**-ter-oh-spazm): painful contractions (cramps) of the intestine
gastr/o	stomach	*gastrectomy* (gas-**TRECK**-toh-mee): surgical removal of part or all of the stomach
gloss/o	tongue	*glossoplegia* (glos-oh-**PLEE**-jee-ah): paralysis of the tongue
hem/o, hemat/o	blood	*hemocyte* (**HEE**-moh-sight): a blood cell
hepat/o	liver	*hepatitis* (**hep**-ah-**TIE**-tis): inflammation of the liver
hyster/o	uterus	*hysterectomy* (**his**-ter-**ECK**-toh-mee): surgically removing the uterus
mamm/o, mast/o	breast	*mammoplasty* (**MAM**-oh-**plas**-tee): surgical alteration of the size of the breast which may involve an increase or a decrease *mastitis* (mass-**TIE**-tis): inflammation of the breast

my/o	muscle	*myoatrophy* (**MY**-oh-**AT**-roh-fee): wasting away of muscle tissue
nas/o, rhin/o	nose	*nasogastric tube* (**nay**-zoh-**GAS**-trick tewb): a tube that is inserted through the nose and extends into the stomach *rhinitis* (rye-**NIGH**-tis): inflammation of the mucous lining (mucosa) of the nose
nephr/o, ren/o	kidney	*nephroptosis* (**nef**-rop-**TOH**-sis): downward displacement of the kidney
neur/o	nerve	*neurectomy* (new-**RECK**-toh-mee): partial or total excision of a nerve
ocul/o, ophthalm/o	eye	*oculogyric* (**ock**-you-loh-**JYE**-rick): pertaining to movements of the eye *ophthalmia* (ahf-**THAL**-mee-ah): abnormal condition of the eye
or/o, stoma, stomat/o	mouth	*oronasal* (**oh**-roh-**NAY**-zal): concerning the mouth and nose *stomatitis* (stoh-mah-**TIE**-tis): inflammation of the mouth
oste/o	bone	*osteectopia* (**os**-tee-eck-**TOH-pee-ah**): displacement of a bone
ot/o	ear	*otalgia* (oh-**TAL**-jee-ah): pain in an ear
pharyng/o	pharynx	*pharyngeal* (fah-**RIN**-jee-al): concerning the pharynx
phleb/o	vein	*phlebostenosis* (**fleb**-oh-steh-**NOH**-sis): narrowing or constriction of a vein
pneum/o, pneumon/o, pulmon/o	lung, air	*pneumectomy* (new-**MECK**-toh-mee): excision of all or part of a lung *pneumatosis* (**new**-mah-**TOH**-sis): abnormal presence of air or gas in the body

proct/o, rect/o	rectum	*proctocele* (**PROCK**-toh-seel): a herniation of the rectal mucosa into the vagina; also called rectocele
splen/o, lien/o	spleen	*splenectomy* (spleh-**NECK**-toh-mee): surgical excision of the spleen *lienitis* (**lie**-eh-**NIGH**-tis): inflammation of the spleen
thorac/o	chest	*thoracotomy* (**thoh**-rah-**KOT**-oh-mee): surgical incision of the chest wall
ureter/o	ureter	*ureterography* (you-**ree**-ter-**OG**-rah-fee): radiographic (x-ray) examination of the ureter
urethr/o	urethra	*urethritis* (**you**-reh-**THRIGH**-tis): inflammation of the urethra
uter/o	uterus	*uteroplasty* (**you**-ter-oh-**PLAS**-tee): plastic surgery of the uterus

FREQUENTLY USED PREFIXES

Prefix	Meaning	Example Word and Definition
a–, an–	absence of, without, not, non–,	*amastia* (ah-**MASS**-tee-ah): nondevelopment of breasts
ab–	away from	*aboral* (ab-**OH**-ral): away from the mouth
ad–	to, toward, near, increase	*adduction* (ah-**DUCK**-shun): drawn toward the median plane of the body
ambi–	both	*ambidextrous* (**am**-bih-**DECK**-strus): ability to use either hand effectively
ante–	before	*anteflect* (**AN**-teh-fleckt): to bend forward
anti–	against	*antimycotic* (**an**-tih-**my**-**KOT**-ick): an agent that prevents the growth of fungi (*myc* = fungus)

aut/o	self	*autogenesis* (**aw**-toh-**JEN**-eh-sis): self-generation
bi–	two, both, double	*bicuspid* (by-**KUS**-pid): having two cusps (points or leaflets)
circum–	around	*circumscribed* (**SER**-kum-skryb'd): confined within a limited space
co–, con–	together, with	*congenital* (kon-**JEN**-ih-tal): refers to condition existing at birth
contra–	against	*contraception* (**kon**-trah-**SEP**-shun): prevention of pregnancy (conception)
de–	from, down, not	*deceleration* (dee-**sell**-er-**AY**-shun): decrease in rate of speed
di–	double, two	*dimorphous* (die-**MOR**-fus): occurring in two forms (*morph* = form)
dia	across, apart, through	*diathermy* (**DIE**-ah-**ther**-mee): heating of body tissues by means of high-frequency electromagnetic radiation
dis–	separate from, apart	*dissect* (die-**SECKT**: to cut apart or separate tissues
dys–	painful, difficult, improper	*dysphasia* (dis-**FAY**-zee-ah): speech impairment
e–, ec–	out, away	*eccentric* (eck-**SEN**-trick): located or moving away from a center
ecto–	on the outer edge	*ectocytic* (**eck**-toh-**SIGH**-tick): outside of the cell
em–	in, within	*empyema* (**em**-pie-**EE**-mah): pus inside a space
en–	in	*encapsulated* (en-**KAP**-sue-**lay**-ted): situated within a capsule
endo–	within	*endocardial* (**en**-doh-**KAR**-dee-al): situated or occurring within the heart
epi–	upon, at, in addition to	*epiotic* (**ep**-ee-**OT**-ick): located upon or above the ear

eu–	good, normal	*eucrasia* (you-**KRAY**-see-ah): state of normal or good health
ex–	out, away from, over	*extremity* (ecks-**TREM**-ih-tee): a distal or end portion; an arm or a leg
exo–	outside	*exogenous* (ecks-**AHJ**-eh-nus): caused by factors outside the body or part
extra–	outside	*extrabuccal* (**ecks**-trah-**BUCK**-al): outside the cheek (*bucca* = cheek)
hemi–	half	*hemifacial* (**hem**-ee-**FAY**-shul): referring to one side of the face
hyper–	above, beyond, excessive	*hypertension* (high-per-**TEN**-shun): condition of blood pressure being consistently above normal
hypo–	below, beneath, deficient	*hypodipsia* (**high**-poh-**DIP**-see-ah): below normal sense of thirst
inter–	between	*intercostal* (**in**-ter-**KOS**-tal): situated between the ribs
intra–	within, inside	*intralobar* (**in**-trah-**LOH**-bar): within a lobe
intro–	into, within	*introflexion* (in-troh-**FLECK**-shun): a bending inward
para–	beside, around, abnormal	*paramedian* (**par**-ah-**MEE**-dee-an): situated near the midline *paraplasm* (**PAR**-ah-plazm): abnormal new growth; malformation
peri–	around, about, in the vicinity of	*perisplenic* (per-ih-**SPLEN**-ick): occurring around the spleen
post–	after, behind in time or place	*postprandial* (post-**PRAN**-dee-al): related to after a meal
pre–	before, in front of	*precostal* (pree-**KOS**-tal): in front of the ribs
pro–	before, forward, in front of	*protrusion* (proh-**TREW**-zhun): the state of pushing forward

re–	again, back	*reflected* (ree-**FLECK**-ted): folded or bent back
retro–	backward, behind	*retrocecal* (**ret**-roh-**SEE**-kal): behind the cecum
semi–	half	*semilunar* (**sem**-ee-**LEW**-nar): half-moon shaped
sub–	under, below	*subjacent* (sub-**JAY**-sent): lying underneath. **Note:** *sub-* changes to *suf-* or *sup-* before words beginning with *f* or *p* (examples: *suffix, suppuration*)
super–, supra–	above, beyond, extreme	*superflexion* (**sue**-per-**FLECK**-shun): extreme flexion (bending) *supraocular* (**sue**-prah-**OCK**-you-lar): above the eye
syn–, sym–	with, together, beside	*syndactyly* (sin-**DACK**-tih-lee): congenital webbing together of two or more fingers or toes **Note:** *syn-* drops the *n* before *s*, changes to *l* before *l* and changes to *m* before *b, m, p,* and *ph*
trans–	across, over, beyond, through	*transection* (tran-**SECK**-shun): a cut made across a long axis
tri–	three	*tripod* (**TRY**-pod): any object having three feet or supports
ultra–	excessive, beyond	*ultraviolet* (uhl-trah-**VIE**-oh-let): beyond the visible spectrum at its violet end

2.1 Review: Suffixes

DIRECTIONS: On the blanks provided, write the meanings of the listed terms.

A. Suffixes related to pathology

1. _____ inflammation
2. _____ tumor
3. _____ enlargement
4. _____ dilatation
5. _____ softening

6. _____ disease
7. _____ abnormal condition
8. _____ paralysis
9. _____ hernia
10. _____ rupture

B. Suffixes related to surgery or treatment

1. _____ fixation
2. _____ binding, fixation
3. _____ creation of opening
4. _____ crushing, friction
5. _____ puncture for aspiration
6. _____ examining instrument
7. _____ incision
8. _____ suture
9. _____ internal examination
10. _____ to mold or shape
11. _____ excision

C. Suffixes related to anatomy and physiology

1. _____ production, development
2. _____ cell
3. _____ immature cell
4. _____ formation
5. _____ origin
6. _____ eating, swallowing
7. _____ speaking

D. Suffixes related to pathology

1. _____ abnormal reduction
2. _____ discharge
3. _____ urine
4. _____ pain
5. _____ excessive flow
6. _____ breaking down, dissolution
7. _____ exaggerated fear
8. _____ downward displacement
9. _____ resembling
10. _____ blood
11. _____ tumor
12. _____ presence of

2.2 Review: Building Blocks

DIRECTIONS: Cover the column on the left while you write the building blocks for the following words.

A.

aden	1. gland _____
arter	2. artery _____
cardi	3. heart _____
cheil	4. lip _____
cost	5. rib _____
cyst	6. sac, bladder _____
derm	7. skin _____
enter	8. intestine _____
gloss	9. tongue _____
hepat	10. liver _____
mamm, mast	11. breast _____
nas, rhin	12. nose _____
neur	13. nerve _____
or, stoma	14. mouth _____
ot	15. ear _____
phleb	16. vein _____
proct, rect	17. rectum _____
thorac	18. chest _____
urethr	19. urethra _____

2.2 Review: Building Blocks

DIRECTIONS: Cover the column on the left while you define the following building blocks.

B.

vessel	1. angi _____
joint	2. arthr _____
head	3. cephal _____
cartilage	4. chondr _____
skull	5. crani _____
cell	6. cyt _____
brain	7. encephal _____
stomach	8. gastr _____
blood	9. hem, hemat _____
uterus	10. hyster _____
muscle	11. my _____
kidney	12. nephr _____
eye	13. ocul, ophthalm _____
bone	14. oste _____
pharynx	15. pharyng _____
lung, air	16. pneum _____
spleen	17. splen, lien _____
ureter	18. ureter _____
uterus	19. uter _____

2.3   Review: Prefixes

DIRECTIONS: Match the meanings in the second column with the prefixes in the first column.

A.

_____ 1. a–, an–	a. two
_____ 2. ab–	b. both
_____ 3. ad–	c. across
_____ 4. ambi–	d. with
_____ 5. ante–	e. without, not
_____ 6. anti–	f. painful
_____ 7. bi–	g. toward
_____ 8. circum–	h. before
_____ 9. co–, con–	i. apart
_____ 10. dia–	j. against
_____ 11. dis–	k. around
_____ 12. dys–	l. away from

B.

_____ 1. e–, ec–	a. on the outside
_____ 2. ecto–	b. upon
_____ 3. endo–	c. below
_____ 4. epi–	d. outside
_____ 5. eu–	e. excessive
_____ 6. ex–	f. inside
_____ 7. exo–	g. half
_____ 8. hemi–	h. within
_____ 9. hyper–	i. out
_____ 10. hypo–	j. between
_____ 11. inter–	k. good
_____ 12. intra–	l. out, away

C.

_____ 1. intra–	a. behind
_____ 2. para–	b. before
_____ 3. peri–	c. across
_____ 4. post–	d. above
_____ 5. pre–	e. within
_____ 6. re–	f. around
_____ 7. retro–	g. three
_____ 8. sub–	h. under
_____ 9. super–	i. after
_____ 10. syn–	j. with
_____ 11. trans–	k. again
_____ 12. tri–	l. abnormal

2.4   Review: Word Building

DIRECTIONS: Build a medical term for each of the following conditions.

1. head pain   _____
2. glandular inflammation   _____
3. excision of the uterus   _____
4. muscle pain   _____
5. hernia of the bladder   _____
6. surgical puncture of the thorax   _____
7. enlargement of the liver   _____
8. inflammation of a lung   _____
9. incision into the intestine   _____
10. surgical removal of a breast   _____

2.5   Review: Word Building

DIRECTIONS: Fill in the blanks with the correct building block or medical term.

1. The root for *nerve* is _____ .
   The suffix meaning *disease* is _____ .
   _____ is a disease condition of a nerve.
2. The root for *bone* is _____ .
   A suffix for *tumor* is _____ .
   _____ is a tumor of the bone.
3. _____ is the root for *tongue*.
   _____ means *inflammation*.
   Inflammation of the tongue is _____ .
4. The suffix _____ means *creation of an opening*.
   The combining form for *chest* is _____ .
   _____ means creating of an opening in the chest.
5. _____ is the root for *rib*.
   _____ is the root for *cartilage*.
   Inflammation of a rib and its cartilage would be referred to as _____ .

CHAPTER 3

General and
Structural Terms

OBJECTIVES

When you have successfully completed Chapter 3, you should be able to:
— List the structural units of the body and explain their relationship.
— Name and define the planes of the body.
— List the body cavities and briefly describe what they enclose.
— Define five body positions.
— Define commonly used directional terms.
— List and demonstrate common terms used to describe body motions.
— Identify the anatomic regions of the abdomen and back.
— List the clinical divisions of the abdomen.
— Analyze the medical terms in this and previous chapters.
— Build medical terms using the building blocks in this chapter.

KEY TERMS

allied health	A term used to describe a wide range of health-related disciplines whose practitioners assist, facilitate, and complement the work of physicians, nurses, and other health professionals
anatomist	A person skilled in the art of dissecting (artificially separating) and identifying the different parts of any animal or plant
anatomy	The science that concerns itself with the structure of animals or plants
clinical	Pertaining to the actual investigation and treatment of disease in living subjects, rather than to theoretical science
cytoplasm	The living portion (protoplasm) of a cell that is within the cell membrane but outside the nucleus
function	The normal, unique activity of any organ or part of a living organism
identification	Establishing the name, features, and characteristics of something, for example, a body part
membrane	A thin, soft, pliable sheet or layer of tissue
pericardial	Pertaining to the membrane that encloses the heart (the pericardium)
physiology	The study of the functions of a living organism and each of its parts or structures
plane	A flat or level surface; in anatomy, one of several imaginary views of the body used to locate structures
pleural	Pertaining to the pleura, the membrane that lines the chest cavity
region	In anatomy, a part or division of the body
structure	Arrangement of parts; of organs; or of constituent tissues, cells, or particles in a substance or body

USING YOUR NEW VOCABULARY

Anyone who enters the field of medicine or allied health must be able to recognize medical terms and to understand their usage in context—that is, in the report, chapter, or paragraph where they are used. To understand the structure (anatomy) and function (physiology) of the human body, you need to know some of the terms anatomists and physiologists use.

This text cannot teach you anatomy or physiology, but it provides brief overviews to introduce each body system. These overviews are intended as introductions or reviews to help you apply your new vocabulary.

POINTS OF REFERENCE

In talking about any physical object or space, it helps to have points of reference. For example, in looking at maps, we can always assume that north is at the top, west on the left, and so forth. Over the years, anatomists have identified and labeled certain structural and functional units of the body, as well as planes, cavities, positions, and motions to serve as reference points.

STRUCTURAL UNITS OF THE HUMAN BODY

The fundamental structural units of the body are cells, tissues, organs, and systems (Figure 3.1).

The human body begins from the union of two cells—the egg (ovum) and the sperm. All the billions of cells in the human body are formed from these two cells by processes of cell division called mitosis and meiosis. Cells unite to form tissues; various kinds of tissue combine to form organs; and, finally, groups of organs working together make up body systems.

The Cell

The *cell* is the basic structural and functional unit of any living organism. Cells have many shapes and sizes, and they perform a variety of functions. The cell contains two main parts, the *nucleus* and the *cytoplasm*, which are enclosed in a thin covering called the *cell membrane*. Not all cells reproduce themselves in exactly the same way, but when cells divide, both the nucleus and the cytoplasm undergo an exact division so that two more identical offspring are formed. Different groups of cells develop different characteristics; for example, nerve cells (neurons) are quite different in shape from skin cells or bone cells.

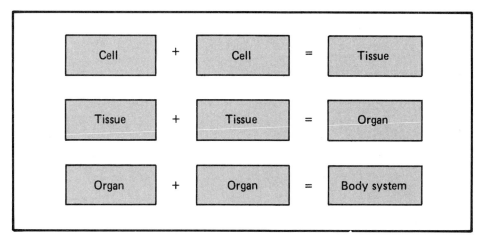

FIGURE 3.1 **Structural units of the human body**

The Tissues

The human body has four basic types of *tissues*, each of which is composed of a group of similar cells and the material that holds them together. The four basic types of tissue are:

- epithelial tissue
- connective tissue
- muscle tissue
- nerve tissue

In brief, *epithelial tissue* is a protective covering of the skin. It also lines hollow organs such as the stomach, the intestines and the air passages. *Connective tissue* supports and connects other tissues, and includes adipose or fat tissue, cartilage, and bone. There are several kinds of *muscle tissue*, which will be described in Chapter 6. The cells of *nerve tissue* are quite different from other cells. They form threadlike outgrowths called *processes*. These nerve fibers, known as axons and dendrites, may be as much as 4 feet long, entending to many parts of the body.

The Organs

When several kinds of tissue combine in performing some special function, they form a structure called an *organ*. For instance, the kidneys, the stomach, the lungs, and the liver are all organs.

The Systems

A *body system* is a group of closely allied organs that are involved in the same functions. Part II of this text is arranged by body systems, which are the:

- integumentary (in-**teg**-you-**MEN**-tah-ree) system
- skeletal (**SKEL**-eh-tel) system
- muscular (**MUS**-kyou-lar) system
- cardiovascular (**kar**-dee-oh-**VAS**-kyou-lar) system
- blood and lymphatic (lim-**FAT**-ick) system
- respiratory (**REH**-spih-rah-**toh**-ree) system
- digestive (die-**JES**-tiv) system
- reproductive (**ree**-pro-**DUCK**-tiv) system
- urinary (**YOU**-rih-**nar**-ee) system
- endocrine (**EN**-doh-krin) system
- nervous (**NER**-vus) system
- special senses

PLANES OF THE BODY

Body planes are imaginary planes that divide the body into sections (Figure 3.2). They serve as a point of reference by naming the direction from which the body is being viewed.

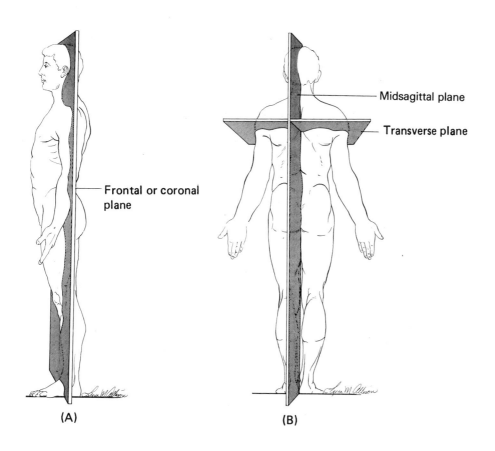

Labels in figure: Frontal or coronal plane, Midsagittal plane, Transverse plane, (A), (B)

FIGURE 3.2   Body planes (From Kinn, *Medical Terminology—Review Challenge*, copyright 1987 by Delmar Publishers Inc.)

The *midsagittal,* or *median, plane* divides the body from head to foot into right and left halves.

The *frontal,* or *coronal, plane* divides the body from head to foot into *anterior* (front) and *posterior* (back) portions.

The *transverse,* or *horizontal, plane* is formed by a crosswise line that divides the body into *superior* (above) and *inferior* (below) portions.

BODY CAVITIES

A cavity is any hollow space. *Body cavities* serve to confine organs and systems that have related functions (Figure 3.3). The two major body cavities are the dorsal *cavity* and the ventral *cavity*. The dorsal cavity is further divided into (1) the *cranial* (skull) *cavity* containing the brain and (2) the *spinal cavity* containing the spinal cord.

The *ventral cavity* has three divisions:

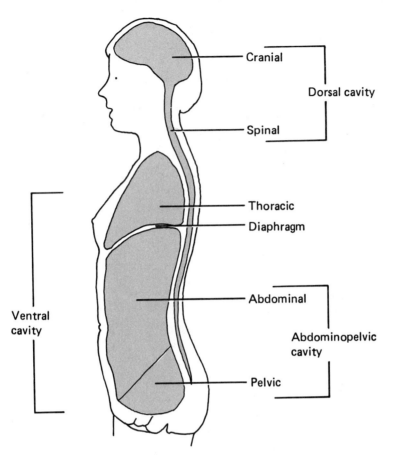

FIGURE 3.3   The body cavities

1. The *thoracic cavity* lies above the diaphragm. It in turn contains (a) two *pleural cavities* which enclose the right and left lungs and (b) a *pericardial cavity* which contains the heart. The area between the two lungs is called the *mediastinum*.

2. The *abdominal cavity*, situated below the diaphragm, contains the digestive organs.

3. The *pelvic cavity*, the space containing the reproductive and excretory systems, lies below the abdomen. Together, the abdominal and pelvic cavities are called the *abdominopelvic cavity*.

THE ANATOMIC POSITION

When you read or hear directions pertaining to the body, you can always assume that the body is being described in its *anatomic position* (Figure 3.4). In this position the

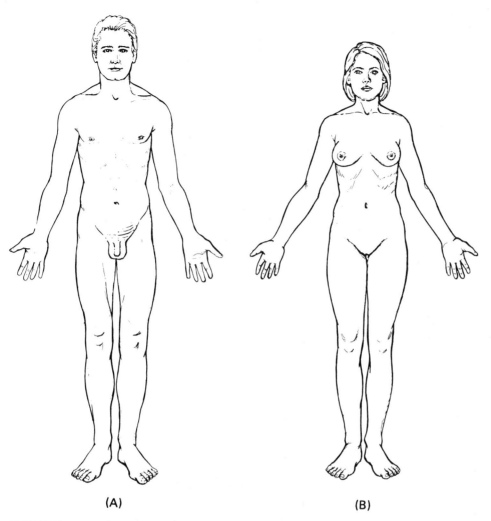

(A)   (B)

FIGURE 3.4 **The anatomic position. The body is erect, facing forward, with arms at the side and palms facing forward**

body is erect, facing forward, with arms at the side and the palms forward. Other positions of the body include:

lateral recumbent	(**LAT**-er-al ree-**KUM**-bent)	Lying on either the right or left side
prone		Lying face down and flat
recumbent		Lying down
supine	(**SUE**-pine)	Lying flat on the back

DIRECTIONAL TERMS

Medicine uses many directional terms. These are generally relative to some assumed base, center, or location.

afferent	(**AF**-er-ent)	Directed toward a center
efferent	(**EF**-er-ent)	Directed away from a center
anterior	(an-**TEER**-ee-or)	Situated in front of or in the forward part of a structure (sometimes *ventral*)
posterior	(pos-**TEER**-ee-or)	Situated behind or in the back part of a structure (also, *dorsal*)
distal	(**DIS**-tal)	Remote, farther from the point of origin than whatever is being compared
proximal	(**PROCK**-sih-mal)	Nearest, closer to point of origin
central	(**SEN**-tral)	Situated at or pertaining to a center
peripheral	(peh-**RIF**-er-al)	Situated away from a center, toward the outer part
inferior	(in-**FEER**-ee-or)	Situated below or directed downward
superior	(sue-**PEE**-ee-or)	Situated above, or directed upward
caudal	(**KAW**-dal)	Toward the cauda or tail; also *inferior*
cephalad	(**SEF**-ah-lad)	Toward the head; situated above or directed upward; also *superior*
external	(ecks-**TER**-nal)	Outside
internal	(in-**TER**-nal)	Inside
lateral	(**LAT**-er-al)	Away from midline; pertaining to a side
medial	(**MEE**-dee-al)	Pertaining to the median or middle; also *mesial*
median	(**MEE**-dee-an)	Situated in the midline of a structure
mesial	(**MEE**-zee-al)	Located near the median line of the body
intermediate	(in-ter-**MEE**-dee-at)	Between median (middle) and lateral (side)
deep		Situated far beneath the surface; the term *deep to*, used in anatomy, means deep in relation to
superficial	(sue-per-**FISH**-al)	Situated near the surface
ventral	(**VEN**-tral)	Pertaining to the belly; *anterior*
dorsal	(**DOR**-sal)	Pertaining to the back; *posterior*
palmar	(**PAL**-mar)	Referring to the palm
plantar	(**PLAN**-tar)	Referring to the sole of the foot

BODY MOTIONS

Like terms of direction, terms that describe body motions are often relative to some assumed point. See Figure 3.5.

abduction	(ab-**DUCK**-shun)	Movement away from the midline

adduction	(ad-**DUCK**-shun)	Movement toward the midline
circumduction	(**ser**-kum-**DUCK**-shun)	Circular movement of a leg or arm or of an eye
flexion	(**FLECK**-shun)	A bending motion that decreases the angle between adjoining long bones
extension	(ecks-**TEN**-shun)	A straightening motion that increases the angle between adjoining bones
hyperextension	(**high**-per-ecks-**TEN**-shun)	Extreme or excessive straightening of a part
lateral rotation	(roh-**TAY**-shun)	Turning away from midline
medial rotation		Turning toward midline
pronation	(proh-**NAY**-shun)	Act of turning the palm or the sole of the foot backward or downward
supination	(**sue**-pih-**NAY**-shun)	Act of turning the palm or the sole of the foot upward

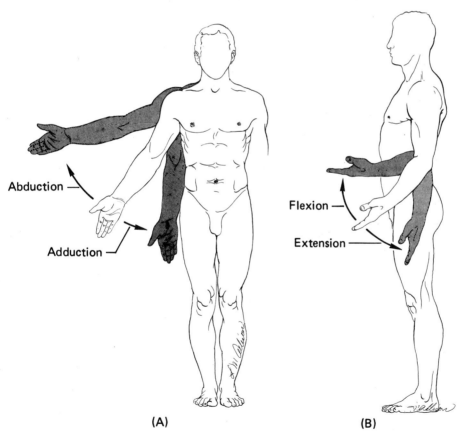

FIGURE 3.5 Directional terms (From Kinn, *Medical Terminology—Review Challenge,* copyright 1987 by Delmar Publishers Inc.)

ANATOMIC REGIONS OF THE ABDOMEN

For purposes of location of the internal organs, the abdomen is divided into nine regions, much like a tic-tac-toe board, by four imginary planes. Two horizontal and two sagittal planes are imagined to be passing through the cavity. The median (middle) region of the upper zone is the *epigastric region*. The lateral regions are the *right hypochondriac* and *left hypochondriac*. The median region of the middle zone is the *umbilical region*, and the lateral regions of the middle zone are the *right* and *left lumbar*, or *lateral regions*. The median region of the lower zone is the *hypogastric* or *pubic region*, and the lateral regions of the lower zone are the *right* and *left iliac*, or *inguinal regions*. See Figure 3.6.

CLINICAL DIVISIONS OF THE ABDOMEN

For purposes of clinical examination and reporting, the abdomen is divided into four corresponding regions called *quandrants*, the umbilicus, or navel, being the intersecting point (Figure 3.7). In reporting, the following abbreviations are used:

Right Upper Quandrant	RUQ
Left Upper Quadrant	LUQ
Right Lower Quadrant	RLQ
Left Lower Quadrant	LLQ

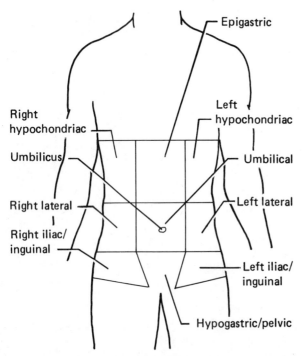

FIGURE 3.6 **Anatomic regions of the abdomen** (From Caldwell and Hegner, *Health Care Assistant*, 4th edition, copyright 1985 by Delmar Publishers Inc.)

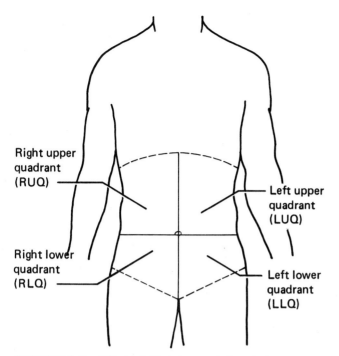

FIGURE 3.7 Clinical divisions of the abdomen (From Caldwell and Hegner, *Health Care Assistant*, 4th edition, copyright 1985 by Delmar Publishers Inc.)

ANATOMIC REGIONS OF THE BACK

The regions of the back are named to correspond to the vertebrae that lie under them:

- Cervical (neck)   (7 vertebrae)
- Thoracic (chest)   (12 vertebrae)
- Lumbar (loin)   (5 vertebrae)
- Sacral (lower back or sacrum)   (5 fused vertebrae)
- Coccygeal (tail bone)   (4 fused vertebrae)

BUILDING BLOCKS

PREFIXES

Word Element	Meaning
ana–	without
dia–	through, complete
epi–	upon
homeo–	similar, same
hyper–	abnormally increased, excessive, too much
hypo–	under, deficient, too little
meta–	change
mito–	thread
proto–	first
trans–	through, across

SUFFIXES

Word Element	Meaning
–osis	condition, abnormal increase
–phragm	fence, wall off
–plasia	to form
–plasm	mold, shape
–stasis	standing
–trophy	nourishment

ROOTS (WITH COMBINING VOWEL)

nucle/o	kernel, nucleus
path/o	disease, abnormal condition
phag/o	eat, swallow
pin/o	to drink
ur/o	urine, urinary tract

BUILDING BLOCKS REVIEW

PREFIXES

Word Element	Meaning
acro–	extremity (a limb)
ambi–	both
ante–	before
bi–	two, double
con–	with, together
eu–	good, normal
inter–	between

SUFFIXES

Word Element	Meaning
–gram	a record
–graphy	the procedure of recording
–meter	measure
–opia	sight condition
–ostomy	surgically formed artifical opening
–ptosis	downward displacement
–stenosis	narrowing

ROOTS (WITH COMBINING VOWEL)

cyt/o	cell
dactyl/o	finger or toe
dermat/o	skin
hemat/o	blood
lith/o	stone
myc/o	fungus
neur/o	nerve
phleb/o	vein
py/o	pus
thorac/o	chest

VOCABULARY

Terms Related to Anatomy and Physiology

adipose	(ADD-ih-pohs)	Pertaining to fat; fatty
cartilage	(KAR-tih-lij)	A specialized, fibrous connective tissue
cytoplasm	(SIGH-toh-plazm)	The essential matter of a cell within the cell membrane and outside the nucleus
diaphragm	(DIE-ah-fram)	The partition dividing the abdominal and thoracic cavities
embryo	(EM-bree-oh)	The developing human organism from about two weeks after fertilization to the end of the seventh or eighth week of gestation
epigastric	(ep-ih-GAS-trick)	Pertaining to the upper and middle region of the stomach
homeostasis	(hoh-mee-oh-STAY-sis)	A maintenance of the normal external environment of an organism.
hypochondriac	(high-poh-KON-dree-ack)	Pertaining to the hypochondrium, the upper lateral abdominal region overlying the ribs
meiosis	(my-OH-sis)	Cell division of sperm or ova
membrane	(MEM-brain)	A soft, thin layer of tissue that covers the inner surface of a body cavity, or divides an organ or space.
metabolism	(meh-TAB-oh-lizm)	The total of the physical and chemical processes necessary to keep the body cells alive
mitosis	(my-TOH-sis)	The continuous process of cell division and cell replacement
nucleus	(NEW-klee-us)	A round body within a cell that contains the chromosomes, or cell "identity"

phagocytosis	(**fag**-oh-sigh-**TOH**-sis)	The process by which phagocytes (a type of white blood cell) ingests bacteria and other foreign particles
pinocytosis	(**pie**-noh-sigh-**TOH**-sis)	The process of absorbing fluids and nutrients by the body cells.
protoplasm	(**PROH**-toh-plazm)	The essential constituent of the living cell
pubic	(**PEW**-bick)	Pertaining to or lying near the pubic bone
thoracic	(thoh-**RAS**-ick)	Pertaining to the chest or thorax
transverse	(trans-**VERS**)	Extending from side to side; at right angles to the long axis of the body
umbilical	(um-**BIL**-ih-kal)	Pertaining to the umbilicus (the navel)

Terms Related to Pathology

anaplasia	(**an**-ah-**PLAY**-zee-ah)	Reverting of cells to a lesser stage of development and their failure to function as mature cells. Characteristic of malignancies (cancers)
aplasia	(ah-**PLAY**-zee-ah)	The failure of an organ or tissue to develop in a normal manner.
atrophy	(**AT**-roh-fee)	Wasting away (without nourishment)
hyperplasia	(**high**-per-**PLAY**-zee-ah)	Increase in the volume of an organ or tissue because of an abnormal increase in the *number* of cells, which remain in their normal arrangement
hypertrophy	(high-**PER**-troh-fee)	Increase in size of an organ or part related to increase in *size* of its constituent cells
hypoplasia	(**high**-poh-**PLAY**-zee-ah)	Incomplete development or underdevelopment of an organ or tissue

3.1   Review: Body Planes

DIRECTIONS: Label the body planes in the figure below.

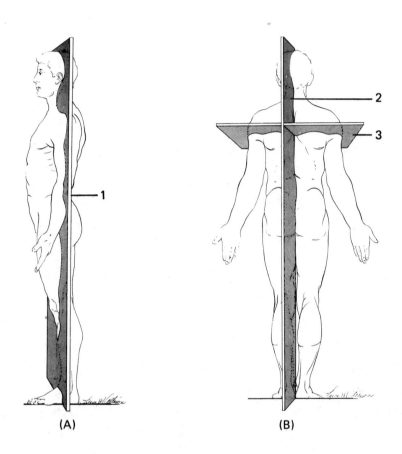

(A)　　　　　　　　(B)

(From Kinn, *Medical Terminology—Review Challenge,* copyright 1987 by Delmar Publishers Inc.)

1. _____

2. _____

3. _____

3.2 Review: Body Cavities

DIRECTIONS: Label the body cavities in the figure below.

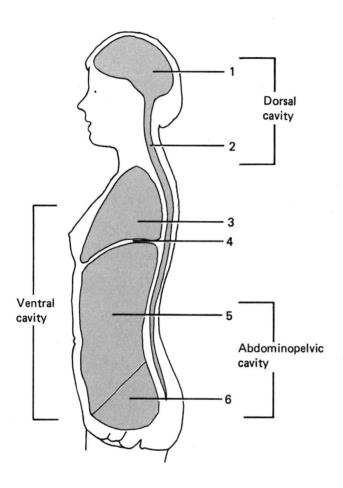

(From Kinn, *Medical Terminology—Review Challenge,* copyright 1987 by Delmar Publishers Inc.)

1. _____   4. _____
2. _____   5. _____
3. _____   6. _____

3.3   Review: Directional Terms

DIRECTIONS: Match the definitions in the right column with the directional terms in the left column.

Directional Term	Definition
____ 1. afferent	A. Toward the head
____ 2. anterior	B. Toward the tail
____ 3. caudal	C. Directed upward
____ 4. central	D. Directed downward
____ 5. cephalic	E. Toward the outer part
____ 6. distal	F. Pertaining to a center
____ 7. efferent	G. Closer to point of origin
____ 8. inferior	H. Farther from point of origin
____ 9. peripheral	I. Situated in back of
____ 10. posterior	J. Situated in front of
____ 11. proximal	K. Away from a center
____ 12. superior	L. Toward a center

3.4   Review: Directional Terms

DIRECTIONS: Match the definitions in the right column with the directional terms in the left column.

Directional Term	Definition
____ 1. deep	A. Referring to sole of foot
____ 2. dorsal	B. Referring to the palm
____ 3. external	C. Pertaining to the back
____ 4. intermediate	D. Pertaining to the belly
____ 5. internal	E. Situated near the surface
____ 6. lateral	F. Situated far beneath the surface
____ 7. medial	G. Between the middle and the side
____ 8. median	H. Referring to the middle
____ 9. mesial	I. Situated in the midline of a structure
____ 10. palmar	J. Pertaining to the middle
____ 11. plantar	K. Pertaining to a side
____ 12. superficial	L. Inside
____ 13. ventral	M. Outside

3.5   Review: Body Motions

DIRECTIONS: Match the definitions in the right column with the body motions listed in the left column.

Body Motions

_____ 1. abduction

_____ 2. adduction

_____ 3. circumduction

_____ 4. extension

_____ 5. flexion

_____ 6. hyperextension

_____ 7. lateral rotation

_____ 8. medial rotation

_____ 9. pronation

_____ 10. supination

Definitions

A. A straightening motion that increases the angle of the joint

B. A turning away from the midline

C. A movement away from the midline

D. A bending motion that decreases the angle of a joint

E. Act of turning the palm of the hand or the sole of the foot upward

F. Turning toward the midline

G. Movement toward the midline

H. Act of turning the palm of the hand or the sole of the foot downward

I. Circular movement of a limb or of the eye

J. Extreme or excessive straightening

3.6   Review: Building Blocks

DIRECTIONS: Cover the column on the left while you define the Building Blocks on the right.

without	1. ana–	_____
cell	2. cyto–	_____
through, across	3. dia–	_____
upon	4. epi–	_____
stomach	5. gastr–	_____
similar, same	6. homeo–	_____
above, excessive	7. hyper–	_____
under, deficient	8. hypo–	_____
change	9. meta–	_____
threadlike	10. mito–	_____
kernel	11. nucle/o	_____
disease	12. –osis	_____
eat, swallow	13. phag/o	_____
fence, wall off	14. –phragm	_____

drink	15. pino–	_____
first	16. proto–	_____
standing	17. –stasis	_____
chest	18. thorac/o	_____
through, across	19. trans–	_____
nourishment	20. –trophy	_____

3.7 Review: Building Blocks

DIRECTIONS: Cover the column on the left while you define the Building Blocks on the right.

skin	1. dermat/o	_____
nerve	2. neur/o	_____
stone	3. lith/o	_____
lung	4. pulmon/o	_____
nourishment	5. –trophy	_____
heart	6. cardi/o	_____
eat, swallow	7. phag/o	_____
kernel, nucleus	8. nucle/o	_____
urine, urinary tract	9. ur/o	_____
disease	10. path/o	_____
larynx	11. laryng/o	_____
mold, shape	12. –plasm	_____
kidney	13. nephr/o	_____
intestine	14. enter/o	_____
blood	15. hemat/o	_____
eye	16. ophthalm/o	_____
vein	17. phleb/o	_____
ear	18. ot/o	_____
narrowing	19. –stenosis	_____
fungus	20. myc/o	_____

3.8 Review: Analyzing Terms

DIRECTIONS: Analyze the following terms by dividing the term into its elements, giving the meaning of each element, and writing a simple definition of the term.

Example

epigastric

epi / gastr / ic
upon/stomach/pertaining to
Pertaining to the upper region of the stomach

1. adipose

_____ / _____

_____ / _____

_____

2. aplasia

_____ / _____

_____ / _____

_____

3. cytoplasm

_____ / _____

_____ / _____

_____

4. hypertrophy

_____ / _____

_____ / _____

_____

5. phagocytosis

_____ / _____ / _____

_____ / _____ / _____

_____

3.9   Review: Building Medical Terms

DIRECTIONS: Fill in the blanks with the appropriate building blocks to build medical terms.

1. Enter/o means intestine.

   A surgeon might make an incision into the intestine.
   This is called enter / _____ / _____ .

2. Surgical removal of part of the intestine is called
   enter / _____ .

3. Cost means rib.
   Beneath the rib is written _____ / _____ / _____

4. Removal of a rib _____ / _____

5. Between the ribs _____ / _____ / _____

6. Gastr is the root for stomach.
   Removal of stomach is written _____ / _____

7. Inflammation of stomach _____ / _____

8. Pain in the stomach _____ / _____

9. Viewing the stomach through a tubular instrument is written
   _____ / _____ / _____

10. Making an incision into the stomach _____ / _____ / _____

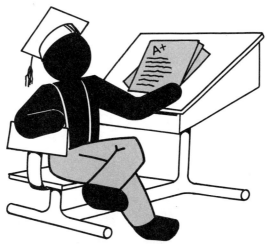

You have now completed the Introduction to Vocabulary Building. Part II will cover the individual body systems and a basic vocabulary for each system.

PART II

BODY SYSTEMS

CHAPTER 4

Integumentary System

OBJECTIVES

When you have successfully completed Chapter 4, you should be able to:
— Discuss the basic functions of the integumentary system.
— Define major terms related to the skin, hair, and nails.
— Build, analyze, and define terms relating to the integumentary system.
— Label the layers and structures of a three-dimensional microscopic view of the skin.

KEY TERMS

albino	(al-**BYE**-noh)	A person born without coloring matter in the skin, hair, and eyes
appendage	(ah-**PEN**-dij)	Anything attached (appended) to a larger or major part; for example, a tail or a limb
bacteria	(back-**TEE**-ree-ah)	A wide group of typically one-celled microorganisms. Singular: *bacterium*
congenital	(kon-**JEN**-ih-tal)	Present at birth (but not necessarily inherited)
corium	(**KOR**-ree-um)	The true skin
dermatologist	(**der**-mah-**TOL**-oh-jist)	A physician who specializes in the diagnosis and treatment of the skin conditions
dermatology	(**der**-mah-**TOL**-oh-jee)	The science of the skin and its diseases
dermis	(**DER**-mis)	The skin. Also, *corium*
epidermis	(**ep**-ih-**DER**-miss)	The outer layer of skin. Sometimes called the cuticle layer
epithelial	(**ep**-ih-**THEE**-lee-al)	Pertaining to or composed of epithelium
fibrous	(**FYE**-brus)	Composed of or containing fibers
follicle	(**FOL**-ih-kal)	A small sac or cavity
integumentary	(in-teg-you-**MEN**-tah-ree)	Relating to the skin
keratin	(**KER**-ah-tin)	An insoluble protein substance found in the skin, hair, tooth enamel, and nails
lanugo	(lah-**NEW**-goh)	The downy hairs that cover the body of a newborn
lubricate	(**LEW**-brih-kayt)	To make smooth or slippery
melanin	(**MEL**-ah-nin)	The pigment that gives color to the hair, skin, and eyes
melanocyte	(**MEL**-ah-noh-sight)	The cell that forms melanin
nostrils	(**NOS**-trilz)	External openings of the nose; *nares*
nutrition	(new-**TRIH**-shun)	The process by which the body obtains and uses food substances
perspiration	(**per**-spih-**RAY**-shun)	The salty secretion of the sweat glands; *sweat*

sebaceous	(seh-**BAY**-shus)	Pertaining to *sebum;* containing the oily matter (sebum) secreted by the sebaceous glands
sebum	(**SEE**-bum)	The secretion of the sebaceous glands of the skin
slough	(sluhf)	The separation of dead tissue from living tissue
subcutaneous	(**sub**-kew-**TAY**-nee-us)	Beneath the skin
sudoriferous	(**sue**-doh-**RIF**-er-us)	Carrying or manufacturing sweat
temperature	(**TEM**-per-ah-chewr)	The degree of heat or cold of a substance or living body measured on a definite scale
ultraviolet	(**uhl**-trah-**VYE**-oh-let)	Beyond the visible spectrum at its violet end, occurring between the violet rays and the roentgen rays

OVERVIEW

The integumentary system (*integument* means covering) consists of the skin, hair follicles, nails, and underlying glands. It is the most visible of the body systems.

The skin serves as a protective covering for the body. It keeps out foreign substances including bacteria and helps hold moisture in the tissues. It also serves as an organ of excretion by getting rid of waste matter through the pores. It shelters the body from harmful ultraviolet rays, while it uses sunshine to form helpful vitamin D. It regulates body temperature, keeping the body cool through perspiration but preventing heat loss when the body is exposed to cold. The skin also acts as a receptor organ for the senses of touch and pain through its vast network of nerve endings.

At times the skin seems magical in its ability to return to normal after suffering minor wounds and blemishes. It accommodates to changes in size that accompany pregnancy and childbirth, loss and gain of body weight. It plays a part in sexual attraction. It even provides a unique personal identification—fingerprints. Close examination of the skin by the physician can provide valuable information regarding the individual's general health.

STRUCTURE OF THE SKIN

The skin is composed of layers called the *epidermis,* or outer layer; the *dermis* (sometimes called the true skin, or *corium*), which lies just under the epidermis; and a supporting underlayer of subcutaneous ("under the skin") tissue that connects it to other body structures (Figure 4.1). Each of these layers is in turn composed of layers which need not concern us now.

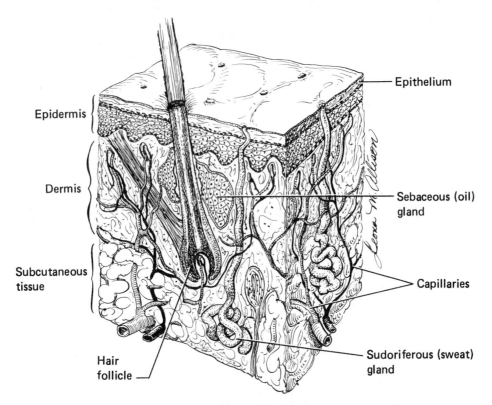

Epidermis

Dermis

Subcutaneous
tissue

Hair
follicle

Epithelium

Sebaceous (oil)
gland

Capillaries

Sudoriferous (sweat)
gland

FIGURE 4.1   Three-dimensional microscopic view of the skin (From Kinn, *Medical Terminology—Review Challenge*, copyright 1987 by Delmar Publishers Inc.)

Epidermis

The *epidermis* (sometimes called the cuticle layer) is composed of epithelial cells. Its outermost layer actually is composed of dead cells that form a tough protein material called *keratin*, which acts as a protective covering. The thickness of this keratin layer varies in different areas of the body. For example, it is thickest at the soles of the feet. The epithelial cells are constantly being renewed, the dead outer keratin being cast off as new cells are formed in the deeper layers and gradually push toward the surface. The thickness of the epidermis varies in different parts of the body, the thinnest being in the eyelids and the thickest covering the back.

Skin has color because of the presence of *melanin*, a pigment that is produced by special cells in the epidermis called *melanocytes*. The differences in skin color among humans is determined by the amount of melanin present. A person with a congenital lack of melanocytes is called an *albino*.

Dermis

The *dermis* is composed of dense connective tissue and forms many of the accessory structures or appendages of the skin. The upper layer of the dermis is composed of fibrous connective tissue within which are the blood vessels, nerve endings, and hair follicles. Underlying the *dermis* is the subcutaneous tissue, a layer of delicate, loosely structured connective tissue containing various amounts of adipose tissue (fat).

SKIN APPENDAGES

The accessory structures of the skin include hair follicles, the nails, sebaceous (oil) glands, and sudoriferous (sweat) glands.

Hair and Nails

Normally, all body surfaces except the palms of the hands and soles of the feet contain hair follicles. Newborn infants are covered by very soft, fine hair called *lanugo*. This soon disappears and is replaced by coarser hair. Growth patterns vary, but few individuals grow hair in all the possible follicles. Males and females have about the same number of hair follicles, but the male usually produces darker, coarser body hair. The male is also more likely to lose hair through baldness.

Certain areas of the body have protective hair. Hairs inside the nostrils, for instance, slow the intake of air, warm air as it is taken in, keep out dust particles and small insects, and prevent the mucus from running out of the nostrils. Eyelashes and eyebrows protect the eyes.

The nails and hair are composed of hard keratin that does not slough off like the soft keratin on the surface of the epidermis. Consequently, the hair and nails must be cut as needed. They have no nerves, but the nailbed does have many nerves and blood vessels, and is quite sensitive. The scalp is also plentifully supplied with blood vessels.

Glands of the Skin

The *sebaceous* (oil) *glands* secrete an oily substance called *sebum* that lubricates the skin and hair. The *sudoriferous* (sweat) *glands* help control body temperature by secreting water on the skin. Evaporation of this secreted water (*perspiration,* or sweat) cools the body during exercise or in hot environments.

Dermatology is the medical specialty dealing with the skin and its disorders. The dermatologist can learn much about a patient's general health by closely examining the skin. The skin may reveal evidence of poor nutrition, allergic conditions, or the presence of infection. A change from the skin's normal color may be significant. Other signs that the physician may note are excessive sweating, dryness, or oiliness. Skin blemishes may signify disease. Patients who are bedridden for a long while sometimes develop skin problems brought about by a decrease in oxygen supply to the tissues. Some common lesions of the skin are shown in Figure 4.2.

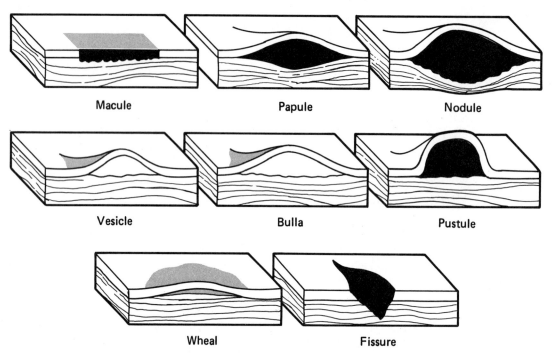

FIGURE 4.2 Skin lesions

BUILDING BLOCKS

ROOTS AND COMBINING FORMS

Word Element	Meaning
acanth/o	thorny, spiny
aden/o	gland
adip/o	fat
alb/o, albin/o	white
caus/o	burn
cry/o	cold
cutane/o	skin
derma, dermat/o, derm/o	skin
diaphor/o	sweat
edema	swelling
epitheli/o	outer skin

BUILDING BLOCKS (continued)

ROOTS AND COMBINING FORMS (continued)

Word Element	Meaning
erythem/o	redness, flushed
erythr/o	red
esthesi/o	sensation, perception
graphia	a writing
hidr/o	sweat
histi/o	tissue
kele	tumor
kerat/o	horny tissue, cornea
leuk/o	white
lip/o	fat, lipid
melan/o	black
myc/o	fungus
necr/o	death
onych/o	nail
pachy/o	heavy, thick
phyt/o	plant
pil/o	hair
scler/o	hard, sclera (white of eye)
seb/o	sebum
squam/o	scale
steat/o	fat, lipid, sebum
sudor	sweat, perspiration
therm/o	heat
trich/o	hair
ungu/o	nail
xanth/o	yellow
xer/o	dry
zoster	girdle, encircling

SUFFIXES

Word Element	Meaning
–algia	pain
–ectasia	dilation, expansion, distention
–emia	blood

SUFFIXES (continued)

Word Element	Meaning
–itis	inflammation
–lysis	loosening, setting free
–oid	resembling
–oma	a swelling or tumor
–rhea	flow

PREFIXES

Word Element	Meaning
de–	lack of
para–	beside, beyond, accessory to

VOCABULARY

General Terms

cicatrix	(sick-**AY**-tricks)	A scar that forms during the healing of a wound
desquamation	(**des**-kwah-**MAY**-shun)	Shedding of the epithelial cells (epidermis)
diaphoresis	(**die**-ah-foh-**REE**-sis)	Excessive sweating or perspiration
eruption	(ee-**RUP**-shun)	A breaking out on the skin, such as a rash, pimple, or blister; also, the breaking through the gums by a tooth
erythema	(er-ih-**THEE**-mah)	Diffused redness of the skin caused by congestion of the capillaries
excoriation	(ecks-**koh**-ree-**AY**-shun)	Superficial damage to the skin, such as that caused by scratching, burns, or chemicals
fissure	(**FISH**-er)	Any cleft, crack, or groove, normal or otherwise
flush		Temporary redness of the face and neck
granulation	(**gran**-you-**LAY**-shun)	The formation of tissue from the

new capillaries that appear on the surface of a wound during the healing process

keloid	(KEE-loyd)	A raised, irregularly shaped scar that forms following surgery or injury and which may continue to grow for an extended time
keratosis	(ker-ah-TOH-sis)	Any horny growth on the skin such as a wart or callus.
laceration	(lass-er-AY-shun)	A ragged or mangled tearing of the flesh
macula	(MACK-you-lah)	A small colored or thickened spot on the skin that is not raised above the surface
milia	(MILL-ee-ah)	Small white nodules in the skin (whiteheads). Plural of milium
mole	(mohl)	A congenital raised, pigmented benign growth on the surface of the skin
nevus	(NEE-vus)	A mole; birthmark
pallor	(PAL-or)	Absence of normal skin color; paleness
pigment	(PIG-ment)	The organic coloring matter formed in body tissues
purulent	(PYOU-rew-lent)	Containing, forming, or consisting of pus; suppurative
vesication	(ves-ih-KAY-shun)	The result or process of blistering
wound	(wewnd)	A laceration or break in normal tissue caused by surgery, violence, or trauma
xeroderma	(zee-roh-DER-mah)	Abnormal roughness or dryness of the skin, sometimes accompanied by discoloration
xerosis	(zee-ROH-sis)	Abnormal dryness that affects the skin and the mucous membranes of the eyes and mouth

Terms Related to Anatomy and Physiology

cuticle	(KYOU-tih-kul)	Alternative term for the epidermis of the skin
integument	(in-TEG-you-ment)	A covering, especially the covering of the body; the skin
lunula	(LEW-new-lah)	A crescent or moon-shaped area; the whitish moon-shaped area at the base of the nail
plantar	(PLAN-tar)	Referring to the sole of the foot. A plantar wart occurs on the sole of the foot
pore	(por)	A small opening; the opening for a sweat gland on the skin
receptor	(ree-SEP-tor)	A receiver; a group of cells that receive stimuli, such as sensory nerve endings.

Terms Related to Pathology

acanthosis	(ack-an-THOH-sis)	An increased thickening of the prickle cell layer of the epidermis
acne	(ACK-nee)	An inflammatory disease of the sebaceous glands accompanied by blackheads and pimples
alopecia	(al-oh-PEE-she-ah)	Loss of hair from areas where it is normally present; baldness
angiitis	(an-jee-EYE-tis)	Inflammation of a blood or lymph vessel
angioedema	(an-jee-oh-eh-DEE-mah)	A condition marked by temporary swelling of the skin or mucous membranes, usually accompanied by intense itching. It may be related to an allergy, to a psychologic state, or to an unknown origin
bulla	(BULL-ah)	A large blister
callus	(KAL-us)	A localized, hardened, thickened

		area of the epidermis caused by pressure or friction
carbuncle	(**KAR**-bung-kal)	A bacterial infection composed of a cluster of boils (*furuncles*), spreading into the subcutaneous tissues
causalgia	(kaw-**ZAL**-jee-ah)	A burning pain caused by injury to a peripheral nerve
cellulitis	(**sell**-you-**LIE**-tis)	Inflammation of cellular tissue
cyanosis	(**sigh**-ah-**NOH**-sis)	A bluish discoloration of the skin and mucous membranes that occurs when the tissues are not receiving sufficient oxygen.
comedo	(**KOM**-eh-doh)	The dried, discolored secretion of an oil gland plugging a pore; a blackhead
decubitus ulcer	(dee-**KYOU**-bih-tus **UHL**-ser)	An open sore (ulceration) caused by prolonged pressure when a patient is allowed to lie in one place for a long time. Also called a bed sore
dermatitis	(der-mah-**TIE**-tis)	Inflammation of the skin
desquamation	(**des**-kwah-**MAY**-shun)	The shedding or scaling off of epithelial cells
diaphoresis	(**die**-ah-foh-**REE**-sis)	Profuse perspiration
ecchymosis	(eck-ih-**MOH**-sis)	A spot where bleeding under the skin or mucous membrane has formed a nonelevated, blue or purplish patch; a bruise
eczema	(**ECK**-zeh-mah)	A noncontagious skin rash characterized by redness, itching, and blistering
epidermolysis	(ep-ih-der-**MOL**-ih-sis)	A loosening of the epidermis, sometimes accompanied by the formation of blisters
epidermophytosis	(ep-ih-**der**-moh-fye-**TOH**-sis)	Infection of the epidermis by fungi or yeasts

furuncle	(**FYOU**-rung-kal)	A bacterial infection involving a hair follicle and/or sebaceous gland; a boil
gangrene	(**GANG**-green)	A necrosis (death) of tissue usually caused by a loss of blood supply
herpes	(**HER**-peez)	An inflammatory skin disease usually caused by the virus *Herpes simplex*, characterized by the formation of clusters of small fluid-filled sacs
hidradenitis	(**high**-drad-eh-**NIGH**-tis)	Inflammation of a sweat gland
hyperplasia	(**high**-per-**PLAY**-zee-ah)	Enlargement of a body part brought about by an increased number of individual normal cells
icterus	(**ICK**-ter-us)	Yellowness of skin and whites of the eyes, mucous membranes, and body fluids caused by an excess of bilirubin (bile pigment) in the blood; jaundice
impetigo	(**im**-peh-**TIE**-go)	A spreading bacterial skin infection evidenced by vesicles (fluid-filled sacs) and pustules (pus-filled sacs)
ischemia	(is-**KEE**-mee-ah)	Local and temporary deficiency of blood in a part resulting from a narrowing or blockage of a blood vessel. Prolonged ischemia can lead to serious or even fatal conditions. For example, prolonged lack of blood flow to a limb leads to gangrene; prolonged lack of blood flow to the heart muscle can kill.
leukoderma	(lew-koh-**DER**-mah)	Small patchy areas of abnormally white skin
leukoplakia	(lew-kah-**PLAY**-kee-ah)	Formation of white patches on the mucous membrane of the cheeks, gums, or tongue which may be pre-cancerous

melanoderma	(**mel**-ah-noh-**DER**-mah)	A generalized or patchy discoloration of the skin caused by an abnormally high level of melanin
melanoma	(**mel**-ah-**NOH**-mah)	A tumor of pigmented cells that may or may not be malignant (cancerous).
mycosis	(my-**KOH**-sis)	A general term for any disease caused by a fungus
nodule	(**NOD**-youl)	A small, solid knot or swelling that can be detected by touch
onychia	(oh-**NICK**-ee-ah)	Purulent (pus-forming) inflammation of the nailbed, frequently resulting in loss of the nail
papule	(**PAP**-youl)	A small, solid, red, raised area on the skin
paronychia	(**par**-oh-**NICK**-ee-ah)	Inflammation around the edge of the nail
pediculosis	(peh-**dick**-you-**LOH**-sis)	Infestation with lice
pemphigus	(**PEM**-fih-gus)	A skin disease characterized by successive crops of large blisters which can prove fatal if neglected
petechiae	(pee-**TEE**-kee-ee)	Pinpoint-size purplish-red spots caused by hemorrhage within the skin or under the mucous membrane
pruritus	(prew-**RYE**-tus)	Severe or chronic itching that may indicate an underlying abnormality
psoriasis	(so-**RYE**-ah-sis)	A chronic (long-lasting) skin disease characterized by red patches covered with silvery scales
purpura	(**PUR**-pyou-rah)	Purplish or brownish-red discolorations of the skin caused by bleeding into the tissues
pustule	(**PUS**-tyoul)	Raised pus-filled area or sac
scabies	(**SKAY**-beez)	A contagious skin disease caused by

		the itch mite, resulting in severe itching and eczema
scleroderma	(sklee-roh-DER-mah)	A chronic disease that causes a hardening and shrinking of the skin and vital organs
seborrhea	(seb-oh-REE-ah)	Excessive secretion of sebum accompanied by greasy skin and dandruff
steatoma	(stee-ah-TOH-mah)	A sebaceous cyst
tinea	(TIN-ee-ah)	A superficial fungal infection of the skin
ulcer	(UL-ser)	An open sore
urticaria	(er-tih-KAY-ree-ah)	A raised, itchy skin reaction, commonly called hives
vesicle	(VES-ih-kal)	A small fluid-filled sac
wart	(wort)	A benign flesh-colored raised area on the skin
wheal	(wheel)	A temporary, smooth, slightly raised area on the skin that is darker or lighter than the surrounding area
xanthoma	(zan-THOH-mah)	A yellowish papule or nodule resulting from deposits of fats

Terms Related to Surgery or Treatment

cryosurgery	(krye-oh-SUR-jer-ee)	Surgery performed by the application of extreme cold
curettage	(kyou-reh-TAHZH)	A scraping procedure used to cleanse the bottom of a cavity after removal of a lesion; the removal of a growth from the wall of a cavity with a spoon-shaped instrument called a *curet*. Also called curettement
electrodesiccation	(ee-leck-troh-des-ih-KAY-shun)	Drying of skin tissue by means of short high-frequency electric sparks

fulguration	(full-gew-RAY-shun)	Destruction of living tissue by long high frequency sparks

4.1 Review: System

1. The skin is composed of two layers, the _____ and the _____ .

2. The outer layer of the _____ , a horny material called _____ , acts as a protective covering.

3. The outer _____ is continually being sloughed off as new cells are formed.

4. Skin color results from the presence of _____ .

5. The _____ is a pigment formed by _____ .

6. A person deficient in _____ is called an albino.

7. A layer of delicate connective tissue forms the undersurface of the _____ .

8. All body surfaces except the _____ and the _____ contain hair follicles.

9. The _____ and _____ are composed of a hard keratin.

10. The oil glands are known as _____ glands and secrete _____ .

11. The sweat glands are called _____ glands.

12. The medical specialty dealing with disorders of the skin is_____ and the specialist is called a/an _____ .

4.2   Review: Building Blocks

DIRECTIONS: Cover the column on the left while you define the following building blocks.

thorny, spiny	1. acanth/o _____
fat	2. adip/o _____
pain	3. −algia _____
cold	4. cry/o _____
skin	5. dermat/o _____
expansion, distention	6. −ectasia _____
blood	7. −emia _____
redness, flushed	8. erythem/o _____
sensation, perception	9. esthesi/o _____
sweat	10. hidr/o _____
horny tissue, cornea	11. kerat/o _____
fat, lipid	12. lip/o _____
black	13. melan/o _____
death of cells or tissues	14. necr/o _____
a swelling, tumor	15. −oma _____
heavy, thick	16. pachy/o _____
plant	17. phyt/o _____
flow	18. −rhea _____
sebum	19. seb/o _____
fat, lipid, sebum	20. steat/o _____
heat	21. therm/o _____
nail	22. ungu/o _____
dry	23. xer/o _____

4.3   Review: Building Blocks

DIRECTIONS: Cover the column on the left while you define the following building blocks.

gland	1. aden/o _____
white	2. alb/o _____
burn	3. caus/o _____
skin	4. cutane/o _____
sweat	5. diaphor/o _____
swelling	6. edema _____
outer skin	7. epitheli/o _____
red	8. erythr/o _____
a writing	9. graphia _____
tissue	10. histi/o _____
tumor	11. kele _____
white	12. leuk/o _____
loosening, setting free	13. –lysis _____
fungus	14. myc/o _____
resembling	15. –oid _____
nail	16. onych/o _____
beside, beyond	17. para– _____
hair	18. pil/o _____
hard, sclera	19. scler/o _____
scale	20. squam/o _____
sweat, perspiration	21. sudor _____
hair	22. trich/o _____
yellow	23. xanth/o _____
girdle, encircling	24. zoster _____

4.4 Review: Skin Structures

DIRECTIONS: Identify the layers and structures of the skin by matching the letters with the correct labels.

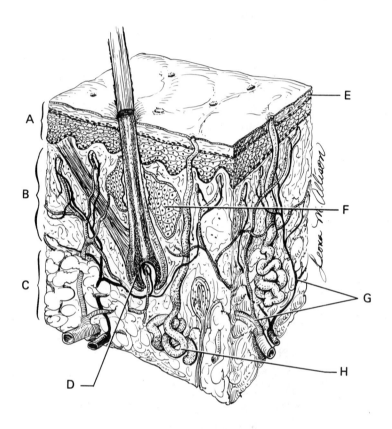

(From Kinn, *Medical Terminology—Review Challenge,* copyright 1987 by Delmar Publishers Inc.)

1. _____ capillaries
2. _____ dermis
3. _____ epidermis
4. _____ epithelium

5. _____ hair follicle
6. _____ sebaceous gland
7. _____ subcutaneous tissue
8. _____ sweat gland

4.5 Review: Vocabulary

DIRECTIONS: If the word is correctly spelled, place a checkmark beside it. If it is incorrectly spelled, write the correct spelling in the space provided.

1. eczema _____
2. gangreen _____
3. impetigo _____
4. comedo _____
5. electrodessication _____
6. nevus _____
7. papule _____
8. curretage _____
9. fissure _____
10. vesical _____
11. laseration _____
12. ischemia _____
13. purolent _____
14. zeroderma _____
15. vesication _____

4.6 Review: Combining Forms

DIRECTIONS: Complete each of the medical terms listed by filling in the blanks.

1. Inflammation of a blood or lymph vessel _____ itis
2. Chronic hardening and shrinking of the connective tissues sclero _____
3. A burning pain _____ algia
4. Bluish discoloration of the skin and mucous membranes _____ osis
5. Redness of the skin _____ ema
6. Inflammation of a sweat gland _____ itis
7. Sebaceous cyst _____ oma
8. Excessive secretion of sebum _____ rhea
9. Any disease caused by a fungus _____ osis
10. Formation of white patches on the mucous membranes _____ plakia

Reading Comprehension 4.1

DIRECTIONS: Underline the medical terms as you go through the reading exercise. Then list and analyze the terms. Some will be completely new to you. Consult a medical dictionary for their meanings. Then re-read the material for better comprehension.

Postoperative Report

Preoperative Diagnosis: Ulcer, left ankle

Postoperative Diagnosis: Same

Operation: Excision of ulcer, left ankle, with skin graft

Procedure: The skin graft was excised from the inner side of the right thigh. The contour of the thigh in this area made it rather difficult to remove a perfectly rectangular piece of skin, but an adequate amount was obtained. The ulcer on the anterior surface of the left ankle was excised down to the fascia. Granulation tissue was removed. The edges of the ulcer were excised and the distal portion was excised to a further distance to attempt to remove as much scar tissue as possible. The scar tissue, however, was everywhere and it was not possible to go beyond it. When the area was debrided, there were several bleeding points which necessitated stick ties with #4–0 silk to arrest the bleeding. Numerous other bleeding points were fulgurated. The graft was then sutured in place over the defect and xeroform gauze pressure dressing applied. A nylon gauze was applied with a pressure dressing over the donor site.

Reading Comprehension 4.2

DIRECTIONS: Underline the medical terms as you go through the reading exercise. Then list and analyze the terms. Some will be completely new to you. Consult a medical dictionary for their meanings. Then re-read the material for better comprehension.

History and Physical Examination

Chief Complaint:
Patient is a 65-year-old white male admitted from the office with fever. He has known multiple myeloma, presently receiving daily interferon therapy.

Present Illness:
Patient's diagnosis was made in November 19— after serum protein electrophoresis was abnormal and bone marrow elevation showed typical myeloma. He was initially treated

with Alkeran and prednisone which were discontinued in February 19—. He was then in remission until December 19— and then was treated with Cytoxan and Decadron. He had progressive disease in March 19— and was started on vincristine, Adriamycin, and Decadron. He then had some shortness of breath and was evaluated by echocardiogram and cardiac ejection fraction in the summer of 19—. These were found to be normal. At that time, however, he did have some abnormal liver function tests and might have had non-A, non-B hepatitis. These resolved. He was admitted in August 19— with acute shortness of breath, pulmonary infiltrates, hypoxemia, and pneumonia. He was intubated and treated with IV antibiotics and aggressive therapy in the ICU. He resolved remarkably well and was discharged at that time on IV antibiotics. He has been followed by Dr. Blank in our office and has been treated with five million units of interferon per day based on a second opinion obtained at Hospital A.

He was last admitted to this hospital on 4/26/— and was found to have a left lower lobe pneumonia that was treated with antibiotics. This pneumonia was resolving and he was discharged on oral antibiotics which have subsequently been discontinued. However, he was seen in the office today by Dr. Blank with a temperature of 102° F. Because of his recent history of pneumonia and his feeling very poorly, he was immediately admitted for evaluation and therapy. He has not had any cough or chest pain. He has had no dysuria or other GU tract symptoms. He has no headache or other symptoms that would suggest meningeal infection. He has, however, had some draining sinuses and he feels that this may be the site of his infection. He has no other new complaints at the present time.

For past history, family history, and social history, see old charts.

Review of Systems: Noncontributory

Physical Examination:

General: Slightly toxic appearing male in no acute distress. He does not appear tachypneic or short of breath at rest.

Vital Signs: BP 120/70; temperature 102° F; pulse 90 and regular; respiratory rate 20.

HEENT: Normocephalic. Scalp showed no abnormalities. Hearing appeared normal. There was a slight sunburn over the face. Eyes showed no icterus. Fundi showed no papilledema. TMs were clear. There was no tenderness to palpation of the sinuses. Tongue normally hydrated, no pharyngitis.

Neck: Supple without lymphadenopathy. Carotid pulses were full and equal. Thyroid was not enlarged. JVP was not increased.

Chest: Clear to A&P.

Heart: No murmurs, rubs, or gallops. There was a regular tachycardia.

Abdomen: No hepatosplenomegaly or abdominal masses.

Rectal: No abnormalities in March, not repeated on this occasion.

GU: Penis, scrotum, and testicles negative.

Extremities: No clubbing, cyanosis, edema.

Neurologic:

1. Longstanding multiple myeloma since 19—, having failed multiple chemotherapy regimens, presently stable on 5 million units interferon per day.
2. Fever and chills. Rule out bacteremia or viremia.

Plan: Patient will be admitted and cultures will be obtained as well as routine x-rays and sinus x-rays. He will immediately be started on IV antibiotics following the cultures. Further recommendations to follow based on his course.

Reading Comprehension Vocabulary

Use the space below to list the medical terms for analysis and definition.

_____

_____

_____

_____

_____

_____

_____

_____

_____

_____

_____

_____

_____

_____

_____

_____

_____

CHAPTER 5

Skeletal System

OBJECTIVES

When you have successfully completed Chapter 5, you should be able to:
— Distinguish the types of bones.
— Define the common markings of bone.
— Name and define the divisions of the skeleton.
— Name the classes of joints.
— Correctly name the bones of the skeleton on a familiar illustration.
— Define, spell, and pronounce the terms in the chapter vocabulary.
— Build medical terms from the word elements in this and previous chapters.

KEY TERMS

cancellous bone	(**KAN**-sell-us bohn)	Spongy bone resembling latticework
circumference	(ser-**KUM**-fer-ens)	The boundary surrounding anything
compact bone	(**KOM**-packt)	Hard or dense bone
femur	(**FEE**-mur)	Thigh bone
intervertebral	(in-ter-**VER**-teh-bral)	Lying between the vertebrae
junction	(**JUNCK**-shun)	The place where any two parts come together
marrow	(**MAR**-oh)	A soft, fatty material that fills the hollow parts of bones. *Yellow marrow* is found in the long bones and consists of mostly fat cells and connective tissue. *Red marrow* is found in cancellous tissue of bones and produces early forms of red and white blood cells.
medullary	(**med**-you-**LAIR**-ee)	Pertaining to the inner or central portion of an organ. From the Latin words for middle and marrow. *Medulla ossium* is bone marrow.
necrosis	(neh-**KROH**-sis)	Localized death of tissue or bone surrounded by healthy parts
projection	(proh-**JECK**-shun)	A jutting out, especially at a sharp angle
sternum	(**STER**-num)	The breast bone

STRUCTURE AND FUNCTION OF THE SKELETAL SYSTEM

The skeletal system includes all of the bones of the body (Figure 5.1). The study of the bones is called *osteology.*

The adult human skeleton consists of 206 bones. Its main function is to provide shape and support to the body. Joints allow movement of the whole body and of individual parts. Many of the bones protect delicate internal organs by forming a surrounding framework. For example, the bones of the skull protect the brain. The skeletal framework also provides points of attachment for muscles. Red blood cells form in the bone marrow, a soft, fatty material that fills the hollow spaces of bones. Bone tissue also serves as a storehouse for the minerals calcium and phosphorus.

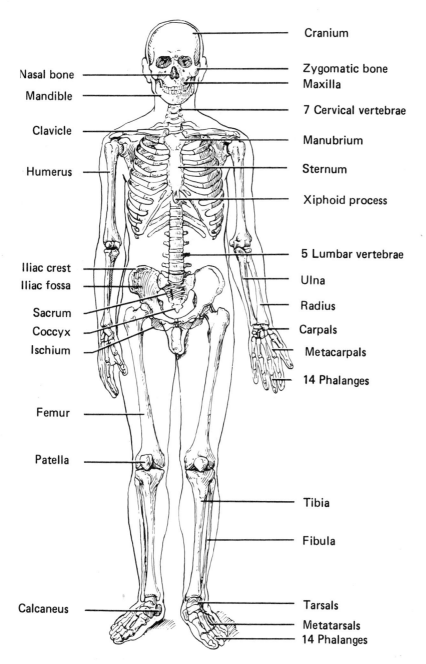

Cranium

Zygomatic bone
Maxilla

Nasal bone

Mandible

7 Cervical vertebrae

Clavicle

Manubrium

Humerus

Sternum

Xiphoid process

5 Lumbar vertebrae

Iliac crest

Ulna

Iliac fossa

Radius

Sacrum

Carpals

Coccyx

Ischium

Metacarpals

14 Phalanges

Femur

Patella

Tibia

Fibula

Calcaneus

Tarsals

Metatarsals
14 Phalanges

FIGURE 5.1   The skeleton (From Kinn, *Medical Terminology—Review Challenge,* copyright 1987 by Delmar Publishers Inc.)

TYPES OF BONES, STRUCTURE, AND BONE MARKINGS

Types of Bones

The many bones in the human body can be classified as belonging to five types (Figure 5.2).

Types	Examples
long	humerus, radius, ulna, femur, tibia, fibula
short	wrist and ankle bones
flat	ribs, sternum, scapulae
irregular	vertebrae, face, and hip bones
sesamoid	small bones, such as the patella, which form in tendons that are subjected to pressure

Structure

Long bones such as the femur have both compact (hard) bone and *cancellous* (spongy) bone. The long, slender part of the bone, the *diaphysis*, or bone shaft, is composed of compact bone. In the center of the shaft is a cavity called the *medullary cavity*, which is filled with *bone marrow*. This cavity is lined with cancellous bone. Its size increases as the bone grows in circumference. The two ends of each long bone, the *epiphyses*, are composed of hard bone on the outside and cancellous bone on the inside.

Surrounding the shaft of the bone is a fibrous membrane, the *periosteum*. It contains blood vessels and bone-forming cells called *osteoblasts*. The periosteum functions in the nutrition, growth, and repair of the bones. The medullary cavity within the bone is lined with a membrane, the *endosteum*, cells called *osteoclasts*, which break down bone during growth so that osteoblasts can re-form it in new shapes. (Here is an example of the difference a single letter makes in medical terms: osteoblasts form bone, osteoclasts erode it.

Bone Markings

Bones have openings, depressions, processes, and projections that are called *markings* and are used as reference points.

OPENINGS. The word *foramen* (foh-**RAY**-men) means a natural opening or passage. A tube-shaped opening is a *canal* or *meatus* (mee-**AY**-tus) such as the ear canal. Cavities within bony structures, especially those within the skull, are called *sinuses* (for example, the paranasal (**par**-ah-**NAY**-zal) sinuses).

DEPRESSIONS. A depression in a bone may be called a:

fossa	(**FOSS**-ah)	a ditch or canal
groove		a long narrow channel
fissure	(**FISH**-ur)	a narrow, deep groove
sulcus	(**SUHL**-kus)	a shallow surface groove
pit		a tiny hollow pocket

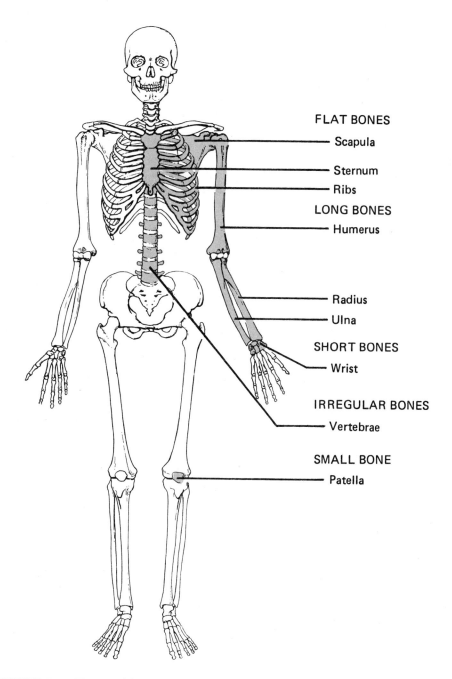

FLAT BONES
— Scapula
— Sternum
— Ribs

LONG BONES
— Humerus

— Radius
— Ulna

SHORT BONES
— Wrist

IRREGULAR BONES
— Vertebrae

SMALL BONE
— Patella

FIGURE 5.2   Types of bones

The names of many specific depressions will be found in a medical dictionary, listed under these general terms.

PROCESSES AND PROJECTIONS. The *head* of a bone is the rounded projection just beyond the narrow part or *neck* of the bone. A *condyle* (**KON**-dial) is a rounded projection on a bone that enters into the formation of a joint. A *process* is a small rounded projection or outgrowth. Other terms used to identify processes are *trochanter*, (troh-**KAN**-ter), *tuberosity*, (**tew**-ber-**AHS**-ih-tee) *spine*, and *crest*.

DIVISIONS OF THE SKELETON

The skeleton has two main divisions, the *axial* (**ACK**-see-al) *skeleton* and the *appendicular* (**ap**-pen-**DICK**-you-lar) *skeleton* (Table 5.1). The axial skeleton, composed of the skull, vertebrae, and thorax, contains 80 bones. The appendicular skeleton is composed of the upper and lower extremities and contains 126 bones.

Axial Skeleton

SKULL. The skull can be divided into the *cranium*, with 8 bones, and the *face* with 15 bones, plus 6 little bones, the *ossicles* in the ears.

VERTEBRAL COLUMN. The 26 bones of the vertebral column are separated by shock-absorbing *intervertebral disks* made up of cartilage and containing a jellylike substance. The vertebrae are identified by location (Figure 5.3) as being the:

- cervical spine   (C_1 to C_7)
- thoracic spine   (T_1 to T_{12})
- lumbar spine   (L_1 to L_5)
- sacrum   (5 fused vertebrae forming one structure)
- coccyx (tail bone) (5 fused vertebre forming one structure)

TABLE 5.1. Divisions of the Human Skeleton			
Axial Skeleton		**Appendicular Skeleton**	
Skull		Upper extremities:	
cranium	8 bones	collarbone, shoulder blade, arm,	
face	15	forearm wrist, hand and fingers	
ear ossicles	6		64 bones
Vertebral column	26	Lower extremities:	
Ribs and sternum	25	hip, thigh, leg, ankle and foot	
Total	80		62 bones
		Total	126

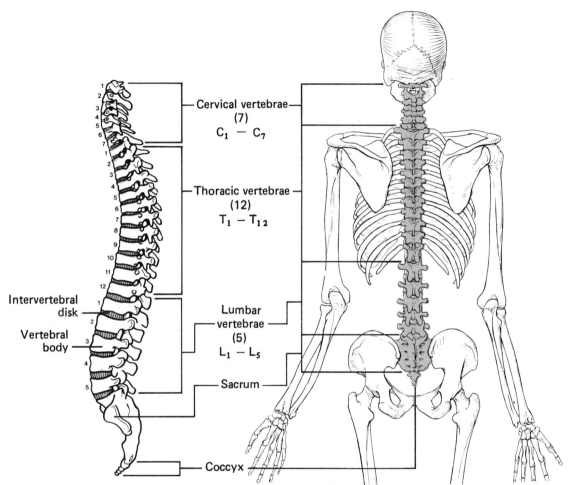

FIGURE 5.3 **The vertebrae** (From Keir, Wise, and Krebs-Shannon, *Medical Assisting: Clinical and Administrative Competencies,* copyright 1986 by Delmar Publishers Inc.)

THORAX. In adults there are twelve pairs of ribs, each pair of which is attached at the spinal column to a thoracic vertebra (Figure 5.4). Starting from the top, the first seven pairs are also attached in front to the *sternum* or breast bone. These seven pairs are called the true ribs. The next three pairs are attached by cartilage to the adjoining rib above and are called false ribs. The last two pairs have free ends and are sometimes called false ribs but are also referred to as floating ribs.

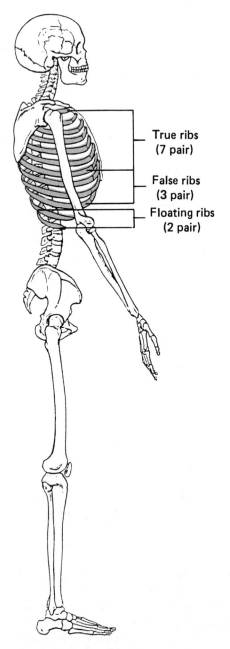

True ribs
(7 pair)

False ribs
(3 pair)

Floating ribs
(2 pair)

FIGURE 5.4   The ribs

The sternum has three parts (Figure 5.5). The broad upper part is called the *manubrium*; the middle portion is the *body;* and the small, lower portion is called the *xiphoid process.*

Appendicular Skeleton

The extremities consist of the structures of the shoulders and arms (upper extremity) and those of the hips and legs (lower extremity). Both the upper and the lower extremities are paired.

UPPER EXTREMITY. *Each* upper extremity has 32 bones (Figure 5.6) and includes:

- clavicle (collarbone)
- scapula (shoulder blade)
- humerus (upper arm bone)
- 2 forearm bones (radius and ulna)
- 8 carpal (wrist) bones
- 5 metacarpal (hand) bones
- 14 phalanges (finger bones)

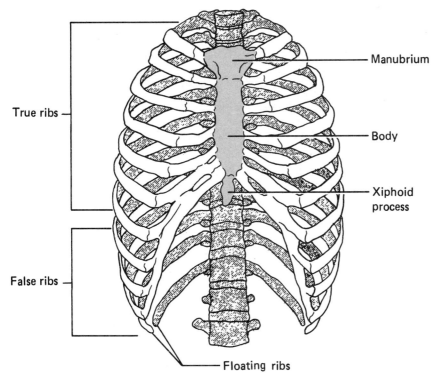

True ribs

False ribs

Manubrium

Body

Xiphoid process

Floating ribs

FIGURE 5.5   The sternum consists of the manubrium, body and xiphoid process

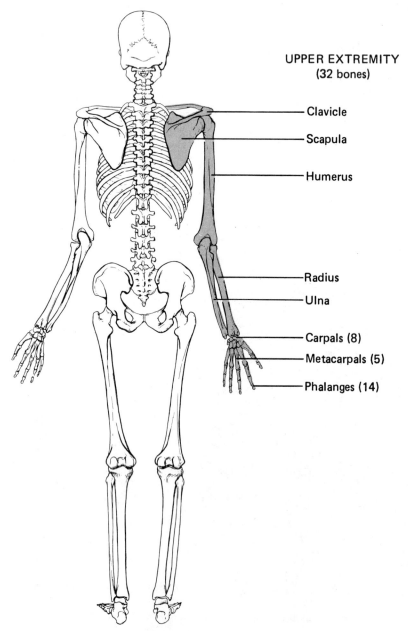

UPPER EXTREMITY
(32 bones)

Clavicle

Scapula

Humerus

Radius

Ulna

Carpals (8)

Metacarpals (5)

Phalanges (14)

FIGURE 5.6   Upper extremity bones

The bones of the hand are shown in Figure 5.7.

LOWER EXTREMITY. *Each* lower extremity has 31 bones (Figure 5.8):

- os coxae (hip bone, or pelvic bone)
- femur (thigh bone)
- 2 leg bones, tibia and fibula
- 7 tarsal (ankle) bones
- 5 metatarsal (foot) bones
- 14 phalanges (toe bones)
- patella (kneecap)

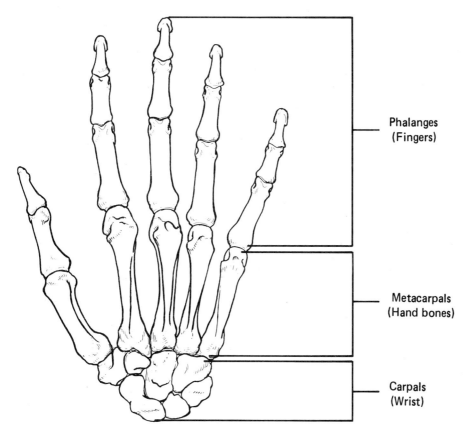

Phalanges
(Fingers)

Metacarpals
(Hand bones)

Carpals
(Wrist)

FIGURE 5.7 Dorsal aspect (back) of the hand

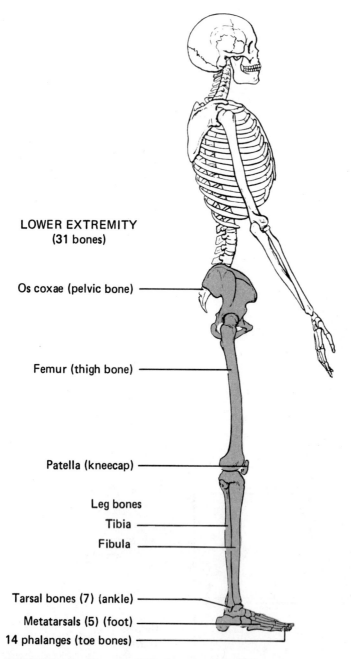

LOWER EXTREMITY
(31 bones)

Os coxae (pelvic bone)

Femur (thigh bone)

Patella (kneecap)

Leg bones
Tibia
Fibula

Tarsal bones (7) (ankle)

Metatarsals (5) (foot)

14 phalanges (toe bones)

FIGURE 5.8   Bones of the lower extremity

JOINTS

Joints are often referred to as *articulations*. Two or more bones may come together or *articulate*, forming a joint. A strong, flexible band of fibrous connective tissue called a *ligament* helps hold bones together at the joints.

Joints may be classified as:

- immovable (*synarthroses*) with no joint cavities, such as the joining of the skull bones

- slightly movable (*amphiarthroses*), for example, the vertebral disks

- freely movable (*diarthroses*)

Diarthroses are also called *synovial* joints, having a cavity between the ends of the bones. The outer layer of this cavity becomes thickened into *ligaments*, and the inner layer is made up of *synovial membrane*, which secretes a sticky fluid that helps prevent friction between the joining bones.

The diarthrotic joints are classified by type of movement:

- Ball and socket: hip, shoulder (Figure 5.9*A*)

- Hinge: elbow, knee, fingers, toes (Figure 5.9*B*)

- Pivot: atlas and axis (first two vertebrae); upper ends of radius and ulna at the elbow (Figure 5.9*C*)

FRACTURES

A *fracture* is any break in the continuity of a bone. It may be caused by physical injury such as a blow or a fall or by disease. The three general classifications of fractures are simple fractures, compound fractures, and comminuted fractures. Further classifications of fractures are shown in Table 5.2.

A *simple fracture* does not cause a break in the skin. A *compound fracture* is one in which the overlying skin has been torn or punctured. Comminuted fractures are those in which the bone is broken in two or more places, splintered, or crushed. For the fracture to heal, the separated pieces of bone must first be placed in their proper position. Medically, this is called *reducing* the fracture. The following table lists just a few of the common types of fractures.

Orthopedics is the branch of medicine that is specially concerned with the preservation and restoration of the function of the skeletal system, its articulations, and associated structures. It is one of the oldest specialties, having its origins in pre-Christian Greece when it concerned the correction of congenital deformities in children (*orth–*, straight; *paedics*, child). Today the specialty deals with trauma and fractures, bone tumors, degenerative diseases such as rheumatoid arthritis, and sports medicine, in addition to congenital malformations. The *orthopedic surgeon*, or *orthopedist*, is the specialist in this branch of medicine.

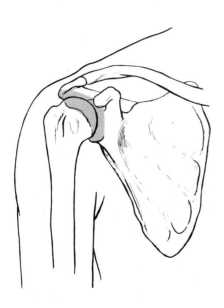

FIGURE 5.9A Ball and socket joint—the shoulder

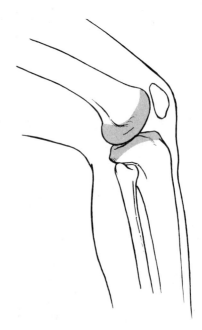

FIGURE 5.9B Hinge joint—knee

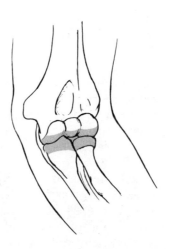

FIGURE 5.9C Pivot joint—upper ends of radius and ulna at elbow

TABLE 5.2. Common Types of Fractures

closed or simple	A fracture that does not produce an open wound
Colles' (**KOL**-eez)	Fracture at lower end of the radius resulting in hand being displaced posteriorly
comminuted (**KOM**-ih-**new**-ted)	Bone is splintered or crushed
complicated (**KOM**-plih-**kay**-ted)	Fracture includes injury to adjacent parts
compound (open)	Fracture comes through skin to outside
depressed (dee-**PREST**)	Skull fracture with a piece of bone being broken and driven inward
greenstick	Fracture in which only one side of bone is broken and the remaining side only bent
impacted	Fracture in which one broken fragment is firmly wedged into the other
incomplete	Fracture that does not include the whole bone
oblique (oh-bleek)	Break extends in a diagonal direction
pathologic (**path**-oh-**LOJ**-ick)	Fracture occurring from mild injury because there is preexisting bone disease
Pott's (pots)	Fracture of the lower part of the leg bone (fibula)
spiral (spy-ral)	Fracture occurring from bone being twisted apart
stellate (**STELL**-ayt)	A fracture with a central point of injury from which cracks radiate
transverse (trans-**VERS**)	A fracture across the long axis of the bone

BUILDING BLOCKS

ROOTS AND COMBINING FORMS

Word Element	Meaning
ankyl/o	crooked, bent, stiff
arthr/o	joint
brachi/o	arm
calcane/o	calcaneus, heel bone
carp/o	carpus, wrist bone
caud/o	tail, lower part of body
cephal/o	head
cervic/o	neck, cervix
chondr/o	cartilage
cleid/o	clavicle, collarbone
cost/o	rib
crani/o	skull
dactyl/o	finger, toe
fasci/o	fascia
ili/o	ilium
ischi/o	ischium
lumb/o	lower back, loin
myel/o	spinal cord, marrow
nas/o	nose
orth/o	straight
oste/o	bone
ped/o	child, foot
pod/o	foot
scapul/o	scapula, shoulder blade
scoli/o	crooked, bent
spondyl/o, vertebr/o	vertebrae

SUFFIXES

Word Element	Meaning
–clasis	break
–desis	to bind together
–oma	tumor
–physis	to grow
–plasty	surgical repair
–porosis	passage

Word Element	Meaning
dia–	complete, through
endo–	in, within
epi–	above, upon
exo–	out, away from
meta–	change, beyond
peri–	around, about
sub–	under

VOCABULARY

General Terms

articulation	(ar-**tick**-you-**LAY**-shun)	The juncture between two or more bones; a joint
brachial	(**BRAY**-kee-al)	Pertaining to the arm
caries	(**KAR**-eez)	The decay and crumbling of soft or bone tissue, or a tooth (dental caries)
cervical	(**SER**-vih-kal)	Pertaining to the neck, or to the neck of an organ such as the uterus
diarthrosis	(**die**-ar-**THROH**-sis)	A movable joint
erythropoiesis	eh-**rith**-roh-poy-**EE**-sis)	The formation of red blood cells
fissure	(**FISH**-ur)	A cleft or groove
fontanel, fontanelle	(fon-tah-**NELL**)	A soft spot, such as the membrane-covered space between the cranial bones in the skull of an infant
foramen	(foh-**RAY**-men)	A general term for a natural opening or passage
fossa	(**FOSS**-ah)	General term for a depression or channel
fracture	(**FRACK**-cher)	The breaking of a bone; a broken bone

kyphosis	(kigh-**FOH**-sis)	Abnormally increased outward curvature of the thoracic spine; the condition of being a hunchback or humpback
lordosis	(lor-**DOH**-sis)	Abnormal forward curvature of the spine; swayback
lumbar	(**LUM**-bar)	Pertaining to the part of the back between the ribs and the pelvis
malar	(**MAY**-lar)	Pertaining to the cheek or cheekbone
medulla	(meh-**DULL**-ah)	The innermost portion of any organ or structure. In reference to bone, the bone marrow is called *medulla ossium.*
parietal	(pah-**RYE**-eh-tal)	In general, pertaining to the walls of a cavity. In relation to the skeletal system, pertaining to the parietal bone, one of two bones that together form the roof and sides of the skull.
pubic	(**PYOU**-bick)	Pertaining to or lying near the pubis
scoliosis	(skoh-lee-**OH**-sis)	Lateral curvature of the spine
sequestrum	(see-**KWES**-trum)	A piece of dead bone, separated from the healthy bone during the process of necrosis
sulcus	(**SUL**-kus)	A general term for a groove or fissure

Terms Related to Anatomy and Physiology

acetabulum	(ass-eh-**TAB**-you-lum)	A large pelvic socket that holds the head of the femur (thigh bone); hip socket
calcaneus	(kal-**KAY**-nee-us)	The heel bone
carpus	(**KAR**-pus)	The joint between the arm and hand; the wrist

cartilage	(KAR-tih-lij)	Gristle. A translucent, whitish connective tissue
clavicle	(KLAV-ih-kal)	The bone that articulates with the sternum and scapula; the collarbone
coccyx	(KOCK-sicks)	The lowest bone of the vertebra; "tailbone"
cranium	(KRAY-nee-um)	The skeleton of the head; the skull
diaphysis	(die-AF-ih-sis)	The shaft or middle part of a long bone
endosteum	(en-DOS-tee-um)	The lining of the medullary cavity of a bone
epiphysis	(eh-PIFF-ih-sis)	The end of a long bone
femur	(FEE-mur)	The long bone extending from the pelvis to the knee; the thigh bone is the longest and strongest bone in the body
fibula	(FIB-you-lah)	The outer and smaller of the two bones of the leg that extend from the knee to the ankle
frontal bone	(FRUN-tal bohn)	A bone of the forehead
humerus	(HYOU-mer-us)	The upper arm bone that extends from the shoulder to the elbow
iliac crest	(ILL-ee-ack krest)	The ridge bordering the ilium
iliac fossa	(ILL-ee-ack FOSS-ah)	A large, smooth, concave area on the inner surface of the ilium
ilium	(ILL-ee-um)	The wide upper portion of the hip bone. (In early childhood it is a separate bone.)
ischium	(IHS-kee-um)	The lower dorsal portion of the hip bone (also a separate bone in early childhood)
ligament	(LIG-ah-ment)	A strong, flexible band of fibrous connective tissue that connects bones or cartilages. Ligaments support and strengthen joints.
mandible	(MAN-dih-bul)	The bone of the lower jaw

manubrium	(mah-**NEW**-bree-um)	The upper portion of the sternum. The manubrium articulates with the clavicles and the first two pairs of ribs.
maxilla	(mack-**SILL**-ah)	The upper jawbone
meniscus	(meh-**NIHS**-kus)	One of the half-moon shaped disks of fibrocartilage found in the knee joint
metacarpus	(**met**-ah-**KAR**-pus)	The part of the hand between the wrist and the fingers. The five metacarpal bones form the framework of the palm of the hand.
metatarsus	(**met**-ah-**TAR**-sus)	The part of the foot between the ankle and the toes. There are five metatarsal bones.
occipital bone	(ock-**SIP**-ih-tal)	The bone of the occiput, in the back part of the skull
patella	(pah-**TELL**-ah)	A triangular bone situated at the front of the knee; the kneecap
periosteum	(**per**-ee-**OSS**-tee-um)	A specialized connective tissue that tightly covers all bones of the body except at their articular surfaces
phalanx; plural, phalanges	(**FAY**-lankz, fah-**LAN**-jeez)	A general term for any finger or toe bone
radius; plural radii	(**RAY**-dee-us, **RAY**-dee-eye)	The shorter of the two bones on the forearm which is on the outer side when the body is in the anatomic position
sacrum	(**SAY**-krum)	The triangular bone located immediately below the lumbar vertebrae is formed by five fused vertebrae
scapula	(**SKAP**-you-lah)	The flat, triangular bone that forms the back of the shoulder; the shoulder blade
sternum	(**STER**-num)	The breast bone. A longitudinal bone consisting of the manubrium,

		the body, and the xiphoid process, which forms the middle of the anterior chest wall
symphysis pubis	(**SIM**-fih-sis **PYOU**-bis)	The junction of the pubic bones on the anterior midline
tarsus	(**TAHR**-sus)	The ankle consisting of seven bones located between the bones of the lower leg and the metatarsus.
temporal bone	(**TEM**-poh-ral)	A bone located on each side of the skull which forms part of its side and base
tibia	(**TIB**-ee-ah)	The shin bone; the inner and larger bone of the two bones of the leg that extend from the knee to the ankle
trochanter	(troh-**KAN**-ter)	Either of the two processes below the neck of the femur
ulna	(**ULL**-nah)	The larger of the two bones of the forearm, which is located on the side opposite that of the thumb
vertebra	(**VER**-teh-brah)	Any one of the thirty-three bones of the spine
xiphoid	(**ZIF**-oyd)	Shaped like a sword. The *xiphoid process* is the lowest portion of the sternum.

Terms Related to Pathology

ankylosis	(**ang**-kih-**LOH**-sis)	The immobilization and fixation of a joint
arthritis	(ar-**THRIGH**-tis)	Inflammation of a joint
dislocation	(**dis**-loh-**KAY**-shun))	The temporary displacement of a bone from its normal position in a joint
exostosis	(**eck**-soss-**TOH**-sis)	A benign (noncancerous) bony growth that projects outward from the surface of a bone

gout	(gowt)	A form of acute arthritis that is caused by excessive uric acid in the blood. It most often starts in the foot or knee.
myeloma	(my-eh-**LOH**-mah)	A tumor originating in cells of the bone marrow
osteoarthritis	(**oss**-tee-oh-ar-**THRIGH**-tis)	A chronic inflammatory disease involving the weight-bearing joints
osteoma	(**oss**-tee-**OH**-mah)	A tumor composed of bone tissue
osteomalacia	(**oss**-tee-oh-mah-**LAY**-she-ah)	Softening of the bones
laminectomy	(**lam**-ih-**NECK**-toh-mee)	The excision of a vertebral posterior arch
ostectomy	(oss-**TECK**-toh-mee)	Surgical excision of bone
osteoplasty	(**oss**-tee-oh-**PLAS**-tee)	Plastic repair of the bones
osteotomy	(**oss**-tee-**OT**-oh-mee)	Surgical cutting through a bone
rheumatoid arthritis	(**REW**-mah-toyd ar-**THRIGH**-tis)	A chronic systemic disease with inflammation of joints
spondylosis	(**spon**-dih-**LOH**-sis)	Ankylosis of a vertebral joint
sprain	(sprayn)	Painful injury to a joint in which the ligaments may be torn
subluxation	(**sub**-luck-**SAY**-shun)	An incomplete or partial dislocation
syndactylism	(sin-**DACK**-tih-lizm)	A webbing of two or more fingers or toes; syndactyly
talipes	(**TAL**-ih-peez)	Clubfoot. A congenital deformity resulting in the foot being twisted out of shape or position

Terms Related to Surgery or Treatment

amputation	(**am**-pyou-**TAY**-shun)	Removal of a limb, part, or organ which may be accidental or performed surgically
arthrectomy	(ar-**THRECK**-toh-mee)	Excision of a joint
arthrocentesis	(ar-throh-sen-**TEE**-sis)	Puncture of a joint space with a

		needle for removal of fluid (aspiration)
arthroclasia	(**ar**-throh-**KLAY**-zee-ah)	The artificial breaking down of ankylosis to allow free movement in a joint
arthrodesis	(**ar**-throh-**DEE**-sis)	Surgical fixation of a joint
arthroplasty	(**AR**-throh-**plas**-tee)	Plastic surgery of a joint
diskectomy	(dis-**KECK**-toh-mee)	Surgical removal of a herniated disk

5.1   Review: System

1. The adult human skeleton has _____ bones.
2. Bone tissue is a storehouse for _____ and _____ .
3. The five types of bones are:

   Type   **Example(s)**

   _____   _____

   _____   _____

   _____   _____

   _____   _____

   _____   _____

4. The bone shaft is called the _____ and is composed of _____ bone.
5. The bone marrow cavity is lined with _____ bone.
6. The epiphyses are composed of _____ bone on the outside and _____ bone on the inside.
7. Surrounding the shaft of the bone is a fibrous membrane called the

   _____ .

8. The two main divisions of the skeleton are the _____ _____ and the _____ _____ .
9. There are _____ pairs of ribs.
10. The three parts of the sternum are:

    a. _____   b. _____   c. _____
11. An articulation is commonly called a _____ .
12. Immovable joints are called _____ .
13. Slightly movable joints are called _____ .
14. Freely movable joints are called _____ .
15. A strong, flexible band of fibrous connective tissue, called a _____ , helps hold bones together at the joints.

5.2   Review: Bones of the Skeleton

DIRECTIONS: Match the lettered structures in the figure with the correct labels. Write the identifying letter in the space provided.

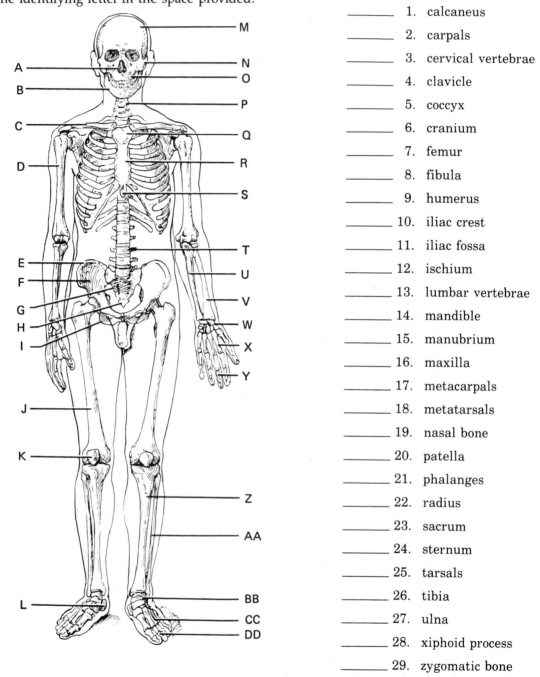

_____ 1. calcaneus

_____ 2. carpals

_____ 3. cervical vertebrae

_____ 4. clavicle

_____ 5. coccyx

_____ 6. cranium

_____ 7. femur

_____ 8. fibula

_____ 9. humerus

_____ 10. iliac crest

_____ 11. iliac fossa

_____ 12. ischium

_____ 13. lumbar vertebrae

_____ 14. mandible

_____ 15. manubrium

_____ 16. maxilla

_____ 17. metacarpals

_____ 18. metatarsals

_____ 19. nasal bone

_____ 20. patella

_____ 21. phalanges

_____ 22. radius

_____ 23. sacrum

_____ 24. sternum

_____ 25. tarsals

_____ 26. tibia

_____ 27. ulna

_____ 28. xiphoid process

_____ 29. zygomatic bone

(From Kinn, _Medical Terminology—Review Challenge,_ copyright 1987 by Delmar Publishers Inc.)

5.3   Review: Fractures

DIRECTIONS: Match the descriptions in the right column with the names of fractures in the left column.

Fracture

_____ 1. closed or simple

_____ 2. Colles'

_____ 3. comminuted

_____ 4. complicated

_____ 5. compound (open)

_____ 6. depressed

_____ 7. greenstick

_____ 8. impacted

_____ 9. incomplete

_____ 10. oblique

_____ 11. pathologic

_____ 12. Pott's

_____ 13. spiral

_____ 14. stellate

_____ 15. transverse

Description

A.   Fracture of the skull in which a fragment is driven inward.

B.   Break extends in a diagonal direction.

C.   Fracture that does not produce an open wound.

D.   Fracture with a central point of injury from which cracks radiate.

E.   Fracture in which one fragment is firmly wedged into the other.

F.   Fracture of the lower end of the radius in which the hand is displaced posteriorly.

G.   Fracture in which the bone has been twisted apart.

H.   Fracture with injury of the adjacent parts.

I.   Fracture across the long axis of the bone.

J.   Fracture of the lower part of the fibula.

K.   Bone is splintered or crushed.

L.   The line of fracture does not include the whole bone.

M.   Fracture occurring from mild injury because of preexisting bone disease.

N.   One side of bone is broken, the other side is only bent.

O.   Fracture having an external wound leading to the break of the bone.

5.4   Review: Building Blocks

DIRECTIONS: Cover the column on the left while you define the following building blocks.

heel bone, calcaneus	1. calcane/o _____
in, within	2. endo– _____
crooked, bent, stiff	3. ankyl/o _____
ilium	4. ili/o _____
spinal column, vertebra	5. rachi/o _____
out, away from	6. exo– _____
lower back, loin	7. lumb/o _____
skull	8. crani/o _____
to grow	9 –physis _____
child, foot	10. ped/o _____
clavicle, collarbone	11. cleid/o _____
bone	12. oste/o _____
under	13. sub– _____
neck, cervix	14. cervic/o _____
fascia	15. fasci/o _____
around, about	16. peri– _____
to bind together	17. –desis _____
change, beyond	18. meta– _____

5.5 Review: Building Blocks

DIRECTIONS: Cover the column on the left while you define the following building blocks.

vertebra	1. spondyl/o _____
complete, through	2. dia– _____
tail, lower part of body	3. caud/o _____
foot	4. pod/o _____
cartilage	5. chondr/o _____
joint	6. arthr/o _____
spinal cord, marrow	7. myel/o _____
shoulder blade	8. scapul/o _____
ischium	9. ischi/o _____
arm	10. brachi/o _____
finger, toe	11. dactyl/o _____
head	12. cephal/o _____
surgical repair	13. –plasty _____
nose	14. nas/o _____
above, upon	15. epi– _____
break	16. –clasis _____
wrist bone, carpus	17. carp/o _____
rib	18. cost/o _____

5.6   Review: Building New Medical Terms

1. The combining form for *bone* is _____ .
   The suffix _____ means *to break*.
   The term _____ means surgical fracture of a bone.
2. The root _____ means joint.
   The suffix _____ means pain.
   A word for *joint pain* is _____ .
3. The prefix _____ means *around*.
   The root _____ means *bone*.
   Write a word meaning *around a bone* _____ .
4. The root _____ means *rib*.
   The prefix _____ means *under*.
   Write a word meaning *under a rib* _____ .
5. The prefix _____ means *together*.
   The suffix _____ means *to grow*.
   _____ means *fusion* or *growing together*.

5.7   Review: Word Building

1. The combining form for *bone marrow* is _____ .
   _____ is a word ending meaning *tumor*.
   A tumor originating in bone marrow is a _____ .
2. _____ is a suffix meaning *softening*.
   The combining form for *bone* is _____ .
   Softening of a bone is expressed as _____ .
3. The suffix for *puncture with a needle* is _____ .
   _____ is the combining form for *joint*.
   Puncture of a joint space with a needle is _____ .
4. The suffix for *surgical fixation* is _____ .
   Surgical fixation of a joint is _____ .
5. _____ is a root meaning *finger or toe*.
   A prefix meaning *together* is _____ .
   _____ is a fusion of two or more fingers or toes.

Reading Comprehension 5.1

DIRECTIONS: Underline the medical terms as you go through the reading exercise. Then list and analyze the terms. Some will be completely new to you. Consult a medical dictionary for their meanings. Then re-read the material for better comprehension.

Medical Imaging

Metastatic Bone Survey:

A PA view of the chest is submitted for evaluation. This is compared to the previous chest film of 1/10/—. No interval change in the appearance of the heart size is noted. Arteriosclerotic changes are again identified in the aorta. There is no evidence of acute infiltrate, atelectasis, or pleural effusions. Callus is seen in the region of the left tenth rib fracture. This is unchanged from the previous study. Old healed deformity is noted of the right fifth rib fracture. Post-inflammatory changes, minimal in nature, are seen at both lung bases.

Impression:

The PA view of the chest is unchanged from the previous study of 1/10/—.

Rib Series:

AP and shallow oblique views were obtained of the ribs. The study demonstrates a healing right fifth rib fracture. There is a subtle lucency transversing the left ninth rib. In addition, there is minimal irregularity of the left eighth rib. This is noted anterolaterally. These changes may reflect small subtle nondisplaced fractures. Follow-up films are suggested. One notes the callus in the region of the left tenth rib fracture, which is better identified on the chest film.

Lytic changes are seen in the distal right humerus. Minimal degenerative changes are seen at both shoulder joints. Small lucencies are seen in the mid left humerus which may represent metastatic disease.

Impression:

1. Possible small left eighth and left ninth rib fractures. Healing left tenth rib fracture. Old right fifth rib fracture. Lytic lesions involving both humeri compatible with metastatic disease.

AP View of the Pelvis and AP View of Both Femurs:

The study demonstrates osteoporosis and mild degenerative changes of the lower lumbosacral spine. Minimal degenerative disease is identified at both hip joints. There is no evidence of fracture or dislocation.

Reading Comprehension 5.2

DIRECTIONS: Underline the medical terms as you go through the reading exercise. Then list and analyze the terms. Some will be completely new to you. Consult a medical dictionary for their meanings. Then re-read the material for better comprehension.

Operative Report

Preoperative Diagnosis: Tear of the right medial meniscus

Postoperative Diagnosis: Same

Procedure: Arthroscopic right medial meniscectomy

Under general anesthesia with the patient in the supine position, the right lower extremity was prepped from the toes to the tourniquet with Betadine. After sterilely draping the extremity free, an anteromedial and anterolateral portal incision was made. The arthroscope was introduced in the knee joint. There was found to be minimal chondromalacia of the patella. Upon entering the medial joint compartment, the medial femoral condyle revealed some very slight erosion posteriorly. It was quite superficial. The tear was confirmed starting at approximately the midsection of the meniscus approximately 2–3 mm from the border extending all the way around to the posterior aspect. There was no plica noted along the medial femoral condyle area. The anterior cruciate ligament was found to be normal. Upon entering the lateral joint compartment, there was found to be almost a completely discoid lateral meniscus. There was only a very small, perhaps 1 × 1 cm opening on its inner border. However, there were no tears, and it appeared quite normal other than the discoid appearance.

At this point, using baskets and rongeurs, the inner border of the unstable portion of the meniscus was trimmed back to a stable rim. This removed approximately from the midsection around the posterior aspect up close to the rim area. This was subsequently trimmed down, also using the full-radius cutter and the small Shutt basket rongeurs.

After all of this had been accomplished, the knee was thoroughly irrigated with normal saline through the arthroscope. At the beginning of the procedure 20 cc of 0.5% Marcaine with epinephrine was instilled into the knee joint. At the end of the knee joint, another 20 cc was placed in the soft tissues. During the procedure with leg elevation, the tourniquet was inflated to 300 mm Hg. After a sterile dressing had been applied, the patient was taken to the recovery room with good circulation to the foot.

Reading Comprehension Vocabulary

Use the space below to list the medical terms for analysis and definition.

_____
_____
_____
_____
_____
_____
_____
_____
_____
_____
_____
_____
_____
_____
_____
_____
_____
_____
_____
_____
_____
_____
_____
_____
_____
_____
_____

CHAPTER 6

Muscular System

OBJECTIVES

When you have successfully completed Chapter 6, you should be able to:
— Name three kinds of muscles.
— List three primary functions of muscles.
— Identify principal muscles on a familiar drawing.
— Define terms related to the muscular system introduced in this chapter.
— Build new medical terms using the word elements in this and previous chapters.

aponeurosis	(ap-oh-new-**ROH**-sis)	A ribbon-like fibrous sheet of connective tissue that attaches muscle to bone or other tissue
insertion of muscle	(in-**SER**-shun)	The place where muscle is attached to a bone in a manner that permits movement
locomotion	(loh-coh-**MOH**-shun)	Movement from one place to another
myocardium	(my-oh-**KAR**-dee-um)	The middle muscular layer of heart wall that contracts to force blood from the heart chambers
origin of muscle	(**OR**-ih-jin)	The place where muscle is attached to bone in a manner permitting little or no movement
peristalsis	(per-ih-**STALL**-sis)	An involuntary, wavelike movement that occurs in hollow passages of the body such as the digestive organs
reflex	(**REE**-flecks)	An involuntary response to a stimulus; also, the nerve connections by which this occurs. Example, the eyeblink reflex
tendon	(**TEN**-don)	Fibrous cord that attaches muscles to bones and other parts
viscera	(**VISS**-er-ah)	Internal organs enclosed within a cavity

OVERVIEW

The study of the muscles is called *myology*. Muscle tissue is responsible for all movement of the body, whether the movement consists of *locomotion* (movement of the body through space); changes in the size of body openings, (for example, the iris of the eye); or the movement of fluids or wastes through body organs. The muscles are all-important in keeping the body erect. They also provide protection to internal organs.

TYPES OF MUSCLE TISSUE

There are three types of muscle tissue: cardiac, smooth (unstriated), and skeletal (striated).

Cardiac Muscle

Cardiac muscle is located in the *myocardium*, the middle layer of the heart, and forms the bulk of the heart wall.

Smooth Muscle

Smooth (unstriated) *muscle* lacks the striated (striped) formation typical of skeletal muscle. It is found in the walls of the *viscera* (hollow organs) and blood vessels, and is not attached to bones or joints. Smooth muscle is also called *visceral* or *involuntary* muscle. Its action occurs without conscious control, and it is involved in such activities as digestion and circulation.

Skeletal Muscle

The so-called musculoskeletal system is composed of bone and *skeletal muscle* (Figures 6.1 and 6.2). Skeletal muscles are *voluntary*; they respond to conscious control as well as moving by *reflex*. They contract quickly and tightly to control movement of the bones and joints of the skeleton. They are involved in such activities as breathing, walking, jumping, twisting, nodding the head, and grasping.

MUSCLE ATTACHMENTS

Muscles may be attached to other muscles, to bones, or to skin. Many muscles are connected to bones by cords of fibrous tissue called *tendons*. Others are attached to each other or to bone by a flattened sheetlike tendon called an *aponeurosis*.

MUSCLE PARTS

The less movable part of the muscle is called the *origin*. Generally, the origin is proximal (closer to) the trunk. The *insertion* is the attachment on the more movable bone, generally the end distal to (farther from) the trunk. The main part of the muscle is its *body* or *belly*. When a muscle contracts, its insertion is pulled toward its origin.

MUSCLE FUNCTIONS

The primary functions of the muscles are (1) movement, (2) maintenance of posture, and (3) heat production. Table 6.1 lists major muscles and their functions. Movement may consist of *locomotion* of the body, contraction of the digestive tract for carrying forward its contents (*peristalsis*), and changes in the sizes of body openings, for example the iris of the eye. A skeletal muscle moves a body part only by pulling across a joint, never by pushing. Although skeletal muscles can only pull, some can move either of their two ends. For muscles of this kind, which attachment is designated as the origin and which as the insertion depends on which end is moving. Muscles also help produce heat by contracting and by complicated chemical changes in cells which release heat as well as

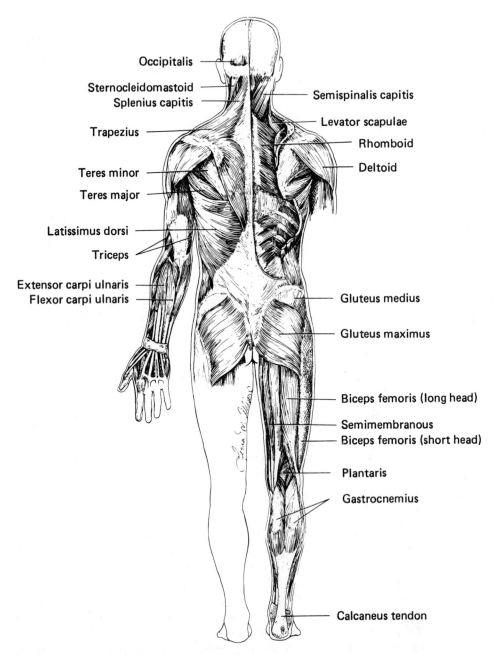

FIGURE 6.1 **Posterior view of the muscles of the body** (From Kinn, *Medical Terminology—Review Challenge*, copyright 1987 by Delmar Publishers Inc.)

Labels on figure:

Occipitalis
Sternocleidomastoid
Splenius capitis
Trapezius
Teres minor
Teres major
Latissimus dorsi
Triceps
Extensor carpi ulnaris
Flexor carpi ulnaris
Semispinalis capitis
Levator scapulae
Rhomboid
Deltoid
Gluteus medius
Gluteus maximus
Biceps femoris (long head)
Semimembranous
Biceps femoris (short head)
Plantaris
Gastrocnemius
Calcaneus tendon

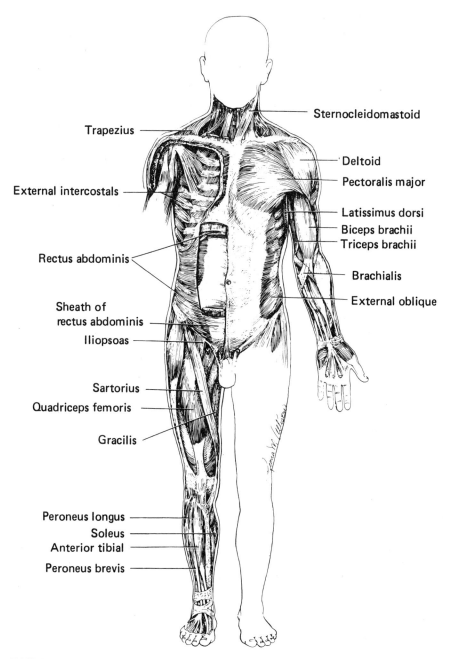

FIGURE 6.2 Anterior view of the muscles of the body (From Kinn, *Medical Terminology—Review Challenge*, copyright 1987 by Delmar Publishers Inc.)

energy. For example, shivering is a way the body forces the muscles to move and produce heat. Treatment of the muscular system is within the practice of orthopedics along with the skeletal system.

TABLE 6.1. Partial List of Muscles

Name	Function
anterior tibial	Elevates and flexes foot
biceps brachii	Flexes arm and forearm and supinates hand
biceps femoris (short head) biceps femoris (long head)	Flexes knee and rotates it outward
brachialis	Flexes forearm
deltoid	Raises and rotates arm
extensor carpi ulnaris	Extends and abducts wrist
external oblique	Contracts abdomen and viscera
external intercostals	Draw ribs together and raise ribs
flexor carpi ulnaris	Flexes and adducts wrist
gastrocnemius	Flexes foot and leg
gluteus maximus	Extends and rotates thigh
gluteus medius	Abducts and rotates thigh
gracilis	Flexes and adducts leg; adducts thigh
iliopsoas	Flexes and rotates thigh
latissimus dorsi	Adducts, extends, and rotates arm
levator scapulae	Elevates posterior angle of scapula
occipitalis	Draws scalp back
pectoralis major	Flexes, adducts, and rotates arm
peroneus longus	Extends, abducts, and everts foot
peroneus brevis	Extends and abducts foot
plantaris	Extends foot

TABLE 6.1. Continued	
Name	**Function**
quadriceps femoris	Extends leg
rectus abdominis	Compresses abdomen
rhomboid	Elevates scapula
sartorius	Flexes and rotates thigh and leg
semimembranous	Flexes and rotates leg; extends thigh
semispinalis capitis	Rotates and draws head backward
soleus	Extends and rotates foot
splenius capitis	Rotates and extends head
sternocleidomastoid	Rotates and depresses head
teres major	Rotates arm inward, draws it down and back
teres minor	Rotates arm outward
trapezius	Draws head back and to the side, rotates scapula
triceps brachii	Extends forearm and arm

BUILDING BLOCKS

ROOTS AND COMBINING FORMS

Word Element	**Meaning**
brachi/o	arm
clon/o	turmoil
duct	carry
erg/o	work
kym/o	wave, quiver
loc/o	place
sarc/o	flesh
scler/o	hardening
spondyl/o	vertebra

ROOTS AND COMBINING FORMS (continued)

Word Element	Meaning
sthen/o	strength
tom/o	incision, cut
ton/o	tension
tort/i	twisted
viscer/o	body organs

SUFFIXES

Word Element	Meaning
–algia	pain
–diastasis	separation
–lysis	destruction
–malacia	softening
–oid	resembling, like
–rhaphy	sewing, suturing
–rhexis	rupture
–tasis	stretching
–trophy	nourishment

PREFIXES

Word Element	Meaning
a–	not, without
ab–	away from
ad–	toward
anti–	against
bi–	two
dys–	bad, difficult, painful
iso–	equal
leio–	smooth
metr–	measure
quadri–	four
syn–	together

VOCABULARY

General Terms

abductor	(ab-**DUCK**-tor)	That which abducts or carries away
active movement	(**ACK**-tiv)	Movement characterized by action
adduction	(ah-**DUCK**-shun)	Drawing toward a body
ambulation	(**am**-byou-**LAY**-shun)	The act of walking
clonic	(**KLON**-ick)	A state of turmoil. Pertaining to the condition of the clonus
clonus	(**KLOH**-nus)	Rapid alternating of muscular contraction and relaxation
deltoid	(**DEL**-toyd)	Resembling a triangle, such as the deltoid muscle
distal	(**DIS**-tal)	Remote; farthest from the point of reference (see *proximal*)
electromyography	(ee-**leck**-troh-my-**OG**-rah-fee)	The process of electrically stimulating muscle so as to record the strength of its muscle contraction; abbreviated EMG
flaccid	(**FLACK**-sid)	Weak, relaxed, soft
isometric	(**eye**-soh-**MET**-rick)	In relation to the muscular system, this means contracting a muscle while holding it fixed so that it becomes more tense but remains constant in length
isotonic	(**eye**-soh-**TON**-ick)	In relation to the muscular system, contracting a muscle against a constant load so that it shortens, as in lifting weights
myoid	(**my**-oyd)	Musclelike
myology	(my-**OL**-oh-jee)	The scientific study of muscles and their parts
myotasis	(my-**OTT**-ah-sis)	Stretching of a muscle
myotome	(**MY**-oh-tohm)	An instrument used in performing myotomy (cutting of muscle)

myotrophy	(my-**OTT**-roh-fee)	The nutrition of muscle tissues
neuromuscular	(**new**-roh-**MUSS**-kyou-lar)	Pertaining to both nerves and muscles
passive movement	(**PASS**-iv)	Movement that is produced without active effort
posture	(**POS**-chur)	The position or bearing of the body
proximal	(**PROCK**-sih-mal)	Closest to the point of reference (see *distal*)
quadriceps	(**KWAHD**-rih-seps)	Four-headed
relaxation	(**ree**-lack-**SAY**-shun)	A lessening of tension or activity
rigor mortis	(**rig**-or **MOR**-tis)	The stiffening that occurs in a dead body
rotation	(roh-**TAY**-shun)	Movement around an axis
striated	(**STRY**-ayt-ed)	Striped
synergist	(**SIN**-er-jist)	An organ that functions cooperatively with another; a medicine that aids or intensifies the action of another
visceral	(**VISS**-er-al)	Pertaining to a viscus (a soft, internal organ such as the stomach or heart)

Terms Related to Anatomy and Physiology

antagonist	(an-**TAG**-oh-nist)	An agent (for example, a muscle) that acts in opposition to the action of another, its agonist
aponeurosis	(**ap**-oh-new-**ROH**-sis)	A ribbon-like sheet of connective tissue that attaches muscle to bone or other tissue
biceps	(**BY**-seps)	A muscle having two heads
diaphragm	(**DIE**-ah-fram)	The partition that separates the abdominal and thoracic cavities
fascia	(**FASH**-ee-ah)	A fibrous membrane that encloses a muscle
gastrocnemius	(gas-trock-**NEE**-mee-us)	The large muscle at the back of the

		lower leg which controls flexion of the foot and knee
insertion	(in-**SER**-shun)	The place where a muscle is attached to the bone which it moves
involuntary muscle	(in-**VOL**-un-**ter**-ee)	Muscle that performs independently of the will
ligament	(**LIG**-ah-ment)	A band of fibrous tissue that binds bones together at a joint
muscle	(**MUS**-el)	A type of tissue that by contraction moves or prevents the movement of an organ or part of the body
myoblast	(**MY**-oh-blast)	An embryonic cell that develops into a cell of the muscle fiber
origin	(**OR**-ih-jin)	The source or beginning of something; the more fixed end or attachment of a muscle (see *insertion*)
pectoralis	(peck-toh-**RAY**-lis)	Pertaining to the breast or chest. The pectoralis muscles are found in the anterior chest.
popliteal	(pop-**LIT**-ee-all, **pop**-lih-**TEE**-al)	Pertaining to the back of the knee
prime mover	(prym **MOO**-ver)	A muscle that acts directly to bring about a desired movement
sphincter	(**SFINGK**-ter)	A circular band of muscle fibers that constricts or closes a natural orifice (body opening)
striated muscle	(**STRY**-ayt-ed)	Skeletal muscle having cross striations (stripes)
synovia	(sih-**NOH**-vee-ah)	A sticky, whitish, lubricating fluid found in the joints, bursa, and tendon sheaths; also called synovial fluid
tendon	(**TEN**-dun)	A fibrous cord that attaches muscles to bones and other parts
tone, tonus	(**TOH**-nus)	In relation to muscle, tone is the

degree of continuous contraction of the muscle fibers that determines its firmness (compare with **clonus**)

voluntary muscle	(**VOL**-un-**tar**-ee **MUS**-el)	Any muscle that is normally controlled by the will

Terms Related to Pathology

amyotrophic lateral sclerosis	(ah-**my**-oh-**TROF**-ick)	A condition marked by muscular weakness and atrophy with degeneration of the nerves in the spinal cord, medulla, and cortex of the brain
asthenia	(as-**THEE**-nee-ah)	lack or loss of strength and energy; weakness
ataxia	(ah-**TACK**-see-ah)	Lack of order; defective muscular coordination
atrophy	(**AT**-roh-fee)	A wasting away; shrinking of a body part
brachialgia	(**bray**-kee-**AL**-jee-ah)	Severe pain in an arm
chondroma	(kon-**DROH**-mah)	A tumor made up of cartilage cells
contracture	(kon-**TRACK**-chewr)	Permanent contraction of a muscle; for example, Dupuytren's contracture of the hand and fingers
convulsion	(kon-**VUL**-shun)	A series of uncontrollable muscular contractions and relaxations of the voluntary muscles
dystonia	(dis-**TOH**-nee-ah)	Impaired muscle tone
fasciitis	(**fass**-ee-**EYE**-tis)	Inflammation of fascia
fibrillation	(**fih**-brih-**LAY**-shun)	quivering or involuntary contraction of muscle
fibromyitis	(**figh**-broh-my-**EYE**-tis)	Inflammation and degeneration of muscle fibers resulting in atrophy
fibrosis	(figh-**BROH**-sis)	Abnormal condition of fibrous tissue
fibrositis	(**figh**-broh-**SIGH**-tis)	Inflammatory hyperplasia of the white fibrous tissue anywhere in

the body, but especially of the locomotor system

leiomyoma	(**lie**-oh-my-**OH**-mah)	A benign tumor derived from smooth muscle; for example, fibroid tumor of the uterus
muscular dystrophy	(**MUS**-kyou-lar **DIS**-troh-fee)	A group of inherited, degenerative diseases involving weakness and atrophy of muscle without involvement of the nervous system
myasthenia gravis	(**my**-as-**THEE**-nee-ah **GRAH**-vis)	A progressive, chronic disease in which fatigue and muscular weakness are the dominant symptoms, caused by a chemical imbalance that inhibits the nerve impulses
myalgia	(my-**AL**-jee-ah)	Tenderness or pain in a muscle or muscles
myitis	(my-**EYE**-tis)	Inflammation of a muscle
myoclonus	(my-**OCK**-loh-nus)	Twitching, shocklike spasms affecting part or all of a muscle or group of muscles
myodiastasis	(**my**-oh-die-**ASS**-tah-sis)	Separation or rupture of a muscle
myoedema	(**my**-oh-eh-**DEE**-mah)	Swelling of a muscle
myofibroma	(**my**-oh-fih-**BROH**-mah)	A tumor containing muscular and fibrous elements
myokymia	(**my**-oh-**KIM**-ee-ah)	Persistent twitching of the muscles
myolysis	(my-**OL**-ih-sis)	Destruction or degeneration of muscle tissue
myoma	(my-**OH**-mah)	A tumor composed of muscle cells or tissue
myomalacia	(**my**-oh-mah-**LAY**-shee-ah)	Softening of a muscle related to disease
myopathy	(my-**OP**-ah-thee)	Any disease or abnormal condition of a muscle
myorrhexis	(**my**-oh-**RECK**-sis)	The rupture of a muscle

myosarcoma	(**my**-oh-sar-**KOH**-mah)	A malignant tumor derived from muscle cells
myosclerosis	(**my**-oh-sklee-**ROH**-sis)	Hardening (sclerosis) of muscle tissue
myositis	(**my**-oh-**SIGH**-tis)	Inflammation of a muscle; myitis
myospasm	(**my**-oh-spazm)	Spasmodic contraction of a muscle
myotonia	(**my**-oh-**TOH**-nee-ah)	Tonic spasm of muscle, wherein the muscle has a decreased ability to relax
paralysis	(pah-**RAL**-ih-sis)	Temporary or permanent loss of sensation or motor function in a part
rigor mortis	(**RIG**-or **MOR**-tis)	The stiffening that occurs in a dead body
shin splints		Pain felt along the front of the lower leg, caused by muscle strain, usually following strenuous exercise
spasm	(spazm)	A sudden, involuntary, and abnormal contraction of a muscle or group of muscles
spasticity	(spass-**TIS**-ih-tee)	Stiff, awkward body movement caused by abnormal contraction of muscles
tendinitis	(**ten**-dih-**NIGH**-tis)	Inflammation of a tendon
tenodynia	(**ten**-oh-**DIN**-ee-ah)	Pain in a tendon
tenosynovitis	(**ten**-oh-sin-oh-**VIE**-tis)	Inflammation of a tendon sheath
torticollis	(**tor**-tih-**KOL**-is)	Wry neck; contraction of cervical (neck) muscles, causing the neck to twist and the head to turn to an unnatural position

Terms Related to Surgery or Treatment

fasciectomy	(**fash**-ee-**ECK**-toh-mee)	Excision of fascia
fascioplasty	(**FASH**-ee-oh-**plas**-tee)	Plastic operation on a fascia
hernioplasty	(**HER**-nee-oh-**plas**-tee)	Surgical repair of hernia
herniorrhaphy	(**her**-nee-**OR**-ah-fee)	Surgical repair of hernia

myoplasty	(**MY**-oh-**plas**-tee)	Plastic surgery of muscle tissue
myorrhaphy	(my-**OR**-ah-fee)	The process of suturing (stitching) a muscle wound
myotomy	(my-**OT**-oh-mee)	The cutting or dissection of a muscle
tendolysis	(ten-**DOL**-ih-sis)	The surgical process of freeing a tendon from adhesions
tenodesis	(ten-**ODD**-eh-sis)	Surgical fixation of the end of a tendon to a bone
tenolysis	(ten-**OL**-ih-sis)	See *tendolysis*.
tenoplasty	(**TEN**-oh-plas-tee)	Operative repair of a tendon

6.1   Review: System

1. The study of muscles is called _____ .
2. The muscular system is composed of _____ muscle.
3. There are two other kinds of muscle:
   a. _____ and b. _____
4. The bulk of the heart wall is composed of _____ muscle.
5. The muscle tissue found in the walls of hollow organs and blood vessels is called
   _____ .
6. Many muscles are connected to bones by _____ .
7. The less movable part of the muscle is called the _____ .
8. The opposite end of the muscle is the _____ .
9. The three primary functions of the muscles are:
   a. _____
   b. _____
   c. _____
10. Treatment of the muscular system is within the practice of _____ .

6.2   Review: Structures

DIRECTIONS: Match the letter of each structure with the correct label. Write the identifying letter in the space provided.

_____ 1. biceps femoris (long head)

_____ 2. biceps femoris (short head)

_____ 3. calcaneus tendon

_____ 4. deltoid

_____ 5. extensor carpi ulnaris

_____ 6. flexor carpi ulnaris

_____ 7. gastrocnemius

_____ 8. gluteus maximus

_____ 9. gluteus medius

_____ 10. latissimus dorsi

_____ 11. levator scapulae

_____ 12. occipitalis

_____ 13. plantaris

_____ 14. rhomboid

_____ 15. semimembranous

_____ 16. semispinalis capitis

_____ 17. splenius capitis

_____ 18. sternocleidomastoid

_____ 19. teres major

_____ 20. teres minor

_____ 21. trapezius

_____ 22. triceps

(From Kinn, _Medical Terminology—Review Challenge,_ copyright 1987 by Delmar
Publishers Inc.)

6.3   Review

DIRECTIONS: Match the lettered structures with the correct labels. Write the identifying letter in the space provided.

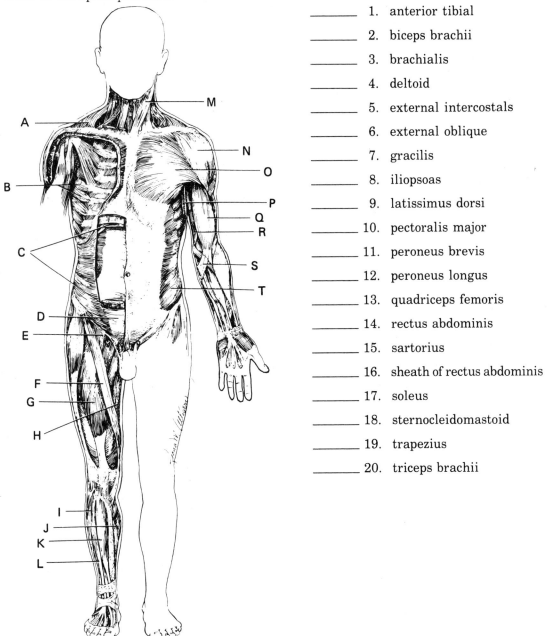

_____ 1. anterior tibial

_____ 2. biceps brachii

_____ 3. brachialis

_____ 4. deltoid

_____ 5. external intercostals

_____ 6. external oblique

_____ 7. gracilis

_____ 8. iliopsoas

_____ 9. latissimus dorsi

_____ 10. pectoralis major

_____ 11. peroneus brevis

_____ 12. peroneus longus

_____ 13. quadriceps femoris

_____ 14. rectus abdominis

_____ 15. sartorius

_____ 16. sheath of rectus abdominis

_____ 17. soleus

_____ 18. sternocleidomastoid

_____ 19. trapezius

_____ 20. triceps brachii

(From Kinn, _Medical Terminology—Review Challenge_, copyright 1987 by Delmar Publishers Inc.)

6.4   Review: Building Blocks

DIRECTIONS: Cover the column on the left while you define the following building blocks.

pain
away
head
smooth
vertebra
stretching
work
softening
tension
stiffness
against
body organs
sewing, suturing
together
hump
two
destruction
twisted

1. –algia _____
2. ab– _____
3. caput _____
4. leio– _____
5. spondyl/o _____
6. –taxis _____
7. ergon _____
8. –malacia _____
9. tonos _____
10. rigor _____
11. anti– _____
12. viscera _____
13. –rrhaphy _____
14. syn– _____
15. kyphos _____
16. bi– _____
17. –lysis _____
18. tortus _____

6.5   Review: Building Blocks

DIRECTIONS: Cover the column on the left while you define the following building blocks.

incision	1. tom/o _____
strength	2. −sthenia _____
place	3. locus _____
carry	4. duct _____
nourishment	5. −trophy _____
resembling, like	6. −oid _____
turmoil	7. klonus _____
rupture	8. −rrhexis _____
not, without	9. a− _____
measure	10. metr− _____
toward	11. ad− _____
bad, difficult, painful	12. dys− _____
to join	13. serere _____
hardening	14. scler/o _____
equal	15. iso _____
wave	16. kyma _____
four	17. quadri− _____
flesh	18. sarc− _____

6.6 Review: Vocabulary

DIRECTIONS: Write the definitions for the following terms.

1. flaccid _____
2. dystonia _____
3. myoma _____
4. ambulation _____
5. myotasis _____
6. fibrillation _____
7. myalgia _____
8. tenodesis _____
9. asthenia _____
10. myitis _____
11. myotrophy _____
12. fibrosis _____
13. myoid _____
14. tenosynovitis _____
15. atrophy _____

6.7 Review: Vocabulary

DIRECTIONS: Write the medical term for the following definitions.

1. _____ A muscle that acts in opposition to the action of another muscle
2. _____ A muscle having two heads
3. _____ The partition that separates the abdominal and thoracic cavities
4. _____ The process of recording the strength of muscle contraction in response to electrical stimulation
5. _____ The place of attachment of a muscle to the bone that it moves
6. _____ Swelling of a muscle
7. _____ Persistent quivering of the muscle fibers
8. _____ Disintegration or degeneration of muscle tissue
9. _____ The process of suturing a muscle wound
10. _____ An instrument used for dissection of a muscle or of muscular tissue
11. _____ Loss or impairment of motor function in a part

12. _____ Pertaining to the posterior surface of the knee
13. _____ The process of turning on an axis
14. _____ A ringlike band of muscle fibers that constricts a passage or closes a natural orifice
15. _____ A fibrous cord by which a muscle is attached to bones and other parts

6.8 Review: Word Building

DIRECTIONS: Fill in the blanks with the appropriate building block or medical term.

1. _____ is the suffix for *process of recording*.

   The root for *muscle* is _____ .

   The process of recording the strength of muscle contraction in response to electrical stimulation is _____ .

2. _____ is a prefix meaning *equal*.

   The root for *measure* is _____ .

   The term meaning of *equal measure* is _____ .

3. A suffix meaning *separation* is _____ .

   _____ is the combining form for *muscle*.

   Separation or rupture of a muscle is called _____ .

4. The combining form for *nerve* is _____ .

   _____ means *pertaining to both nerves and muscles*.

5. _____ is a suffix meaning *embryonic cell*.

   An embryonic muscle cell is called (a) (an)_____.

6. A prefix meaning *not* or *without* is _____ .

   _____ is a suffix meaning *pertaining to nourishment*.

   The combining form for *muscle* is _____ .

   The term meaning pertaining to the lack of nourishment to a muscle is

   _____ .

7. _____ is a suffix meaning *pain*.

   The root term for *arm* is _____ .

   _____ means pain in an arm.

8. The suffix for *tumor* is _____ .

   The prefix meaning *smooth* is _____ .

   _____ is the combining form for *muscle*.

   A benign tumor derived from smooth muscle is a _____ .

9. _____ is a suffix meaning *rupture*.

   The word for rupture of a muscle is _____ .

10. _____ is a prefix meaning *together*.

The root for *work* is _____ .

The word _____ pertains to working together.

Reading Comprehension 6.1

DIRECTIONS: Underline the medical terms as you go through the reading exercise. Then list and analyze the terms. Some will be completely new to you. Consult a medical dictionary for their meanings. Then re-read the material for better comprehension.

Magnetic Resonance Imaging (MRI)

MRI, Left Knee:

History:
Status post-fall with possible lateral meniscal tear.

Technique:
High resolution T1-weighted sagittal, axial, and coronal images were performed (three sequences).

Findings:
The lateral meniscus is normal in morphology and signal intensity without evidence of tear. The adjacent articular cartilage and subchondral marrow are homogeneous and normal throughout. The medial meniscus is normal in size and morphology but demonstrates mild (grade I) intrasubstance signal within the posterior horn. There is no evidence of associated meniscal tear. The anterior cruciate ligament is well seen and intact. However, the posterior cruciate ligament appears markedly thickened and has intermediate to slightly increased signal intensity within it, suggestive of a partial tear. The medial and lateral collateral ligaments are also intact. The patellofemoral joint appears unremarkable with the exception of some subchondral sclerosis in the lateral facet of the patella. This is nonspecific and may represent some early degenerative change or chondromalacia. There is no evidence of a knee joint effusion or abnormal periarticular cyst.

Impression:

1. Probable incomplete tear of posterior cruciate ligament.
2. Mild (Grade I) intrasubstance degeneration within the posterior horn of the median meniscus.
3. No evidence of meniscal tear.
4. Mild degenerative change or early chondromalacia within the lateral patellar facet.

Reading Comprehension 6.2

DIRECTIONS: Underline the medical terms as you go through the reading exercise. Then list and analyze the terms. Some will be completely new to you. Consult a medical dictionary for their meanings. Then re-read the material for better comprehension.

Consultation

Consulting Physician: ——

Referring Physician: ——

Reason for Consultation/History

This patient is admitted to the hospital for elective surgery to the right shoulder. He underwent repair of a torn right rotator cuff under A. Blank, M.D. Surgery was performed on 12/18/—. The patient developed a generalized rash, pruritic in nature. He also has complained of slight chest pain over the past 12 hours. Concomitantly the patient has been quite anxious and distraught over the generalized pruritus and chest pain and overall "feeling badly." Of note is the patient's blood pressure, which is quite elevated in the past 12 hours to levels of 230/120.

Past Medical History:

The patient is an active young adult male who plays football for the state college. He was told of hypertension approximately six years earlier. No particular followup was advised. He is on no medications for hypertension. He has no history of diabetes, no history of heart disease per se. He has been in good health.

Family History:

There is a strong family history of heart disease as well as hypertension. His father has had coronary artery bypass and is known to have hypertension. The patient has had no similar type episodes in the past.

Physical Examination:

General: On examination at this time the patient is a somewhat distraught young adult male.

Vital Signs: Blood pressure 210/110. Pulse 80 and regular. Afebrile.

Chest: He is complaining of slight chest pain. Chest is clear to P&A without rales or rhonchi.

HEENT: The face is somewhat reddened. Fundi appear within normal limits. No evidence of exudates or hemorrhages. No oral lesions are noted.

Neck: Neck veins are flat. Carotids are free of bruits.

Heart: Heart rate is 80. Normal sinus rhythm without murmurs, PVCs, or rubs

Extremities: Lower extremities reveal no evidence of phlebitis clinically.

Laboratory Data: White count 9,000; hemoglobin 17 gm; hematocrit 48. Urinalysis was negative thus far.

Impression:

1. Status post repair of torn right rotator cuff.
2. Exogenous obesity.
3. Acute anxiety syndrome.
4. Allergic drug reaction secondary to either morphine or Ancef.
5. Hypertension, etiology unknown, duration unknown.

Recommendations:

Recommendations are to treat the patient's anxiety and pruritus with Vistaril IM. Lab data is recommended including catecholamines, metanephrines, and VMA studies for the purpose of the patient's hypertension as well as the hypertensive IVP. Also will place patient on Benadryl 50 mg tid in view of his rash. Chest x-ray and EKG are ordered also. Doubt at this time, if any serious cardiac or embolic phenomena are occurring; however, the patient's hypertension certainly could be further evaluated.

Will follow the patient in the hospital.

—— , M.D.

Reading Comprehension Vocabulary

Use the space below to list the medical terms for analysis and definition.

CHAPTER 7

Circulatory, Lymphatic, and Immune Systems

OBJECTIVES

When you have successfully completed Chapter 7, you should be able to:
— Name the chambers of the heart.
— Trace the circulation of the blood through the heart.
— Differentiate between the three types of blood vessels.
— Describe the function of the lymphatic system.
— Analyze and define terms related to the circulatory system.
— Explain the importance of the immune system.
— Write the meanings of the building blocks in this and previous chapters.
— Use the building blocks to build new medical terms.

atherosclerotic	(**ath**-er-oh-sklee-**ROT**-ick)	Having to do with a buildup of fatty deposits in an artery; for examples, *atherosclerotic plaque* is the material that forms the deposits.
atrium	(**AY**-tree-um)	The upper chamber of the heart; plural *atria*.
axillary	(**ACK**-sih-**lar**-ee)	Pertaining to the armpit
bradycardia	(**brad**-ee-**KAR**-dee-ah)	A slow heartbeat
cervical	(**SER**-vih-kal)	Pertaining to the neck
dysrhythmia	(dis-**RITH**-mee-ah)	An abnormality or irregularity in rhythm
endocarditis	(**en**-doh-**KAR**-**DIE**-tis)	Inflammation of the membrane that lines the heart
erythrocyte	(eh-**RITH**-roh-sight)	Red blood cell
excretory organ	(**ECK**-skreh-toh-ree)	An organ that expels waste material from the body
fragment	(**FRAG**-ment)	A part that is incomplete or broken off from a larger part
hematologist	(**hem**-ah-**TOL**-oh-jist)	One who specializes in the study of blood
hormone	(**HOR**-mohn)	The substance secreted by the ductless glands; for example, the pancreas secretes the hormone insulin.
infarction	(**IN**-fark-shun)	An area of tissue that has died because its blood supply was interrupted; or, the process of forming the dead area
inguinal	(**ING**-gwih-nal)	Pertaining to the region of the groin, which lies between the thigh and the trunk
inherent	(in-**HAIR**-ent)	Belonging to anything naturally, not as a result of circumstance or external forces
interstitial	(**in**-ter-**STISH**-al)	Having to do with spaces between the tissues of an organ or between the cells that form a tissue; for example, interstitial fluid
ischemia	(is-**KEY**-mee-ah)	Temporary deficiency of blood supply to a tissue or organ

leukocyte	(**LEW**-koh-sight)	White blood cell
lymphatics	(lim-**FAT**-icks)	The lymph vessels, including lymph nodes and the fluid they circulate; the lymphatic system
lymphocyte	(**LIM**-foh-sight)	A type of white blood cell formed in the lymph nodes
lymphoid tissue	(**LIM**-foyd)	Resembling lymph tissue
mediastinal	(**mee**-dee-as-**TIE**-nal)	Relating to the area of the chest that lies between the lungs (the mediastinum)
monocyte	(**MON**-oh-sight)	A type of white blood cell
myocardial	(my-oh-**KAR**-dee-al)	Concerning the middle layer of the walls of the heart (the myocardium)
node	(nohd)	A knot or swelling; for example, lymph nodes
nutrient	(**NEW**-tree-ent)	Food or any substance that supplies the body with nourishment
oncologist	(ong-**KOL**-oh-jist)	A physician specializing in treating tumors
oxygenation	(**ock**-sih-jeh-**NAY**-shun)	The process by which oxygen is supplied to an organ or tissue
pericarditis	(**per**-ih-kar-**DIE**-tis)	Inflammation of the pericardium
pericardium	(per-ih-**KAR**-dee-um)	The sac of serous membrane that encloses the heart
plethora	(**PLETH**-oh-rah)	Fullness
plethysmograph	(pleh-**THIZ**-moh-graf)	A device used to monitor the amount of blood contained in or passing through a body part
propel	(proh-**PELL**)	To drive forward or onward
reflect	(ree-**FLECKT**)	To turn back upon itself
respiratory	(reh-**SPIH**-rah-**toh**-ree)	Pertaining to respiration (breathing)
rhythmic	(**RITH**-mick)	Recurring at measurable, predictable intervals (see dysrhythmia)
septum	(**SEP**-tum)	A wall separating two cavities; for example, the nasal septum divides the two chambers of the nose
subclavian	(sub-**KLAY**-vee-an)	Under the clavicle (collarbone)

tachycardia	(tack-ee-**KAR**-dee-ah)	Abnormally rapid heart action
tunica adventitia	(**TEW**-nih-kah ad-ven-**TISH**-ee-ah)	The outermost layer of the wall of an artery
tunica intima	(**TEW**-nih-kah **IN**-tih-mah)	The innermost layer of the wall of an artery
tunica media	(**TEW**-nih-kah **MEE**-dee-ah)	The muscular middle layer of an artery
ventricle	(**VEN**-trih-kal)	A lower chamber of the heart

OVERVIEW

The circulatory system consists of (1) the heart, (2) the blood vessels, (3) the blood, and (4) the lymphatics.

The heart is a uniquely specialized muscle that is basically a pump. As it beats, it propels the blood through the vessels to all parts of the body. Situated between the lungs, the heart has four major chambers: the right and left *atria* (singular, *atrium*) on top, and the right and left *ventricles* below. The atria are divided into left and right halves by the *interatrial septum* and the ventricles by the *interventricular septum*.

Figure 7.1 shows the flow of blood through the heart and the vessels that supply it. Blood returning from all parts of the system enters the *right atrium* via the *inferior* and *superior venae cavae* and passes through the *tricuspid valve* to the *right ventricle*. It is then pumped through the *pulmonary semilunar valve* to the *lungs* via the *pulmonary arteries* so that it can be oxygenated. The lungs remove accumulated carbon dioxide and replace it with oxygen. From the lungs the blood returns to the heart via the *pulmonary veins* through the *left atrium*, the *bicuspid valve*, and the *left ventricle*. It is pumped out of the heart by way of the *aorta* after passing through the *aortic semilunar valve*. It then is pumped to tissues and organs through a system of smaller vessels.

Arteries, arterioles, and *capillaries* are the successively smaller vessels that carry blood to the tissues. The return trip begins by way of capillaries, then by way of tiny *venules,* and finally by way of increasingly larger *veins.*

Through this system of vessels, the blood carries nutrients from the digestive tract and oxygen from the respiratory organs *to* the body cells, and it returns waste matter *from* these cells to the excretory organs. The blood also carries hormones from the *endocrine glands*, which help to regulate body processes, and *antibodies* that protect against infection. The blood also assists in regulating body temperature by distributing heat to all body parts.

Red blood cells, or *erythrocytes*, carry oxygen, nutrients, and other substances to tissues and organs. Various types of white blood cells (*leukocytes*) function to combat infection. Both kinds of cells are carried by the *plasma*, the fluid portion of the blood. The pressure of blood pumping through the arteries squeezes some of the fluid from the blood out of the capillaries where it flows among the body cells. This escaped fluid is

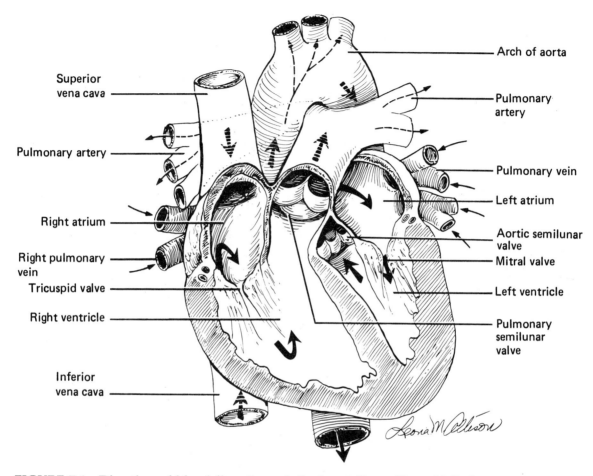

Superior vena cava

Pulmonary artery

Right atrium

Right pulmonary vein

Tricuspid valve

Right ventricle

Inferior vena cava

Arch of aorta

Pulmonary artery

Pulmonary vein

Left atrium

Aortic semilunar valve

Mitral valve

Left ventricle

Pulmonary semilunar valve

FIGURE 7.1   **Direction of blood flow through the heart** (From Kinn, *Medical Terminology—Review Challenge*, copyright 1987 by Delmar Publishers Inc.)

called *interstitial fluid.* Some of the interstitial fluid returns to the vascular system through the capillaries at the ends of venules. Excess interstitial fluid is picked up by the lymphatic capillaries.

Within the heart itself, blood circulates through a system of arteries known as the coronary circulation (Figure 7.2). When these coronary arteries become blocked by a deposit called *atherosclerotic* plaque, the heart muscle may be starved of oxygen, become ischemic, and die. Other tissues are also deprived of oxygen. Coronary artery disease is the number one killer of adults in the United States. Other common diseases of the heart and circulatory system are *myocardial infarction* (heart attack); infectious diseases such as *endocarditis* and *pericarditis*, and *hypertension* (high blood pressure). Cardiac *dysrhythmias*

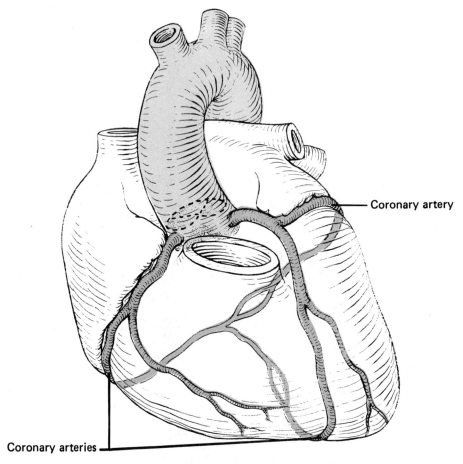

Coronary artery

Coronary arteries

FIGURE 7.2 Coronary artery system of the heart

are electrical disorders of the heart rhythm; for example, *bradycardia* is a slow heart rate and *tachycardia* is a rapid heart rate.

THE HEART

Location

The adult heart is about the size of a man's closed fist and lies in the *mediastinum*, the part of the chest cavity between the lungs. About two-thirds of the heart lies to the left of the midline (Figure 7.3). The broad, top part of the organ is called its *base*; the lower, pointed end that rests on the diaphragm is called the *apex*. If this seems confusing

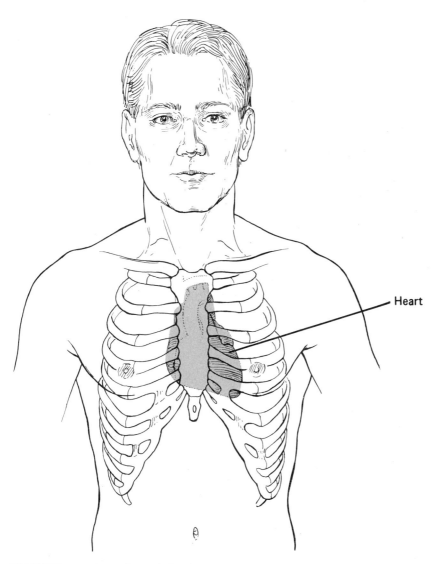

Heart

FIGURE 7.3   Location of the heart in relation to the anterior wall of the thorax

because you think of a base as being on the bottom, picture the heart as a triangle standing on its tip; the apex is down, the broad part, or base, is up.

Structure

The heart is a hollow muscular organ. Its wall is composed of three layers: The *endocardium* is the innermost layer. The *myocardium*, the middle layer, forms the greater part of the muscular wall. The outer layer, the *epicardium*, is a serous membrane that is reflected at the upper portion of the heart to form a sac, the *pericardium*, which surrounds the heart. It is composed of two main layers: the outer *fibrous* layer is the parietal *pericardium* and the inner *serous* layer is the *visceral pericardium*. Between the two layers of the pericardium is a potential space, the *pericardial* cavity, which contains a serous fluid that reduces friction as the heart beats.

Conduction System of the Heart

The rhythmic beat by which the heart pumps blood is maintained by a series of electrical impulses. The conduction system of the heart is made up of specialized fibers and nodal tissue that initiate and distribute these impulses throughout the myocardium.

The *sinoatrial node* (*S-A node*) is responsible for the rhythmic contractions of the heart and is known as its *pacemaker*. (Artificial devices known as pacemakers derive their name from this structure.) It is located in the upper part of the right atrium. The contractions that originate in the S-A node spread through the muscle of both atria and send impulses along the fibers of the conduction system to the *atrioventricular node* (*A-V node*) at the base of the right atrium. As the impulse reaches the other side of the A-V node, it spreads into a group of fibers that make up the *A-V bundle* (formerly called the bundle of His). The A-V bundle enters the upper part of the interventricular septum and divides into right and left branches. The ends of these bundle branches, the *Purkinje fibers*, spread throughout the ventricular musculature.

BLOOD VESSELS

There are three kinds of blood vessels

- Arteries carry blood from the heart to tissues and organs.
- Veins return blood from tissues and organs to the heart.
- Capillaries connect the arteries and veins by way of venules.

Arteries and veins have three layers of tissue. The *tunica intima*, the innermost layer, surrounds the *lumen*, or hollow portion of the vessels. The tunica intima consists of *epithelial tissue*. The *tunica media*, the middle layer, consists of elastic connective tissue and smooth muscle. The *tunica adventitia*, the outer layer, consists of fibrous connective tissue.

Arteries

Arteries have thicker walls than veins or capillaries. The *aorta*, which carries blood from the left ventricle of the heart, is the largest artery in the body. Slightly smaller arteries branch out from the aorta, becoming smaller and smaller. The very smallest are called *arterioles*.

Capillaries

Blood flows from the arterioles into even smaller vessels called *capillaries*. The walls of capillaries consist of only one layer of cells. The exchange of oxygen, nutrients, and wastes between the blood and the body cells takes place through the capillaries by way of the interstitial fluid.

Veins and Venules

Blood flows from the capillaries into the smallest of the veins, the *venules*, to begin its return to the heart. *Veins* have thinner walls than arteries and are subject to less pressure. The veins are equipped with valves to prevent backflow of blood. A breakdown in this valvular system may result in *varicose veins*.

BLOOD

Although you may think of blood as a fluid, it is now considered to be a type of connective tissue whose cells are suspended in a liquid intercellular material called *plasma*. The formed elements, the *cells*, include the red cells (*erythrocytes*), the white cells (*leukocytes*), and cellular fragments called *platelets*. The average amount of blood in a normal adult is 4 to $5\frac{1}{2}$ quarts, depending on the size of the individual.

Erythrocytes

The process of forming erythrocytes (red blood cells) is *erythropoiesis*. The average healthy male has about 5,400,000 red blood cells per cubic millimeter of blood. The average healthy female has a few less—about 4,800,000. The red cells are responsible for the transport of oxygen and nutrients to the body cells. A deficiency of red cells results in a condition called *anemia*.

Leukocytes

There are many varieties of leukocytes (white blood cells) and they are formed in large quantities, but they are the body's first line of defense and many leukocytes die in the battle. The number of white cells in the blood of a normal healthy adult at any one time averages 7,000 per cubic millimeter. An increase in the number of white blood cells is called *leukocytosis*, and a decrease is *leukopenia*. The white blood cell count is a key diagnostic tool for the physician.

In their role of defending the body against infection, the variety of white cells called *phagocytes* are able to devour bacterial and other foreign matter. This process is called *phagocytosis*. Unfortunately for the leukocytes, they are destroyed by the ingested toxins. The pus that forms at a site of infection is a collection of dead and disintegrating leukocytes.

Platelets

There are about 250,000 platelets per cubic millimeter of blood. Platelets are involved in the clotting process and are called *thrombocytes*. Their job begins whenever the body experiences a cut, whether accidental or intentional. A series of chemical changes occurs and the clotting process that will stop the flow of blood and seal off the wound begins. The hardened clot becomes the scab that eventually falls off.

LYMPHATICS

The lymphatic system is closely associated with the cardiovascular system and follows approximately the same course through the body. Its network of vessels (Figure 7.4) assists in circulating body fluids by carrying excess fluid away from the *interstitial spaces* and returning it to the main portion of the vascular system via the *subclavian* veins. While this tissue fluid is passing through the lymphatic vessels, it is called *lymph*. Lymph tissue is found throughout the body in nodes, the thymus gland, the spleen and other tissues.

The lymphatic vessels resemble veins in structure but have thinner walls and a greater number of valves. They originate in tissue fluid as blind-ended capillaries. Scattered along the lymphatic vessels at various places are little beanlike masses called *lymph nodes* (sometimes called lymph glands). The nodes vary in size from that of a pinhead to that of a lima bean. The nodes generally occur in groups or chains along the larger lymphatic vessels. The major locations of groups are the *cervical* (neck) region, the *axillary* region, the *inguinal* region, the bend of the elbow, the *pelvic cavity*, the *abdominal* cavity, and the *thoracic* cavity.

Ordinarily, lymph nodes are a line of defense. Lymphocytes produced by the lymph nodes and spleen play apart in immunity. The system filters out bacteria and other foreign particles from the lymph as it passes through. Sometimes, however, the lymphatics become a pathway for the spread of cancer cells or bacteria.

SPLEEN

Closely related to the function of the lymph nodes is the *spleen*, which is made up largely of *lymphoid* tissue. Its appearance is said to resemble a large lymph node (Figure 7.5). The spleen is located on the left side of the upper abdominal cavity, below the diaphragm and above the left kidney (the *left hypochondriac region*). Specialized blood cells called *lymphocytes* and *monocytes* are manufactured in the spleen. The spleen can serve as a blood reservoir and is sometimes referred to as a "blood bank." The spleen also destroys worn-out red blood cells. The spleen is not essential to life. When the spleen is surgically removed, other organs take over its function.

THYMUS

In children, the *thymus* gland, consisting of lymphatic tissue, is located within the mediastinum behind the upper part of the sternum. It performs functions similar to those of the lymph nodes. At puberty the thymus begins to atrophy, and in later life it is largely replaced by fat and connective tissue.

Cardiologists and internists are specialists concerned with the medical management of heart disease and vascular disease. Surgical management of these diseases is divided between cardiac or thoracic surgeons and vascular surgeons. Blood diseases are the domain of the hematologist or the oncologist.

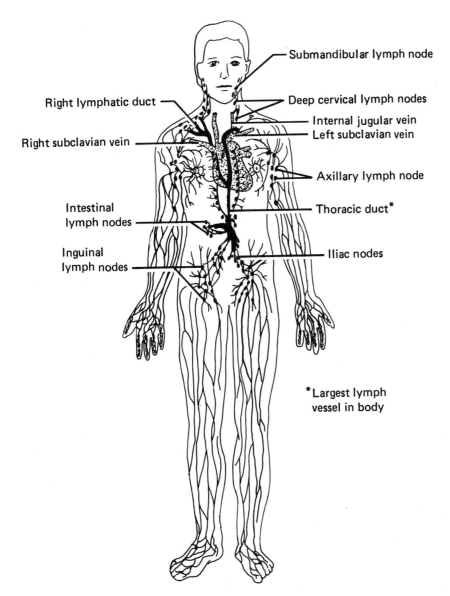

Submandibular lymph node

Deep cervical lymph nodes

Right lymphatic duct

Internal jugular vein

Left subclavian vein

Right subclavian vein

Axillary lymph node

Intestinal lymph nodes

Thoracic duct*

Inguinal lymph nodes

Iliac nodes

*Largest lymph vessel in body

FIGURE 7.4 **The lymphatic system** (From Creager, *Human Anatomy and Physiology,* copyright 1983 by Wadsworth, Inc. Reprinted by permission of the publisher)

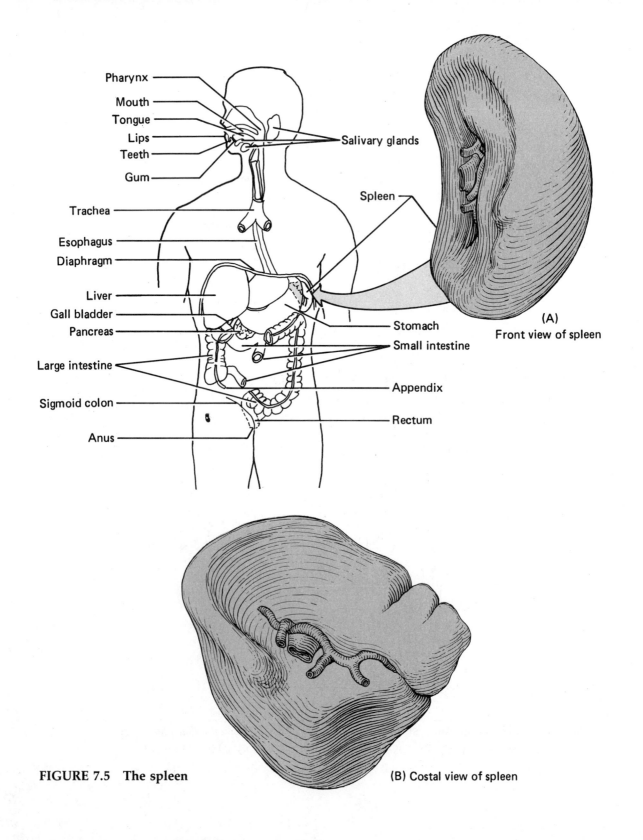

Pharynx

Mouth

Tongue

Lips

Teeth

Gum

Trachea

Esophagus

Diaphragm

Liver

Gall bladder

Pancreas

Large intestine

Sigmoid colon

Anus

Salivary glands

Spleen

Stomach

Small intestine

Appendix

Rectum

(A)
Front view of spleen

FIGURE 7.5   The spleen

(B) Costal view of spleen

IMMUNE SYSTEM

Function

The immune system protects the body from harmful natural substances by a process called *the immune mechanism*. Specialized cells recognize the presence of foreign proteins, including pathogens such as bacteria and the toxins they release. These foreign substances, which are called *antigens*, are destroyed. The skin, the respiratory system, the spleen and the thymus gland, and lymphocytes produced in the lymph nodes and the thymus (in children) are all involved in the immune mechanism. Among the specialized cells involved are lymphocytes known as T cells and B cells.

In reaction to an antigen, the body forms substances called *antibodies*. The antibodies activate a set of enzymes that attack the antigens directly. The immune response also brings about localized changes that help prevent the spread of the antigens. After an infection or other antigen invasion has been dealt with, some of the antibodies formed in the process remain in the blood.

Immunity

The state of being protected from a disease as a result of the antigen/antibody response is called immunity. This state may be brought about in several ways (see next section). Each antigen that attacks the body requires a separate immune process; there is no such thing as generalized immunity. Some pathogens change their structure so often that the body cannot become immune to them. The common cold is an example.

Lymphocytes and macrophages, both leukocytes or white cells, function in the immune mechanism. The macrophages are scavenger cells that can clear foreign particles from tissues. The pus that forms in an infected wound is actually composed of scavenger cells that have been sent to the area by the immune system and have "died in battle" with the invading pathogens.

Types of Immunity

Immunity may occur in several ways (Table 7.1), including intentional stimulation of a mild immune response in the process known as vaccination.

Naturally acquired active immunity occurs when an individual is exposed to a live pathogen, develops a disease, and becomes resistant to that pathogen as a result of a primary immune response. Immunity to a specific disease can be induced by a vaccine, a drug that contains a carefully monitored quantity of live or killed pathogens. This is known as *artificially acquired active immunity*.

During pregnancy, certain antibodies pass from the maternal blood through the placental membrane and into the fetal bloodstream. The fetus acquires some immunity against any pathogens for which the mother has developed active immunities. Thus, the fetus will have a *naturally acquired passive immunity* which may remain effective for 6 months to a year after birth. It is believed that breast milk also contains substances that strengthen the immune system or induce immunity.

By receiving an injection of gamma globulin, a person develops an *artificially acquired passive immunity*. This type of immunity is called passive because the antibodies involved are not produced by the individual's own cells. Such immunity is relatively short-term, seldom lasting more than a few weeks.

TABLE 7.1. Types of Immunity

Type	How Acquired	Response
Naturally acquired active immunity	Exposure to a live pathogen	Person develops the disease and becomes immune to that pathogen
Artificially acquired active immunity	Vaccination	Vaccine stimulates the immune response without the person's developing the disease
Naturally acquired passive immunity	Antibodies pass from the mother to the fetus through the placenta	Infant has immunity for about six months
Artificially acquired passive immunity	Injection of antibodies such as gamma globulin into the person	Short-term immunity but person is susceptible to the pathogens in the future

Disorders of Immune System

Immune disorders are only beginning to be understood. The processes involved are very complex.

Allergy. An *allergy* is an abnormal or excessive reaction of the immune system to a foreign substance that causes no reaction in most individuals. Allergens are substances that may enter the body through a number of routes. They may be inhaled, ingested, absorbed through the skin, or injected. Allergies are accompanied by uncomfortable and often harmful effects on the body. *Anaphylaxis* is a life-threatening allergic reaction that may occur upon exposure to an allergen. For example, a person who is severely allergic to bee venom may die from a bee sting—sometimes in minutes.

Autoimmune Diseases. Sometimes the immune system fails to recognize the body's own tissues. It develops unwanted antibodies, leading to such diseases as rheumatoid arthritis, autoimmune thyroiditis, or systemic lupus erythematosus (SLE).

Immune Deficiency Syndromes. Immune deficiency syndromes are in a sense the reverse of allergies. Instead of being hyperactive, the immune response is reduced or absent. These syndromes may be either inherited or acquired. Acquired immune deficiency syndrome (AIDS) is a major health threat that currently has no cure. It is thought to be caused by the human immunodeficiency virus (HIV). AIDS is transmitted when HIV in blood, semen, and possibly other body fluids of an infected person in some way enters the bloodstream of another person.

Tissue Rejection

A major problem in organ transplantation is rejection of transplanted tissue or organs. In this instance, the immune system becomes harmful. Rejection of organ transplants may sometimes be avoided by the use of drugs that suppress the immune system, but this leaves the patient without protection against infection.

≡ BUILDING BLOCKS

ROOTS AND COMBINING FORMS

Word Element	Meaning
aden/o	gland
angi/o	vessel
arteri/o	artery
ather/o	fatty substance
atri/o	atrium
cardi/o	heart
cyan/o	blue
erythr/o	red
gen/o	producing
leuk/o	white
lymph/o	lymph
my/o	muscle
path/o	disease
phag/o	eat, swallow
phleb/o	vein
ser/o	serum
sin/o	sinus
sphygm/o	pulse
splen/o	spleen
steth/o	chest
thromb/o	clot
thym/o	thymus gland
vas/o	vessel, duct
ven/i, ven/o	vein
ventricul/o	ventricle
viscer/o	internal organs

SUFFIXES

Word Element	Meaning
–cyte	cell
–gram	something written or recorded
–graphy	process of recording
–megaly	enlargement
–penia	deficiency
–philia	attraction for
–poiesis	formation
–ptysis	spitting
–sclerosis	hardening
–spasm	sudden contraction of muscles
–version	a turning

PREFIXES

Word Element	Meaning
auto–	self
brady–	slow
ecto–	out; outside
endo–	in; within
epi–	above; upon; on
inter–	between
macro–	large
peri–	surrounding
sanguin–	bloody
semi–	half
syn–	together, with
tachy–	fast, rapid

VOCABULARY

General Terms

allergen	(AL-er-jen)	Any substance capable of causing an allergic reaction
angiospasm	(AN-jee-oh-spazm)	Spasmodic contraction of blood vessels
asplenia	(ah-SPLEE-nee-ah)	Absence of the spleen

autograft	(**AW**-toh-graft)	A graft transferred from one part of a patient's body to another part
bicuspid	(by-**KUS**-pid)	Having two cusps or points; the bicuspid valve
cardioversion	(**KAR**-dee-oh-**ver**-zhun)	Conversion of an abnormal cardiac rhythm to a normal sinus rhythm
circulatory system	(**SIR**-kyou-lah-tor-ee)	The cardiovascular system consisting of the heart and blood vessels (arteries, arterioles, capillaries, venules, and veins) and the lymphatic system
hemoptysis	(hee-**MOP**-tih-sis)	Spitting (expectoration) of blood arising from the oral cavity, larynx, trachea, bronchi, or lungs
immunity	(ih-**MEW**-nih-tee)	Natural or acquired protection from a disease
immunoglobulin	(**im**-you-noh-**GLOB**-you-lin)	A protein that is known to have antibody capability
interferon	(**in**-ter-**feer**-on)	A chemical produced within the body that protects against viral infection
interventricular	(**in**-ter-ven-**TRICK**-you-lar)	Situated between ventricles
parietal	(pah-**RYE**-eh-tal)	Pertaining to, or forming, the wall of a cavity or hollow organ.
pathogen	(**PATH**-oh-jen)	A disease-producing microorganism or substance
sanguineous; sanguinous	(sang-**GWIN**-ee-us) (**SANG**-gwih-nus)	Containing blood or involving bloodshed
semilunar	(**sem**-ee-**LEW**-nar)	Shaped like a crescent, or half-moon
septum	(**SEP**-tum)	A partition; a wall separating two cavities
serosanguineous	(**see**-roh-san-**GWIN**-ee-us)	Containing or pertaining to both serum and blood
tricuspid	(try-**KUS**-pid)	Having three points or cusps; such as the tricuspid (right atrioventricular) valve of the heart

vaccine	(vack-**SEEN**)	Substance used for immunization against infectious disease
visceral	(**VIS**-er-al)	Pertaining to the viscera (internal organs)
viscosity	(vis-**KOS**-ih-tee)	The degree of stickiness or gumminess of a fluid

Terms Related to Anatomy and Physiology

antibody	(**AN**-tih-**bod**-ee)	A protein substance in the blood developed in response to an antigen that interacts specifically with that antigen (see *antigen*)
antigen	(**AN**-tih-jen)	Any foreign substance, such as a bacterial toxin, capable of stimulating the body to form antibodies that interact specifically with that antigen
aorta	(ay-**OR**-tah)	The main trunk of the arterial system of the body
apex	(**AY**-pecks)	The pointed extremity of a cone-shaped structure; the pointed end of the heart
arteriole	(ar-**TEE**-ree-ol)	A terminal branch of an artery
artery	(**AR**-ter-ee)	One of the vessels carrying blood from the heart to the tissues
atrioventricular (A-V) node	(ay-tree-oh-ven-**TRICK**-you-lar)	Part of the conduction system of the heart
atrium	(**AY**-tree-um) pl. atria (**AY**-tree-ah)	The upper chamber of each half of the heart; plural, *atria*
blood pressure		The pressure exerted by the blood on the wall of any vessel as the heart contracts and relaxes
capillary	(**KAP**-ih-**lar**-ee)	Any of the minute vessels that connect the arterioles and venules
coagulation	(koh-**ag**-you-**LAY**-shun)	Clotting of the blood

coronary artery	(**KOR**-ah-nar-ee)	One of a pair of arteries that branch off from the ascending aorta and encircle the heart like a crown, carrying blood to the myocardium (*corona* mens crown)
coronary veins		Vessels that receive blood that has passed through the capillaries of the myocardium and carry it to a larger vessel, the coronary sinus, from which it empties into the right atrium
corpuscle	(**KOR**-pus-al)	Formed element of the blood (an old term for blood cell still used sometimes)
diastole	(die-**ASS**-toh-lee)	The normal period of dilatation in the heart cycle during which the cavities fill with blood.
diastolic pressure	(die-ah-**STOL**-ick)	The blood pressure during diastole; the point of least pressure in the arterial vascular system
endocardium	(**en**-doh-**KAR**-dee-um)	The membrane lining the inner surface and cavities of the heart
endothelium	(**en**-doh-**THEE**-lee-um)	A form of epithelium that lines the blood and lymphatic vessels
epicardium	(**ep**-ih-**KAR**-dee-um)	The innermost layer of the pericardium
erythrocyte	(eh-**RITH**-roh-sight)	A mature red blood cell
erythropoiesis	(eh-**rith**-roh-poy-**EE**-sis)	The formation of red blood cells
hemoglobin	(**hee**-moh-**GLOW**-bin)	The iron-containing pigment of the red blood cells that carries oxygen from the lungs to the body tissues (*heme* = iron)
leukocyte	(**LEW**-koh-sight)	White blood cell; there are several types of leukocytes.
lumen	(**LEW**-men)	The hollow portion within a tube or tubular organ

lymph	(limf)	A transparent alkaline fluid found in the lymphatic vessels and derived from the tissue fluids
lymph node	(limf nohd)	Accumulations of lymphatic tissue formed into a knot or node, situated at intervals along the lymphatic vessels
lymphocyte	(**LIM**-foh-sight)	A type of white blood cell. Lymphocytes normally make up 25 to 50 percent of the white cells in the blood
macrophage	(**MACK**-roh-fayj)	Specialized cells that function as scavengers to clear foreign particles from tissues
myocardium	(my-oh-**KAR**-dee-um)	The middle layer of the walls of the heart
pacemaker	(**PAYS**-may-ker)	The normal cardiac pacemaker is the sinoatrial (S-A) node. It automatically generates impulses that spread to other regions of the heart. Also, an artificially implanted device to control heart rhythm.
palpation	(pal-**PAY**-shun)	Touching with the hands on the external surface of the body in order to feel the structures underneath
palpitation	(pal-pih-**TAY**-shun)	A rapid, vigorous action of the heart that is perceptible and may be disturbing to the patient
pericardium	(per-ih-**KAR**-dee-um)	The double membranous sac enclosing the heart
plasma	(**PLAZ**-mah)	The liquid part of the lymph and of the blood
pulse	(puhls)	The normally rhythmic dilating (expanding) of an artery as it receives the increased volume of blood caused by a heart contraction; can be felt by palpation

pulse pressure		The difference between the systolic and the diastolic pressure
Purkinje fibers	(pur-**KIN**-jee)	Specialized cardiac muscle fibers lying beneath the endocardium that form the electrical impulse-conducting system of the heart
serum	(**SEE**-rum)	The watery portion of the blood after coagulation. The term also refers to the clear fluid that seeps out (exudes) protectively in response to injury or inflammation
sinoatrial (S-A) node	(**sigh**-noh-**AY**-tree-al)	Node at the juncture of the superior vena cava and the right cardiac atrium, known as the pacemaker of the heart
sinus rhythm		Normal cardiac rhythm regulated by the S-A node
spleen		A large glandlike upper abdominal organ that functions in the formation, storage, and filtration of blood
systole	(**SIS**-toh-lee)	That part of the heart cycle in which the heart is in contraction
systolic pressure	(sis-**TOL**-ick)	Maximum blood pressure that occurs during contraction of the ventricles (systole)
thymus	(**THIGH**-mus)	A ductless gland located in the mediastinal cavity of infants and children that normally disappears during puberty
tunica adventitia	(**TEW**-nih-kah ad-ven-**TISH**-ee-ah)	The outer layer of an artery or of any tubular structure
tunica intima	(**TEW**-nih-kah **IN**-tih-mah)	The lining layer of an artery
tunica media	(**TEW**-nih-kah **MEE**-dee-ah)	The muscular middle layer of an artery

valve		In the circulatory system, a membranous fold in a vessel that prevents the contents passing through it from flowing backward (reflux)
vein	(vain)	Vessel carrying blood from the tissues toward the heart
ventricle	(VEN-trih-KAL)	A small cavity; either of the two lower chambers of the heart
venule	(VEN-youl)	A tiny vein continuous with a capillary and leading to a vein

Terms Related to Pathology

acute bacterial endocarditis	(en-doh-kar-DIE-tis)	Inflammation of the lining membrane of the heart that begins abruptly and progresses rapidly
anaphylaxis	(an-ah-fih-LACK-sis)	An extreme allergic reaction of the body to a foreign protein or drug
anemia	(ah-NEE-mee-ah)	Condition resulting from reduction in number of circulating red blood cells (RBCs), in the amount of hemoglobin, or in the volume of packed red cells
aneurysm	(AN-you-rizm)	A sac formed by localized abnormal expansion (dilatation) of a blood vessel, usually an artery
angina pectoris	(an-JIE-nah, AN-jih-nah, PECK-tor-is)	Severe pain and constriction about the heart, caused by an insufficient supply of blood to the heart
arrhythmia	(ah-RITH-mee-ah)	Irregularity or variation from the normal rhythm of the heartbeat
arteriosclerosis	(ar-tee-ree-oh-sklee-ROH-sis)	Thickening, and loss of elasticity of the walls of arteries
asystole	(ah-SIS-toh-lee)	Absence of heartbeat; cardiac standstill
atherosclerosis	(ath-er-oh-sklee-ROH-sis)	A common form of arteriosclerosis in which fatty deposits

		(atherosclerotic plaque) are formed within the arteries
bradycardia	(brad-ee-KAR-dee-ah)	A slow heartbeat evidenced by slowing of the pulse rate under 60 beats per minute
cardiac tamponade	(tam-pon-AID)	Acute compression of the heart resulting from accumulation of excess fluid in the pericardium
cardiac arrest		Sudden stoppage of cardiac function, with disappearance of arterial blood pressure
congestive heart failure	(kon-JES-tiv)	A clinical syndrome (combination of symptoms) that occurs when the heart cannot adequately pump blood so that blood "backs up" in the lungs and other tissues, leading to edema (swelling)
cor pulmonale	(kor pull-moh-NAY-lee)	Hypertrophy or failure of right ventricle secondary to disease of the blood vessels of the lung or chest wall
ecchymosis	(eck-ih-MOH-sis)	A spot where bleeding has occurred in the skin or mucous membrane forming a blue or purplish patch; a bruise
embolus	(EM-boh-lus)	A mass of undissolved matter which can be air, fat, or a blood clot present in the circulating blood stream
epistaxis	(ep-ih-STACK-sis)	Hemorrhage from the nose; nosebleed
erythrocytosis	(eh-rith-roh-sigh-TOH-sis)	Abnormal increase in the number of red blood cells in circulation
hemophilia	(hee-moh-FILL-ee-ah)	A hereditary deficiency in clotting or coagulation time with a consequent tendency to bleed
hypertension	(high-per-TEN-shun)	Abnormally high blood pressure
hypotension	(high-poh-TEN-shun)	Abnormally low blood pressure

leukemia	(**lew**-**KEE**-mee-ah)	Excessive increase in white blood cells (leukocytes). A cancerous disease of the blood-forming organs characterized by malignant leukocytes invading the bloodstream and bone marrow
lymphadenopathy	(lim-**fad**-eh-**NOP**-ah-thee)	Diseased condition of the lymph glands
lymphocytopenia	(**lim**-foh-**sigh**-toh-**PEE**-nee-ah)	Fewer than the normal number of lymphocytes in the blood
lymphocytosis	(**lim**-foh-sigh-**TOH**-sis)	An excess of lymph cells
lymphoma	(lim-**FOH**-mah)	A general term for growth of new tissue in the lymphatic system
lymphosarcoma	(**lim**-foh-sar-**KOH**-mah)	A malignant disease of lymphatic tissue
mitral valve prolapse (MVP)		A condition in which a cusp of the mitral valve prolapses into the left atrium
occlusion	(ah-**KLEW**-zhun)	The closure, or obstruction, of a passage. *Coronary occlusion:* Obstruction of a coronary vessel by thrombosis or as a result of spasm, leading to myocardial ischemia and ordinarily known as a heart attack.
pericarditis	(**per**-ih-kar-**DIE**-tis)	Inflammation of the pericardium
phlebitis	(fleh-**BY**-tis)	Inflammation of a vein
phlebosclerosis	(**fleh**-boh-sklee-**ROH**-sis)	Fibrous hardening of a vein's walls
splenitis	(spleh-**NIGH**-tis)	Inflamed condition of the spleen
splenomegaly	(**spleh**-noh-**MEG**-ah-lee)	Enlargement of the spleen
tachycardia	(**tack**-ee-**KAR**-dee-ah)	Abnormal rapid heart action
thrombophlebitis	(**throm**-boh-fleh-**BY**-tis)	Inflammation of a vein with formation of a thrombus (clot) in an extremity, most frequently a leg.
thrombus	(**THROM**-bus)	A blood clot that remains at the site of formation and obstructs a blood

		vessel or a cavity of the heart. (When it becomes migratory, it is called an *embolus*.)
thymitis	(thigh-**MIY**-tis)	Inflammation of the thymus gland
varicose vein	(**VAR**-ih-kos vain)	Enlarged, twisted superficial vein, most commonly occurring in the lower extremity and in the esophagus
vasoconstriction	(**vas**-oh-kon-**STRICK**-shun)	Contraction of blood vessels

Terms Related to Diagnostic Procedures

angiocardiography	(an-jee-oh-**kar**-dee-**OG**-rah-fee)	X-ray of the heart and great vessels after intravenous injection of contrast material
arteriography	(ar-tee-ree-**OG**-rah-fee)	X-ray of arteries after injection of contrast material into the bloodstream
cardiac catheterization	(**KAR**-dee-ack **kath**-eh-ter-eye-**ZAY**-shun)	A procedure used in diagnosing heart disorders by passing a small plastic tube into the heart through a blood vessel and withdrawing samples of blood for testing
echocardiography	(eck-oh-**kar**-dee-**OG**-rah-fee)	The use of ultrasound to visualize internal cardiac structures as a diagnostic procedure
echogram	(**ECK**-oh-gram)	The record made by echography
electrocardiogram	(ee-**leck**-troh-**KAR**-dee-oh-gram)-	A recording of the electrical activity of the heart (ECG or EKG)
electrocardiography	(ee-**leck**-troh-**kar**-dee-**OG**-rah-fee)	The making and study of electrocardiograms
venography	(vee-**NOG**-rah-fee)	X-ray of the veins after introduction of contrast material

Terms Related to Surgery or Treatment

endarterectomy	(**end**-ar-ter-**ECK**-toh-mee)	Surgical removal of the lining of a blocked or diseased artery

lymphadenectomy	(lim-**fad**-eh-**NECK**-toh-mee)	Surgical removal of a lymph node
lymphadenotomy	(lim-**fad**-eh-**NOT**-oh-mee)	Surgical incision of a lymph node
pericardiectomy	(**per**-ih-**kar**-dee-**ECK**-toh-mee)	Excision of part or all of the pericardium
phlebotomy	(fleh-**BOT**-oh-mee)	Surgical opening of a vein to withdraw blood
splenectomy	(spleh-**NECK**-toh-mee)	Surgical excision of the spleen
splenotomy	(spleh-**NOT**-oh-mee)	Incision of the spleen
thymectomy	(thigh-**MECK**-toh-mee)	Surgical removal of the thymus gland
valvotomy	(val-**VOT**-oh-mee)	Incision into a valve
vasodilatation	(**vas**-oh-die-lah-**TAY**-shun)	Increase in the caliber of blood vessels
venipuncture	(**VEN**-ih-**punk**-chur)	Puncture of a vein for any purpose. Usually refers to drawing of blood for diagnostic purposes.

7.1   Review: System

1. Included in the circulatory system are the

   _____   _____

   _____   _____

2. The heart has _____ chambers, namely, the _____

   _____

3. Trace the circulation of the blood through the heart and lungs:

4. The blood transports _____ from the digestive tract,
   _____ from the respiratory organs to the body cells, and
   _____ from the body cells to the excretory organs.

5. The fluid portion of the blood is called _____ .

6. The circulatory system of the heart itself is called _____ .

7. The wall of the heart has three layers, which are:

   a. _____   b. _____   c. _____

8. The rhythmic contractions of the heart are controlled by the

   _____ .

9. The three kinds of blood vessels are:

   a. _____   b. _____   c. _____

10. Name five major locations of groups of lymph nodes:

    a. _____   d. _____

    b. _____   e. _____

    c. _____

7.2   Review: Building Blocks

DIRECTIONS: Cover the column on the left while you write the building blocks for the terms in the right column.

ather/o	1. fatty substance _____
gen/o	2. producing _____
sanguin–	3. bloody _____
vas/o	4. vessel, duct _____
angi/o	5. vessel _____
–megaly	6. enlargement
tachy–	7. fast, rapid _____
lymph/o	8. lymph _____
auto–	9. self _____
–penia	10. deficiency _____
–graphy	11. process of recording _____
–cyte	12. cell _____
erythr/o	13. red _____
phag/o	14. eat, swallow _____
leuk/o	15. white _____
phleb/o	16. vein _____
sero–	17. serum _____
–poiesis	18. formation _____
sphygm/o	19. pulse _____
viscer/o	20. internal organ _____

7.3 Review: Building Blocks

DIRECTIONS: Cover the column on the left while you define the following building blocks.

out, outside	1. ecto– _____
something written	2. –gram _____
between	3. inter– _____
muscle	4. my/o _____
gland	5. aden/o _____
disease	6. path/o _____
hardening	7. –sclerosis _____
sinus	8. sino _____
together	9. syn– _____
within, in	10. endo– _____
surrounding	11. peri– _____
artery	12. arteri/o _____
spitting	13. –ptysis _____
large	14. macro– _____
spleen	15. splen/o _____
thymus gland	16. thym/o _____
vein	17. ven/i, ven/o _____
sudden contraction of muscles	18. –spasm _____
slow	19. brady– _____
attraction for	20. –philia _____

7.4 Review: Vocabulary

DIRECTIONS: Define the following terms:

1. arteriole _____
2. atrium _____
3. autograft _____
4. coagulation _____
5. epistaxis _____
6. hemoglobin _____
7. lumen _____
8. lymphocytosis _____
9. phlebitis _____
10. septum _____
11. splenomegaly _____
12. venography _____

7.5 Review: Vocabulary

DIRECTIONS: Write the medical term for each of the following definitions.

1. _____ Severe allergic reaction of the body to a foreign protein or drug
2. _____ Localized abnormal dilatation of a blood vessel, usually an artery
3. _____ The main trunk of the arterial system of the body
4. _____ Absence of heartbeat; cardiac standstill
5. _____ Sudden stoppage of cardiac function, with disappearance of arterial blood pressure
6. _____ A recording of the electrical activity of the heart
7. _____ Inflammation of the membrane that lines the heart
8. _____ A mature red blood cell or corpuscle
9. _____ An area of dead tissue following loss of blood supply
10. _____ Local and temporary deficiency of blood supply to a tissue or part
11. _____ Surgical incision of a lymph node
12. _____ Rapid, vigorous action of the heart that is perceptible and often disturbing to the patient
13. _____ Containing blood or involving bloodshed
14. _____ Normal cardiac rhythm regulated by the S-A node
15. _____ A blood clot that obstructs a blood vessel or a cavity of the heart

7.6   Review: Building Medical Terms

1. The combining form for gland is _____ .
   A suffix for disease condition is _____ .
   _____ means a disease condition of a gland.

2. A word element meaning white is _____ .
   A word element meaning cell is _____ .
   A _____ is a white blood cell.

3. The combining form for heart is _____ .
   A suffix meaning enlargement is _____ .
   Enlargement of the heart is referred to as _____ .

4. The combining form _____ means eat or swallow.
   The word element for cell is _____ .
   A cell that eats or swallows other cells or bacteria might be called a
   _____ .

5. A combining form for blood is _____ .
   The suffix meaning spitting is _____ .
   _____ means the spitting up of blood.

7.7   Review: Word Building

DIRECTIONS: Fill in the blanks with the appropriate building block or medical term.

1. _____ is a combining form for *vein*.
   A suffix meaning *hardening* is _____ .
   Fibrous hardening of the walls of a vein is _____ .
   Surgical opening of a vein to withdraw blood is _____ .

2. The prefix meaning *rapid* is _____ .
   The combining form for *heart* is _____ .
   An abnormally fast heartbeat is called _____ .

3. _____ is a prefix meaning *within*.
   The combining form for *artery* is _____ .
   _____ is a suffix meaning *surgical excision*.
   Surgical excision of the lining of an artery is _____ .

4. The combining form for *lymph node* is _____ .
   Surgical excision of a lymph node is _____ .

5. The term for *red blood cell* is _____ .
   _____ is a word ending meaning *abnormal increase*.
   An abnormal increase in the number of red blood cells in the circulating blood is
   _____ .

Reading Comprehension 7.1

DIRECTIONS: Underline the medical terms as you go through the reading exercise. Then list and analyze the terms. Some will be completely new to you. Consult a medical dictionary for their meanings. Then re-read the material for better comprehension.

History and Physical Examination

Chief Complaint:

74-year-old male admitted for right-sided weakness.

History of P.I.:

The patient states that he had an occipital headache last night, slept poorly, and then noticed problems focusing his eyes this morning. This afternoon the patient's family reports that he was unable to move his right arm and right leg, could not walk, the right side of his face was drooped and his speech was markedly slurred. This prompted the emergency room visit and admission.

Since that time (3 hours), the patient has slowly improved with almost total resolution of symptomatology.

Past History:

The patient's history is interesting in that he has a prosthetic valve, I think a Cutter-type valve, in the aortic area, placed in 1972 for rheumatic fever with aortic stenosis and congestive heart failure. He was catheterized at that time also. Since that time the patient has slowly developed anginal-type symptoms with chest heaviness, relieved by nitroglycerin, occurring several times per month up until several months ago when he developed more angina, taking a few nitroglycerin per day. At that time he was started on long-acting Isordil and he has since required only two nitroglycerin per week. He has never had a M.I. and no longer has any symptoms of congestive heart failure except for shortness of breath on exertion. He sleeps flat and denies any increased nocturia. The patient also suffers from longstanding headaches, bitemporal at times, quite severe and pounding, not always related to his nitrites. Recent sed. rates were found to be normal and it is not thought that he has temporal arteritis.

The patient has no past history of diabetes or hypertension.

Prior surgeries include prosthetic valve, cholecystectomy, appendectomy, hernia repairs ×3 and fistula-in-ano repair.

Medicines include Isordil 40 mg t.i.d., digoxin 0.25 mg per day and Coumadin 5 mg five days a week.

Allergies: None known.

Social History:

The patient is retired. He has two children. He does not drink and has not had a cigarette for years.

Family History:
    Father died of pneumonia at 92. Mother died of cancer at 72. Family history is strongly positive for carcinoma and strokes. One brother has myocardial problems.

Review of Systems:

General: The patient denies any weight change, any severe lightheaded spells or blackout spells. No fevers or chills.

HEENT: See above for history of headaches. The patient wears glasses. He states that he has not seen double but his vision has been impaired recently, and he states he has much difficulty describing how and what the symptoms are. The patient also has hearing problems and wears an aid.

Endocrine: No history of thyroid disorders or diabetes.

Cardiorespiratory: No history of asthma, wheezing, emphysema or cough. No TB history.

GI: No bowel habit changes. No tarry stool. The patient does have some black stool because he takes iron and vitamins. No indigestion or history of hepatitis.

GU: Slight narrowing of the stream. No increased discomfort, dysuria, or bleeding.

Musculoskeletal: No serious arthritides.

Hematologic: No bleeding disorders except that the patient is coumadinized.

Neurologic: The patient states that he had polio as a child, with some paralysis of the right leg and arm for one year. This was accompanied by St. Vitus' dance and rheumatic fever. The patient states that this totally resolved until this present episode.

Physical Examination:

General Appearance: On physical exam today, the patient appears as a well-developed, well-nourished, elderly male lying in bed in no distress.

Vital Signs: B.P. 140/90   P. 70 & regular   Resp. 12.

Skin: Clear

Head & Neck: Head normocephalic. Eyes: Pupils equal and reactive to light and accommodation. Extraocular movements within normal limits. Sclerae are clear. Fundi are benign bilaterally. Nose, mouth, throat: Tongue protrudes midline, no inflammation noted. The patient has no facial asymmetry on smiling or puffing his cheeks. Neck supple, no neck vein distention. Carotids full. Coarse bruit heard bilaterally, probably coming from the aortic valve radiation. No thrills are palpable.

Chest: Anterior chest scar, well-healed, from previous surgery, linear, along the sternum.

Lungs: Lungs are clear to auscultation and percussion except for a few basilar rales.

Back: No CVA or spine tenderness.

Heart: Regular rhythm at 70, PMI at the midclavicular line, fifth intercostal space. S1 and S2 loud and crisp from the prosthetic valve, especially the S2 sound. There is a coarse Grade II/VI systolic ejection murmur along the left sternal border radiating to the neck.

Abdomen: A well-healed scar is noted. No hepatosplenomegaly is appreciated. Bowel sounds are active. The abdomen is nontender.

Genitalia: Normal male. Femoral arteries full bilaterally. Valve click heard over the artery.

Extremities: Distal pulses strong in the feet. No clubbing, cyanosis or edema noted.

Neurologic: Cranial nerves II through XII as stated above and grossly normal. Deep tendon reflexes +2/4 and equal in the biceps, +1/4 and equal in the patellas. Toes are downgoing bilaterally. The patient moves all four extremities equally. Motor strength normal.

Assessment:

1. Transient ischemic attack versus cerebrovascular accident. Rule out embolism from the aortic prosthesis versus left carotid artery disease.
2. Aortic prosthesis on Coumadin, status post aortic stenosis, congestive heart failure and underlying rheumatic heart disease.
3. Arteriosclerotic cardiovascular disease with angina.

Plan: The patient will be hospitalized and monitored. The patient will be followed closely for any signs of severe CNS bleeding. Aortic valve evaluation will be carried out with echocardiogram. Carotids will be evaluated with OPG. The head will be evaluated with a CAT scan. Pro. times and other lab data are now pending. Rule out any over/under-coumadinization.

Reading Comprehension Vocabulary

Use the space below to list the medical terms for analysis and definition.

———————————
———————————
———————————
———————————
———————————
———————————
———————————
———————————
———————————
———————————
———————————
———————————
———————————
———————————
———————————
———————————
———————————
———————————
———————————
———————————
———————————
———————————
———————————
———————————
———————————
———————————

CHAPTER 8

Respiratory System

OBJECTIVES

When you have successfully completed Chapter 8, you should be able to:
— List the structures of the upper respiratory system.
— Briefly describe the function of the respiratory system.
— Recall the meanings of the Building Blocks introduced in this chapter.
— Analyze the terms in the chapter vocabulary.
— Recall the terms for given definitions.
— Identify the structures in an anatomical drawing of the respiratory system.
— Build new medical terms using the Building Blocks introduced in this and previous chapters.

cartilage	(**KAR**-tih-lij)	The dense connective tissue found at the end of most bones, particularly the smooth substance covering the joint surface of the bones; gristle.
friction	(**FRICK**-shun)	Act of rubbing one object against another
lubricate	(**LEW**-brih-kayt)	To make smooth or slippery
mucosa	(myou-**KOH**-sah)	Mucous membrane
orifice	(**OR**-ih-fis)	An opening—either an entrance or exit—to any body cavity
paranasal	(par-ah-**NAY**-zal)	Situated near or beside the nasal cavities
potential	(poh-**TEN**-shal)	Existing in possibility; for example, potential space
respiration	(res-pih-**RAY**-shun)	The continuously repeated process of taking in air (inspiration) and expelling air (expiration)
sinus	(**SIGH**-nus)	A cavity within a bony structure; an abnormal channel or passage leading to an abscess

OVERVIEW

The respiratory system supplies the body cells with oxygen and removes the waste product carbon dioxide. The process of inhaling and exhaling air to and from the lungs is called *external respiration*. The body's use of oxygen and production of carbon dioxide is called *internal respiration*. Individual cells also use oxygen and produce carbon dioxide (*cellular respiration*). Respiration is absolutely necessary for life, and most people will panic if their breathing is interfered with even momentarily.

STRUCTURE AND FUNCTION

The respiratory system (Figure 8.1) is generally divided into upper and lower tracts. The *upper respiratory tract* includes the nose, the pharynx (throat), the larynx (voice box), the trachea (windpipe), and the bronchi, which branch into tiny bronchioles. These structures are sometimes referred to as the *airway*. The lower respiratory system is generally considered to consist of the lungs and the structures that form them.

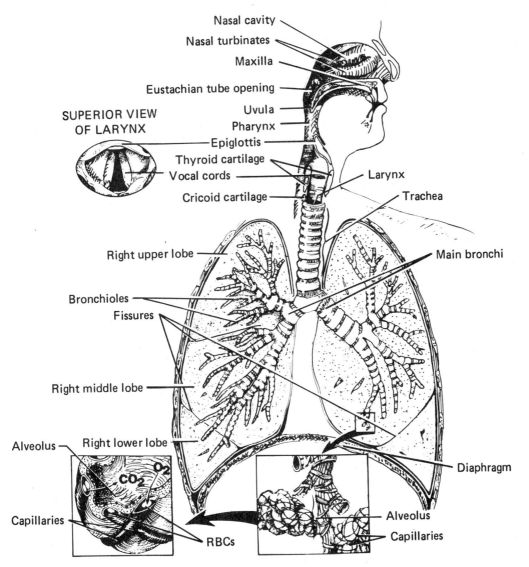

Nasal cavity
Nasal turbinates
Maxilla
Eustachian tube opening
Uvula
Pharynx

SUPERIOR VIEW
OF LARYNX
Epiglottis
Thyroid cartilage
Vocal cords
Cricoid cartilage

Larynx
Trachea

Right upper lobe

Main bronchi

Bronchioles
Fissures

Right middle lobe

Alveolus
Right lower lobe

CO_2 O_2

Diaphragm

Capillaries

Alveolus
Capillaries

RBCs

FIGURE 8.1 **The respiratory tract, with an inset view of the larynx and enlargements of an alveolus** (From Kinn, *Medical Terminology—Review Challenge*, copyright 1987 by Delmar Publishers Inc.)

The Nose

Air is taken into the body through the *nares*, or nostrils. It then passes through the *nasal cavities* (Figure 8.2) into the *nasopharynx*, the first of three designated divisions of the *pharynx*. The two nasal cavities are separated by the cartilaginous *nasal septum*. The

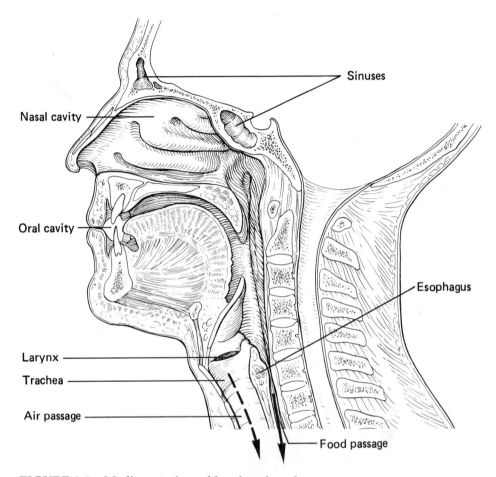

FIGURE 8.2 Median section of head and neck

lining of the nasal cavities secretes mucus and contains blood vessels. The hairs in the nasal cavities filter large particles of dust from the inhaled air. The air is also moistened and warmed as it passes through the nasal *concha*, three small bones on the lateral walls of the nasal cavity that resemble the shape of a concha shell. The conchae are sometimes called *turbinates*.

Associated with the nasal cavities are four pairs of *paranasal sinuses*, air-filled cavities in the frontal, ethmoid, sphenoid, and maxillary bones. The nose drains the sinuses and the tear ducts.

The Pharynx

The pharynx has three designated areas: (1) the *nasopharynx*, (2) the *oropharynx*, and (3) the *laryngopharynx*, (Figure 8.3). The place where the nasal cavity opens into the nasopharynx is called the *choana*. The oropharynx and the laryngopharynx together are a common passageway for both food and air. The pharynx is important in swallowing as well as in breathing.

The Larynx

Immediately below the pharynx is the *larynx,* or voice box. The larynx is composed of several sections of cartilage the largest of which is the *thyroid cartilage.* This cartilage, which is often prominent in men, is commonly known as the "Adam's apple." The larynx contains the vocal cords (Figure 8.4) and controls the movement of air from the lungs in the production of sound. The larynx also keeps food from entering the respiratory tract.

The Trachea

After passing through the larynx, air reaches the *trachea,* a tubelike passage that is 4 to 5 inches long in adults. Sixteen to 20 C-shaped rings of cartilage keep this passageway open. The trachea is sometimes called the windpipe.

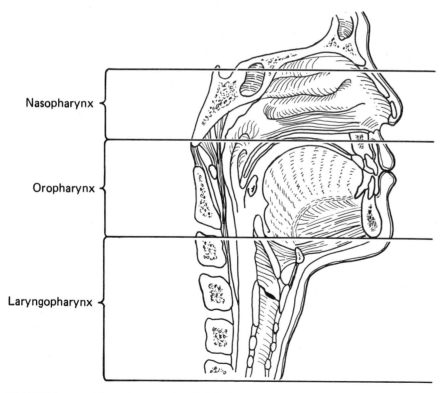

FIGURE 8.3 **The pharynx is divided into three sections**

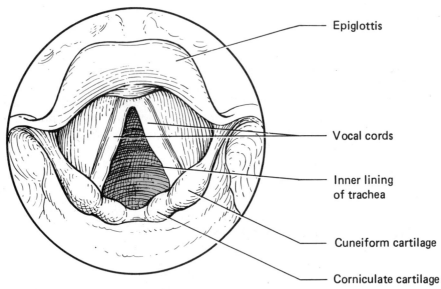

Epiglottis

Vocal cords

Inner lining
of trachea

Cuneiform cartilage

Corniculate cartilage

FIGURE 8.4   Larynx, trachea, bronchi and lungs

The Bronchial Tree

Near the center of the chest, the trachea divides into right and left *bronchi* (singular, *bronchus*) leading to the right and left *lungs*, (Figure 8.5). Each bronchus divides and subdivides into smaller *bronchial tubes,* and *bronchioles,* in a treelike pattern. The bronchioles end in *alveolar ducts, alveolar sacs,* and finally the *pulmonary alveoli,* the tiny structures of the lungs where oxygen from the inspired air is exchanged for carbon dioxide from the bloodstream.

The Lungs

The *lungs* are the organs in which oxygen/carbon dioxide exchange takes place. The right lung has three lobes and the left lung only two. Each lobe is further divided into *segments.* A double-layered serous sac called the *pleura* encloses each lung. The inner layer of the pleura, the layer closest to the lungs, is called the *visceral pleura.* The outer layer, called the *parietal pleura,* lines the chest cavity.

The so-called *potential space* between the visceral and parietal pleurae is called the *pleural cavity.* It contains a thin film of serous fluid (pulmonary surfactant) which lubricates the adjacent pleural surfaces. This lubrication reduces friction as the pleural surfaces rub one another during breathing.

The lungs lie within the *thoracic cavity* and are separated from the abdominal cavity below by the *diaphragm,* which is sometimes called the muscle of respiration (Figure 8.6).

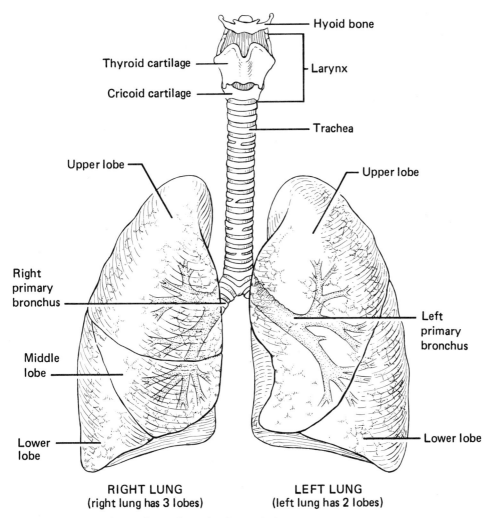

Hyoid bone

Thyroid cartilage

Cricoid cartilage

Larynx

Trachea

Upper lobe

Upper lobe

Right primary bronchus

Left primary bronchus

Middle lobe

Lower lobe

Lower lobe

RIGHT LUNG
(right lung has 3 lobes)

LEFT LUNG
(left lung has 2 lobes)

FIGURE 8.5   View of vocal cords through laryngoscope

Patients with lung disease are generally referred to *pulmonary care physicians*. Pulmonary care is a subspecialty within internal medicine. Diseases of the lungs and airway that require surgery are the province of *thoracic surgeons*. Allied health professionals called *respiratory therapists* work interactively with physicians in providing respiratory care.

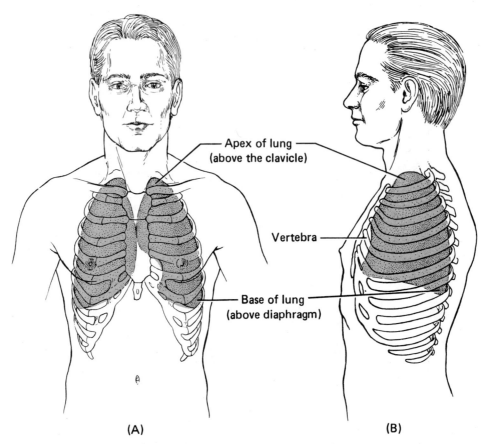

FIGURE 8.6   Positioning of the lungs in the thoracic cavity

☰ BUILDING BLOCKS

ROOTS AND COMBINING FORMS

Word Element	Meaning
actin/o	ray
atel/o	imperfect
bronch/o	bronchus
chondr/o	cartilage
coni/o	dust
cost/o	rib
cyan/o	blue
hydr/o	water

Word Element	Meaning
labi/o; cheil/o	lip
laryng/o	larynx
lingu/o	tongue
mes/o	middle
nas/o	nose
or/o	mouth
orth/o	straight
osm/o	odors
ot/o	ear
pharyng/o	pharynx
phren/o	diaphragm; also mind
pleur/o	pleura
pneum/o, pneumon/o	lung, air
ptyal/o	saliva
py/o	pus
rhin/o	nose
spir/o	breathe
sten/o	contracted, narrow
steth/o	chest
thorac/o	chest
trachel/o	neck
trache/o	trachea

SUFFIXES

Word Element	Meaning
–capnia	carbon dioxide
–centesis	surgical puncture
–dynia	pain
–ectasis	expansion
–osmia	smell
–phonia	voice; sound
–pnea	breathing
–ptysis	spitting
–sphyxia	pulse
–staxis	hemorrhage

VOCABULARY

General Terms

anosmia	(an-**OZ**-mee-ah)	Absence of the sense of smell
anoxia	(an-**OCK**-see-ah)	Absence or lack of oxygen
apnea	(ap-**NEE**-ah)	Temporary stoppage of breathing
asphyxia	(ass-**FICK**-see-ah)	A condition that occurs when no oxygen can be inspired; suffocation
auscultation	(**aws**-kuhl-**TAY**-shun)	The act of listening for sounds within the body
bronchogenic	(brong-koh-**JEN**-ick)	Originating in a bronchus
costochondral	(**kos**-toh-**KON**-dral)	Pertaining to a rib and its cartilage
eupnea	(youp-**NEE**-ah)	Easy or normal respiration
expectoration	(eck-**speck**-toh-**RAY**-shun)	Coughing up and spitting out mucus or phlegm from the lungs, bronchi, and trachea
hyperventilation	(**high**-per-**ven**-tih-**LAY**-shun)	A prolonged period of abnormally fast and deep-breathing, resulting in a lowering of the blood carbon dioxide level. An emotionally upset person may hyperventilate, become dizzy, and faint.
hypoxia	(high-**POCK**-see-ah)	A deficiency of oxygen in the inspired air
infiltration	(in-fill-**TRAY**-shun)	The passage of a substance into a cell, tissue or organ
lingual	(**LING**-gwal)	Pertaining to the tongue
oral	(**OH**-ral)	Pertaining to the mouth
paranasal	(**par**-ah-**NAY**-zal)	Situated near or beside the nasal cavities
parietal	(pah-**RYE**-eh-tal)	Pertaining to the wall of a cavity or hollow organ
percussion	(per-**KUSH**-un)	In medicine, the act of striking a body part with short, sharp blows to obtain a sound that helps in

		diagnosing the condition of the underlying parts or organs
resonant	(**REZ**-oh-nant)	Pertaining to a vibrant sound heard on percussion
stertor	(**STER**-tor)	Snoring

Terms Related to Anatomy and Physiology

alveolus	(al-**VEE**-oh-lus)	A small, saclike pouching; pulmonary alveoli are tiny air sacs within the lungs
aspiration	(**ass**-pih-**RAY**-shun)	The removal of fluids or gases from a cavity by suction; also, the accidental drawing of a foreign body into the nose, throat, or lungs by suction during inspiration
bronchiole	(**BRONG**-kee-ol)	One of the finer subdivisions of the bronchial tree
bronchus	(**BRONG**-kus)	Any of the larger air passages of the lungs
choana	(**KOH**-ay-nah)	The paired openings between the nasal cavity and the nasopharynx; posterior nares
concha	(**KONG**-kah)	One of the three bones on the lateral wall of each nasal cavity; also called nasal turbinates. Also, a term used in anatomy to designate a structure or part that resembles a shell in shape.
diaphragm	(**DIE**-ah-fram)	The musculomembranous partition that separates the abdominal and thoracic cavities. The diaphragm contracts with each inspiration of air and relaxes with each expiration of air. The muscle of respiration.
epiglottis	(ep-ih-**GLOT**-is)	The lidlike structure covering the entrance to the larynx. It prevents food from entering the larynx and trachea during swallowing.

eustachian tubes	(you-**STAY**-kee-an)	The auditory tubes extending from each middle ear to the pharynx. Important in maintaining equal air pressure on both sides of the eardrum.
exhalation	(**ecks**-hah-**LAY**-shun)	The act of breathing out; see *expiration*.
expiration	(**ecks**-pih-**RAY**-shun)	Expelling air from the lungs; the act of breathing out
glottis	(**GLOT**-is)	The sound-producing apparatus of the larynx consisting of the two vocal folds and the space between them
inhalation	(**in**-hah-**LAY**-shun)	The drawing of air or other substances into the lungs; inspiration
inspiration	(**in**-spih-**RAY**-shun)	The act of drawing air into the lungs; inhalation
larynx	(**LAR**-inks)	The organ of voice, located at the upper end of the trachea below the root of the tongue (the voice box)
lobe	(lohb)	A well-defined part of an organ; for example, the large divisions of the lungs are called lobes.
mediastinum	(**mee**-dee-as-**TIE**-num)	The area of the chest between the two lungs behind the sternum and in front of the vertebral column
mucous membrane	(**MYOU**-kus)	In the respiratory system, the membrane lining passages and cavities communicating with the air
nares	(**NAY**-reez)	The external openings of the nose; nostrils
nasopharynx	(**nay**-zoh-**FAR**-inks)	The part of the pharynx that lies above the level of the soft palate
palate	(**PAL**-at)	The partition separating the nasal and oral cavities. The roof of the mouth. *Hard palate:* The anterior

		portion of the palate, which is underlaid by bone. *Soft palate:* A posterior extension of the palate
pharynx	(**FAR**-inks)	The passageway by which air moves from the nasal cavity to the larynx and food moves from the mouth to the esophagus
pleura	(**PLEWR**-ah)	The serous membrane covering the lungs and lining the thoracic cavity
respiration	(**res**-pih-**RAY**-shun)	Breathing; the continuous repetition of inspiration and expiration
segment	(**SEG**-ment)	A portion of a larger body or structure; for example, one of the smaller divisions of the lobes of the lungs
septum	(**SEP**-tum)	A dividing wall or partition; for example, the *nasal septum* separates the two nasal cavities
sinus	(**SIGH**-nus)	In the respiratory system, one of four pairs of air cavities in the cranial bones
trachea	(**TRAY**-kee-ah)	The tubelike structure, formed by rings of cartilage, that extends from the larynx to the bronchial tubes

Terms Related to Pathology

allergic rhinitis	(ah-**LER**-jick rye-**NIGH**-tis)	Any allergic reaction of the nasal mucosa; nasal inflammation related to allergy
asthma	(**AZ**-mah)	A condition characterized by wheezing respirations due to constriction or spasm of the bronchi
atelectasis	(**at**-ee-**LECK**-tay-sis)	Incomplete expansion of the lungs at birth; collapse of the adult lung
bradypnea	(brad-ihp-**NEE**-a)	Abnormally slow breathing
bronchiectasis	(**brong**-kee-**ECK**-tah-sis)	Chronic dilatation of one or more bronchi

bronchitis	(brong-**KYE**-tis)	Inflammation of one or more bronchi
Cheyne-Stokes respiration	(**CHAIN** stohks)	Breathing characterized by rapid, deep respirations followed by a period of diminished respirations or none
dysphonia	(dis-**FOH**-nee-ah)	Any impairment of voice; difficulty in speaking
dyspnea	(**DISP**-nee-ah)	Difficult, painful, or labored breathing
edema	(eh-**DEE**-mah)	The presence of abnormally large amounts of serous fluid in the body tissues; the swelling caused by this condition
emphysema	(**em**-fih-**SEE**-mah)	A chronic disease of the lungs in which the destruction of alveoli (the air sacs) prevents the proper exchange of gases
empyema	(**em**-pie-**EE**-mah)	Accumulation of pus within a cavity especially in the pleural space
epistaxis	(**ep**-ih-**STACK**-sis)	Hemorrhage from the nose; nosebleed
hemothorax	(**hee**-moh-**THOH**-racks)	A collection of blood or bloody fluid in the pleural cavity
hypercapnia	(**high**-per-**KAP**-nee-ah)	Abnormal increase of carbon dioxide in the blood
hyperpnea	(high-perp-**NEE**-ah)	Abnormal increase in the depth or rate of respiration
hypoxemia	(**high**-pock-**SEE**-mee-ah)	Deficient oxygenation of the blood
laryngostasis	(lar-ing-**GOS**-tah-sis)	Croup; a condition resulting from acute obstruction of the larynx caused by allergy, foreign body, infection, or new growth
orthopnea	(**or**-thop-**NEE**-ah)	Difficulty breathing except when in an upright position
pertussis	(per-**TUS**-iss)	Whooping cough; an acute

infectious disease of infants characterized by recurrent spasms of coughing ending in a whooping inspiration

pleurisy	(**PLEW**-rih-see)	Inflammation of the pleura
pleurodynia	(**plew**-roh-**DIN**-ee-ah)	Pain in the intercostal muscles
pneumoconiosis	(**new**-moh-**koh**-nee-**OH**-sis)	A disease of the lungs due to deposition of dust in the lungs, frequently caused by working in coal mines
pneumonia	(new-**MOH**-nee-ah)	Inflammation of one or both lungs
pneumothorax	(**new**-moh-**THOH**-racks)	The abnormal presence of air or gas in the pleural space
rales	(rahlz)	Abnormal respiratory sounds heard with a stethoscope and indicating some pathologic condition
rhinitis	(rye-**NIGH**-tis)	Inflammation of the mucous membrane of the nose
rhinorrhea	(**rye**-noh-**REE**-ah)	Discharge of a thin nasal mucus; runny nose
silicosis	(sil-ih-**KOH**-sis)	A form of pneumoconiosis resulting from inhalation of silica dust
tachypnea	(**tack**-ip-**NEE**-ah)	Excessively rapid respirations; also, a respiratory neurosis marked by rapid, shallow respiration
tracheostenosis	(**tray**-kee-oh-steh-**NOH**-sis)	Contraction or narrowing of the trachea

Terms Related to Diagnostic Procedures

bronchoscopy	(brong-**KOS**-koh-pee)	Examination of the interior of the bronchi through an instrument called a bronchoscope
laryngoscopy	(**lar**-ing-**GOS**-koh-pee)	Examination of the interior of the larynx using a laryngoscope
Lung scan		A process that uses inhaled or injected radioactive material to

| | | create images of the lung tissue for diagnostic purposes |
| pulmonary function tests (PFTs) | | A series of tests that can help determine the cause of shortness of breath and other breathing difficulties |

Terms Related to Surgery or Treatment

laryngectomy	(lar-in-JECK-toh-mee)	Surgical removal of the larynx
lobectomy	(loh-BECK-toh-mee)	Surgical removal of a lobe of any organ or gland; for example, surgical removal of one or more lobes of a lung
pneumocentesis	(new-moh-sen-TEE-sis)	Surgical puncturing of a lung in order to drain fluids
pneumonectomy	(new-moh-NECK-toh-mee)	The surgical removal of lung tissue, especially of an entire lung
rhinoplasty	(RYE-noh-plas-tee)	A plastic reshaping of the nose which may be cosmetic, restorative, or reconstructive
septectomy	(sep-TECK-toh-mee)	Excision of all or a part of the nasal septum
thoracentesis	(thoh-rah-sen-TEE-sis)	Surgical puncture of the chest wall for removal of fluid from the pleural cavity
thoracotomy	(thoh-rah-KOT-oh-mee)	A surgical cut made in the wall of the chest
tracheostomy	(tray-kee-OS-toh-mee)	A surgical (cut) incision made in the trachea so that a tube can be inserted to provide an airway if the trachea is damaged or blocked
tracheotomy	(tray-kee-OT-oh-mee)	Incision of the trachea through the skin and muscles of the neck; note the difference the s in tracheostomy makes.

8.1 Review: System

DIRECTIONS: Cover the left column while you complete the statements on the right side.

pulmonary care physicians
The medical management of lung disease is referred to _____ .

thoracic surgeons
Surgical diseases of the lungs and airway are the province of _____ .

inspiration, expiration
Breathing is absolutely necessary to survival. The two processes in breathing are _____ and _____ .

inspiration
The word that means breathing *in* is _____ .

expiration
The word that means breathing *out* is _____ .

respiration
Together these two processes are called _____ .

upper respiratory tract, lungs
The respiratory system consists of the _____ _____ and the _____ .

nares or nostrils, nasal cavities
Air is taken into the body through the _____ and passes through the _____ into the nasopharynx.

sinuses
Air-filled cavities are called _____ .

four
There are _____ pairs of paranasal sinuses

three
The pharynx has _____ divisions.

oropharynx, laryngopharynx
The first division is the nasopharynx. The other divisions are the _____ and the _____ .

larynx
Immediately below the pharynx is the _____ .

larynx, air
The _____ contains the vocal cords and controls the expulsion of _____ from the lungs in production of sound.

trachea
The medical term for "windpipe" is the _____ .

pulmonary alveoli
The final structures of the bronchial trees are the _____ where gas exchange takes place.

lobes	The main divisions of the lungs are called _____ .
three, two	The right lung has _____ lobes, and the left lung has _____ lobes.
segments	Each lobe is further divided into _____ .
pleura	Each lung is enveloped in a double-layered serous sac called the _____ .
visceral pleura	The inner layer is the _____ .
parietal pleura	The outer layer is the _____ .
pleural cavity	The space between the two layers is known as the _____ and contains a thin film of serous fluid called pulmonary surfactant.

8.2   Review: Building Blocks

DIRECTIONS: Write the meanings of the following building blocks.

1. actin/o _____
2. –capnia _____
3. –centesis _____
4. cost/o _____
5. labi/o _____
6. –osmia _____
7. –phonia _____
8. pleur/o _____
9. –pnea _____
10. –ptysis _____
11. spir/o _____
12. –staxis _____
13. steth/o _____
14. trache/o _____
15. viscer/o _____

8.3   Review: Building Blocks

DIRECTIONS: Supply the combining forms for the following words.

1. straight   _____
2. dust   _____
3. saliva   _____
4. diaphragm   _____
5. chest   _____
6. imperfect   _____
7. blue   _____
8. nose   _____
9. breathe   _____
10. odors   _____
11. lung, air   _____
12. neck   _____
13. pus   _____
14. narrow   _____
15. water   _____

8.4   Review: Vocabulary

DIRECTIONS: Supply the corresponding medical terms for the following definitions.

1. _____ A collection of blood in the pleural cavity
2. _____ Cessation of breathing
3. _____ Deficient oxygenation of the blood
4. _____ Plastic surgery of the nose
5. _____ Pain in the intercostal muscles
6. _____ Absence or lack of oxygen
7. _____ Difficult or labored breathing
8. _____ Excess of carbon dioxide in the blood
9. _____ Chronic dilatation of the lung
10. _____ Difficulty breathing except in an upright position
11. _____ Incomplete expansion of the lungs at birth
12. _____ Deficiency of oxygen in inspired air
13. _____ Surgical puncture of the chest wall for drainage of fluid
14. _____ Small saclike dilatation
15. _____ Abnormally slow breathing

8.5 Review

Check your knowledge of the respiratory system anatomy by identifying the numbered structures in the figure.

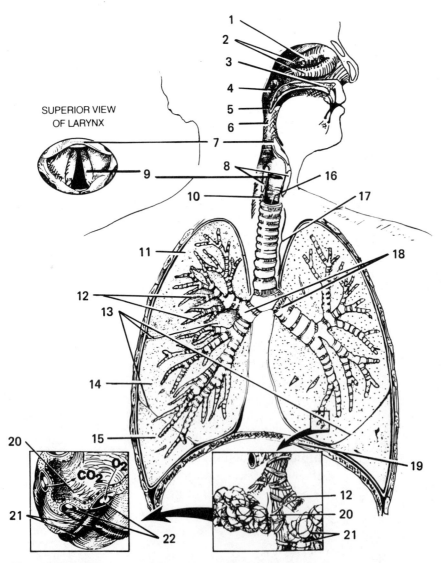

SUPERIOR VIEW OF LARYNX

(From Kinn, *Medical Terminology—Review Challenge*, copyright 1987 by Delmar Publishers Inc.)

1. _____   12. _____
2. _____   13. _____
3. _____   14. _____
4. _____   15. _____ _____
5. _____   16. _____
6. _____   17. _____
7. _____   18. _____
8. _____   19. _____
9. _____   20. _____
10. _____   21. _____
11. _____   22. _____

8.6 Review: Word Building

DIRECTIONS: Fill in the blanks with the appropriate building block or medical term.

1. A prefix meaning *near* or *beside* is _____ .

   _____ is a combining form meaning *nose*.

   Something situated near or *beside* the nose is said to be

   _____ .

2. _____ refers to a sense of smell.

   A prefix meaning *not* or *without* is _____ .

   _____ means absence of a sense of smell.

3. The prefix _____ means *good* or *normal*.

   The building block for *respiration* is _____ .

   _____ means easy or normal respiration.

4. _____ is a combining form for *mouth*.

   _____ means pertaining to the mouth.

5. Any one of the larger air passages of the lung is called a _____ .

   _____ is a suffix meaning *origin*.

   The word for originating in one of the larger air passages of the lung is

   _____ .

6. A suffix meaning *voice* or *sound* is _____ .

   _____ is a prefix meaning *bad* or *difficult*.

   Difficulty in speaking is expressed as _____ .

7. _____ is a suffix meaning *hemorrhage*.

   The prefix _____ means *upon* or *over*.

   The term _____ means hemorrhage from the nose.

8. The combining form meaning *dust* is _____ .
   The combining form _____ means *lung*.
   The suffix _____ describes an *abnormal condition*.
   _____ is a disease caused by deposition of dust in the lungs.

9. _____ is a suffix meaning *flow* or *discharge*.
   The combining form _____ means *nose*.
   _____ is the discharge of a thin nasal mucus.

10. The combining form for *trachea* is _____ .
   The suffix _____ describes the *surgical creation of an artificial opening*.
   A _____ is the surgical creation of an airway during obstruction of the trachea.

Reading Comprehension 8.1

DIRECTIONS: Underline the medical terms as you go through the reading exercise. Then list and analyze the terms. Some will be completely new to you. Consult a medical dictionary for their meanings. Then re-read the material for better comprehension.

Disorders of the Respiratory System

The upper respiratory system is subject to many types of infection and inflammation. While there are many more serious disorders that affect the respiratory system, the common cold causes a greater loss of production hours each year than any other human affliction. A head cold with an acute catarrhal condition of the nasal mucous membrane and a profuse discharge from the nostrils is known medically as *coryza*. *Allergic coryza* is commonly known as *hay fever*. Hundreds of different viruses can cause coryza.

- *Pharyngitis* is a red, inflamed throat.
- *Laryngitis* is an inflammation of the larynx, or voice box.
- *Tonsillitis* is an inflammation of the tonsils and is frequently caused by streptococci. It can affect any age group but is more common in children.
- *Sinusitis*, an inflammation of a sinus, may occur in one or all of the paranasal sinuses. Sinusitis can be an isolated occurrence or a long-term disorder.

Bronchitis is the result of inflammation of the mucous membrane lining the trachea and bronchial tubes. Older people often develop a chronic bronchitis accompanied by a cough. *Influenza*, or "flu," is caused by one of many strains of influenza virus and is characterized by inflammation of the mucous membrane of the respiratory system.
Pneumonia is an infection of the lung. It is usually caused by bacteria but can be caused by a virus. *Tuberculosis* is an infectious disease caused by bacteria. It can affect

any organ or tissue of the body but is most common in the lung. *Diphtheria* is a very infectious disease but has almost been eradicated.

Chronic obstructive pulmonary disease (COPD) is a term applied to any disorder that interferes with the mechanical exchange of gases in the lungs. The causes of COPD may range from asthma to emphysema.

Asthma produces an intermittent form of airway obstruction due to spasms of the bronchi and an increase in sticky secretions. The asthmatic patient typically has paroxysms of dyspnea, which may produce a wheezing sound to the breathing. Chronic bronchitis or asthma may eventually result in *emphysema*, a permanent change in the alveoli of the lungs. The extent of this change will determine the extent of the patient's disability.

Cystic fibrosis, a hereditary disease, is the most serious lung problem affecting children in this country. Both parents must be carriers if an infant is to have this disease.

asthma _____

bronchitis _____

COPD _____

coryza _____

cystic fibrosis _____

emphysema _____

laryngitis _____

pharyngitis _____

pneumonia _____

sinusitis _____

tonsillitis _____

tuberculosis _____

Reading Comprehension 8.2

DIRECTIONS: Underline the medical terms as you go through the reading exercise. Then list and analyze the terms. Some will be completely new to you. Consult a medical dictionary for their meanings. Then re-read the material for better comprehension.

Community Hospital Report of Operation

Date:	Patient:
Preoperative Diagnosis:	Bronchogenic carcinoma, right lower lobe, superior segment.
Postoperative Diagnosis:	Same, Stage I
Procedure:	Bronchoscopy, brush biopsy superior segment, right lower lobe, washings.

Indications:

This 71-year-old retired executive presents with a mass lesion of the right lower lobe, posterior-superior segment, which measures approximately 1 1/2 cm in diameter with irregular margins. There are no calcifications and it has the characteristics of carcinoma. The patient has no history or physical findings suggestive of systemic spread. The hilum and mediastinum appear to be negative on x-ray.

The operative procedure of bronchoscopy under local anesthesia with brush biopsy was fully explained to the patient and he accepted all the risks and attendant potential complications. As the lesion is so peripheral, it was somewhat doubtful that we would be able to obtain fluoroscopic visualization to more significantly direct the biopsy forceps into the lesion. Therefore, decision was made to proceed with a brush biopsy.

Procedure:

With the patient in the seated position in the operating theatre, the nasopharynx and pharynx were sprayed in the usual manner with 1% Xylocaine, which is the IV form without Paraben. The bronchoscope was introduced through the left nostril with no unusual problem, dropped down to the larynx where additional Xylocaine was dripped and subsequently the trachea was entered. Additional Xylocaine was dripped in 2 cc aliquots at the carina and down both left and right mainstem bronchi. Total Xylocaine utilized during the entire procedure was 14 cc.

Excellent anesthesia was obtained. The patient was quite cooperative during the entire procedure. Indeed, I did allow him to visualize his own carina through the bronchoscope which he appreciated. On the left side, the left upper and left lower lobe bronchi and segments and subsegments were perfectly clear. The mucosa was pale and demonstrated no abnormalities. The carina was sharp and moved freely with respirations and on coughing. On the right side, the right upper lobe bronchus was visualized including segments and subsegments and these were clear. Middle lobe bronchus in the usual take-off anteriorly and the medial and lateral segments appeared to be clear as was the take-off. The right lower lobe, the superior segmental orifice, and the basilar orifices were clear as were the segments.

The bronchoscope was then directed into the superior segmental bronchus and the brush was advanced to the limits and a good specimen obtained for brushings. Three slides were made and immediately dropped into the fixative. 5 cc aliquots of normal saline were then dropped into the right lower lobe and bronchus intermedius and all material returned was suctioned off and presented and submitted for culture for TB, fungus, and routine plus cytology. There was no specific lesion to be biopsied and there was no specific mucosal abnormality on either side or in the trachea. The bronchoscope was then removed with no unusual problems. The larynx demonstrated equal vocal cord activity and no laryngeal lesions. The sponge, instrument, and needle counts were correct. The patient tolerated the procedure quite well and was returned to the room in good condition. Plans are to maintain a mask for at least 8 hours with added oxygen. The patient will be kept NPO for an additional two hours and subsequently returned to his regular diet.

The bronchoscopy thus demonstrated no evidence of involvement of the take-off of the lower lobe bronchus, of the middle lobe bronchus, nor of the superior segmental bronchus of the right lower lobe. Remainder of the right side was clear. A specific mucosal biopsy was not obtained from any particular site.

Reading Comprehension Vocabulary

Use the space below to list the medical terms for analysis and definition.

_____
_____
_____
_____
_____
_____
_____
_____
_____
_____
_____
_____
_____
_____
_____
_____
_____
_____
_____
_____
_____
_____
_____
_____
_____
_____
_____
_____
_____

CHAPTER 9

Digestive System

OBJECTIVES

When you have successfully completed Chapter 9, you should be able to:
— List the principal organs of the digestive system.
— Briefly describe the function of the digestive system.
— Define the building blocks introduced in this chapter.
— Analyze the principal terms in the vocabulary.
— Identify the structures on a diagram of the digestive system.
— Build new medical terms using the building blocks introduced in this and previous chapters.

absorption	(ab **SORP** shun)	The taking in of something. The body *absorbs* liquids when they pass through a body surface such as the lining of the intestine
alimentary	(al-ih-**MEN**-tah-ree)	Pertaining to food or nutrition
bolus	(**BOH**-lus)	A large dose. In relation to digestion, a mass of masticated (chewed) food that is swallowed and passes through the esophagus to the stomach
buccal cavity	(**BUCK**-ahl **KAV**-ih-tee)	The mouth. Formed by the insides of the cheeks, the tongue and its muscles, and the roof of the mouth
digestion	(die-**JEST**-yun)	The physical and chemical breaking down of complex foodstuffs into simpler substances that can be absorbed into the bloodstream and used by the body
distal	(**DIS**-tal)	Farther from the point of origin than whatever is being compared; remote
gastroenterology	(**gas**-troh-**en**-ter-**OL**-oh-jee)	The branch of medicine concerned with the function and diseases of the stomach and intestines
hydration	(high-**DRAY**-shun)	The taking in of water by tissue or the addition of water to a substance
mastication	(mass-tih-**KAY**-shun)	Chewing
peristalsis	(**per**-ih-**STALL**-sis)	A wavelike, muscular contraction, found in tubular structures or organs, that propels the contents forward, particularly in the esophagus and intestines
proximal	(**PROCK**-sih-mal)	Nearest; closer to the point of attachment or point of origin
reservoir	(**REZ**-er-vwahr)	A place or cavity for the storage of fluids
rhythmic	(**RITH**-mick)	Recurring at measured, predictable intervals

OVERVIEW

The digestive system (Figure 9.1) consists of the organs that ingest and digest food and excrete solid waste from the body. It is composed of the *digestive tract*, which includes the mouth, pharynx, esophagus, stomach, and intestines, and the *accessory organs* of digestion. The accessory digestive organs or structures are the teeth, salivary glands, liver, gallbladder, and pancreas. Food is ingested, or taken in, through the mouth and is digested, or broken down physically and chemically, as it passes through the digestive tract, often called the *gastrointestinal tract* or *GI tract* and sometimes called the *alimentary canal*. Nutrients made available by digestion are absorbed into the bloodstream in the small intestine, and solid waste is eliminated, or excreted, by the large intestine.

Gastroenterology, a branch of medicine within the larger field of internal medicine, is concerned with the medical problems of the stomach and intestines. Surgical procedures related to this system are often done by a general surgeon.

PRIMARY DIGESTIVE ORGANS

Mouth, Tongue, and Palate

The *mouth* (Figure 9.2) is an opening through which food enters the body and also a cavity, called the *oral* or *buccal cavity*, where food is chewed and prepared for swallowing. The mouth is bordered by the cheeks and contains the tongue, the hard palate, the soft palate, and the teeth, to be discussed later in this chapter.

The *tongue* is a thick, muscular organ covered by mucous membrane and is involved in taste, chewing, swallowing, and speech. It occupies the floor of the mouth, nearly filling the oral cavity when the mouth is closed. The taste buds are located on the upper surface of the tongue.

The *palate* forms the roof of the mouth and is composed of the hard palate and the soft palate. The *hard palate* is a bony structure that separates the oral cavity from the nasal cavity above it. It is located in the anterior part of the mouth. The *soft palate*, located behind the hard palate, is composed of muscle tissue and extends posteriorly and downward, ending in a cone-shaped process called the *uvula*. When we swallow, muscles draw the soft palate and the uvula upward. This action closes the opening between the nasal cavity and the pharynx and prevents food from entering the nasal cavity.

Pharynx

The *pharynx* is what most of us call the throat. It is a passageway for both air and food and is divided into the nasopharynx, oropharynx, and laryngopharynx. Food enters through the mouth, is chewed, and swallowed, and passes through the pharynx into the esophagus.

The *nasopharynx* lies above the level of the soft palate and shares openings with the posterior nares and the *auditory*, or *eustachian*, tubes. The *oropharynx* lies between the soft palate and the upper edge of the epiglottis. The *epiglottis* is the structure that hangs over the entrance to the larynx (voice box) and prevents food from entering the larynx and trachea (windpipe) when we swallow. The *laryngopharynx* lies below the upper edge of the epiglottis and opens into both the larynx and esophagus.

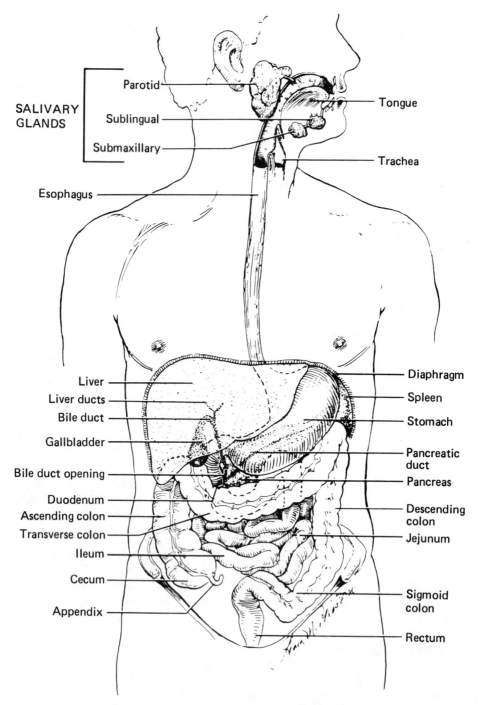

FIGURE 9.1 **The digestive system** (From Kinn, *Medical Terminology—Review Challenge*, copyright 1987 by Delmar Publishers Inc.)

Labels in figure:

SALIVARY GLANDS
- Parotid
- Sublingual
- Submaxillary

Tongue

Trachea

Esophagus

Liver
Liver ducts
Bile duct
Gallbladder
Bile duct opening
Duodenum
Ascending colon
Transverse colon
Ileum
Cecum
Appendix

Diaphragm
Spleen
Stomach
Pancreatic duct
Pancreas
Descending colon
Jejunum
Sigmoid colon
Rectum

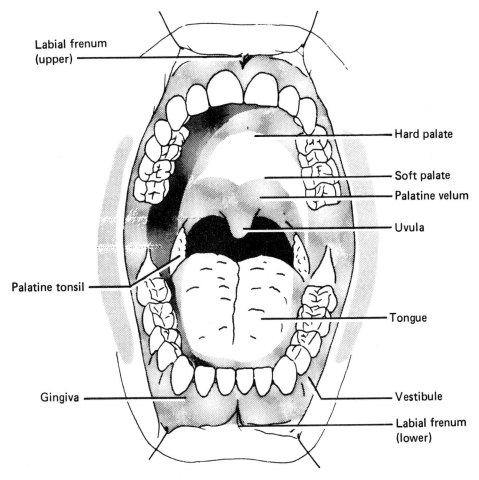

Labial frenum (upper)

Hard palate

Soft palate

Palatine velum

Uvula

Palatine tonsil

Tongue

Gingiva

Vestibule

Labial frenum (lower)

FIGURE 9.2 The mouth (From Anderson and Burkard, *The Dental Assistant*, 5th edition, copyright 1987 by Delmar Publishers Inc.)

Esophagus

The *esophagus* is a tubular structure that extends from the pharynx to the stomach. It is located in the thoracic cavity, is about 10 to 12 inches long, is composed of muscular tissue, and is lined with mucous membrane. It carries food from the throat to the stomach. Food is moved along by wavelike, rhythmic, muscular contractions called *peristalsis*. Peristalsis begins in the esophagus and continues in the stomach and intestines. The mucus produced by the mucous membrane lining the esophagus provides lubrication for the movement of food during peristalsis.

Stomach

The *stomach* (Figure 9.3) is a pouchlike organ shaped like a J. It is located in the upper part of the abdominal cavity, which is separated from the thoracic cavity by the diaphragm. The stomach serves as a reservoir, performs digestive functions, and consists of three parts—the fundus, the body, and the pylorus.

The upper, rounded part of the stomach is the *fundus*. The main and largest part is the *body*, and the lower part is the *pylorus* or *pyloric antrum*.

The stomach also has two *sphincters*, a ringlike muscular structure that can constrict openings. Each sphincter guards a stomach opening. Food enters the stomach from the esophagus through the *cardiac sphincter*, and it leaves the stomach and empties into the small intestine through the *pyloric sphincter*.

The stomach serves as a temporary reservoir while stomach acids, enzymes, and the churning action of the stomach wall break down the bolus of food into a semifluid material called *chyme*.

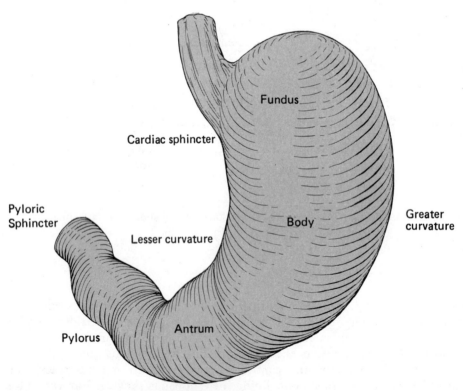

FIGURE 9.3 Front view of the stomach

Small Intestine

The *small intestine* is a coiled, tubular structure about 20 feet long that fills most of the abdominal cavity. It is here that digestion is completed and nutrients are absorbed. The proximal end of the small intestine connects with the distal region of the stomach, and this is where chyme enters the small intestine. There are three major sections of the small intestine: the duodenum, the jejunum, and the ileum.

The first 10 inches (25 cm) of the small intestine, into which the pancreatic duct and and bile duct open, is called the *duodenum*. The duodenum attaches to the pyloric end of the stomach. It is a common site for peptic ulcers.

The *jejunum*, about 8 feet long, is the second section, and the remaining 12 to 13 feet of the small intestine is called the *ileum*. The jejunum and ileum are involved in the mechanical and chemical breakdown of chyme and in the absorption of nutrients. The walls of the small intestine have little fingerlike projections called *villi* through which nutrients are absorbed into the bloodstream. The small intestine opens into the large intestine through the *ileocecal valve*.

Large Intestine

The *large intestine*, or *large bowel*, is about 5 feet (1.5 m) long and is larger in diameter than the small intestine. It is located in the lower part of the abdominal cavity and, like the small intestine, is a tubular structure. Its main divisions are:

- the *cecum*, to which the appendix is attached
- the *colon*, which has ascending, transverse, descending, and sigmoid portions
- the *rectum*, which opens as the *anus* for elimination

The anus is controlled by the *anal sphincter*, which permits voluntary control of the evacuation of solid waste (*feces*).

The main function of the large intestine is the reabsorption of water from digestive waste before it is eliminated from the body. This helps the body maintain hydration, which ensures that adequate water remains in the tissues.

ACCESSORY DIGESTIVE ORGANS

Teeth

The *teeth* are located in the mouth (oral cavity) and help break food down into smaller pieces by chewing (mastication). A *tooth* consists of three parts: the anatomic crown, the anatomic root, and the pulp cavity.

The bulk of a tooth consists of dentin. In the *anatomic crown* portion, which is exposed in the oral cavity, the dentin is covered with *enamel*. In the *anatomic root* portion, which anchors the tooth, the dentin is covered with a bonelike material called cementum. The *pulp cavity*, in the central region of the tooth, is filled with the *pulp*, a soft tissue composed of connective tissue containing blood vessels, lymph vessels, and nerves. Continuous with the pulp cavity is a canal through the root to an opening at the base called the *apical foramen*. Since the function of the teeth is the initial physical breakdown of food by mastication, and because we humans eat many different types of food, we have developed teeth with several different structural forms that adapt to handling food in various ways. The teeth also give form to the mouth and enhance our appearance.

Salivary Glands

There are three pairs of salivary glands as shown in Figure 9.4.

- The *parotid glands* are located just below and in front of each ear, at the angle of the jaw.
- The *submandibular glands* are located far back under either side of the tongue; they open into the floor of the mouth.
- The *sublingual glands* are located below the tip of the tongue and open into the floor of the mouth.

The salivary glands secrete *saliva*, which contains the enzyme *ptyalin*, necessary for breaking down starches, and mucus, which holds the food together in a bolus and facilitates swallowing. Saliva also helps to soften the food, and while dissolving some of it, allows the taste buds to be stimulated.

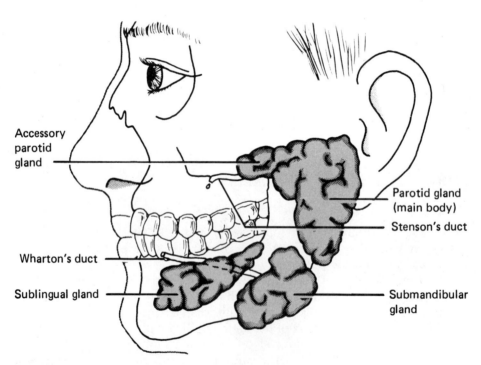

FIGURE 9.4 The salivary glands (From Anderson and Burkard, *The Dental Assistant,* 5th edition, copyright 1987 by Delmar Publishers Inc.)

Liver and Gallbladder

The *liver* is the largest gland in the body. It is dark red, weighs about 3 pounds, and is composed of four lobes, the right lobe being the largest. It is situated in the abdominal cavity directly under the diaphragm, on the right side of the body, Figure 9.5. The liver is a vital organ with many functions, including the secretion of *bile*, important in the digestion of fat.

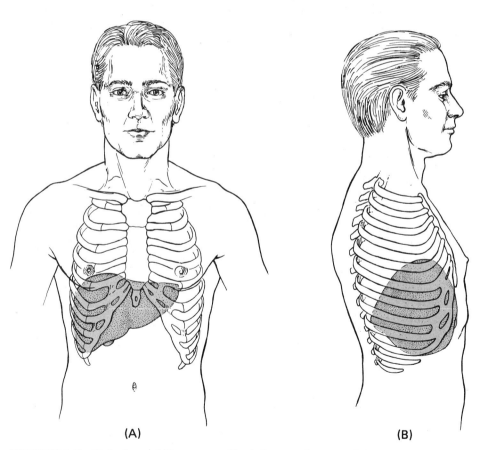

(A)   (B)

FIGURE 9.5   Relation of liver to wall of thorax, front and lateral views

The *gallbladder* is a small sac located on the inferior surface of the liver under the right lobe, Figure 9.6. It concentrates and stores bile, which is secreted by the liver and released into the duodenum when fat enters the small intestine through a duct system. *Hepatic ducts* carry bile from the liver to the *cystic duct*, which leads to the gallbladder. Here it is concentrated and stored. Both the hepatic duct and the cystic duct are connected with the *common bile duct* leading to the duodenum.

Pancreas

The *pancreas*, is both an exocrine and an endocrine gland and is an accessory digestive organ. It is located behind the stomach on the left side of the body and is attached to the duodenum by a duct that carries digestive juices to the intestine. These juices aid in the digestion of proteins, starches, and fats. The pancreas produces *insulin*, a hormone produced in the *islands of Langerhans*, sometimes called the *islets*. Insulin helps control carbohydrate metabolism (see Chapter 13).

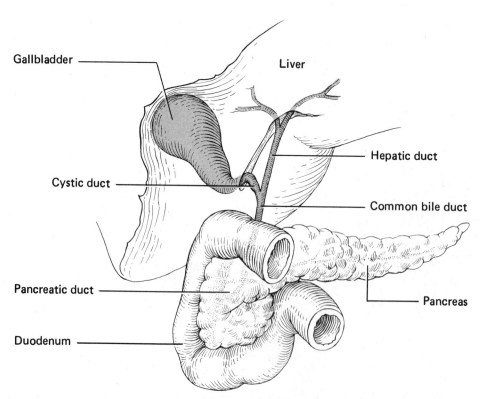

FIGURE 9.6   Relation of gallbladder and bile duct to duodenum and pancreas

BUILDING BLOCKS

ROOTS AND COMBINING FORMS

Word Element	Meaning
aliment/o	food or nutritive material
an/o	anus
append/o	appendix
bil/i	bile; gall
bucc/o	cheek
card/i	pertaining to the heart
cec/o	cecum
cheil/o	lip
chol/e	bile; gall
cholecyst/o	gallbladder
choledoch/o	common bile duct
chym/o	to pour
col/o	colon; large intestine
duoden/o	duodenum
enter/o	small intestine
esophag/o	esophagus
gastr/o	stomach
gingiv/o	gum
gloss/o	tongue
hepat/o	liver
ile/o	ileum
labi/o	lip
laryng/o	larynx
lingu/o	tongue
muc/o	mucus
nas/o	nose
or/o	mouth
palat/o	palate
pancreat/o	pancreas
phag/o	eat; swallow
pharyng/o	pharynx; throat
phas/o	speech
proct/o	anus/rectum
pylor/o	pylorus/pyloric sphincter

ROOTS AND COMBINING FORMS (continued)

Word Element	Meaning
rect/o	rectum
sial/o	saliva
ventr/o	belly, or front of body

SUFFIXES

Word Element	Meaning
–cele	hernia
–emesis	vomiting
–itis	inflammation
–logy	study or science of
–osmia	smell
–plasty	surgical repair
–stalsis	contraction

PREFIXES

Word Element	Meaning
apo–	separation or derivation from
epi–	upon
meso–	middle
peri–	surrounding

VOCABULARY

General Terms

apical	(AP-ih-kal)	Pertaining to or located at an apex
bolus	(BOH-lus)	A large dose. In relation to digestion, a mass of chewed food that is swallowed and passes through the esophagus to the stomach
buccal	(BUCK-ahl)	Pertaining to or directed toward the cheek, as in buccal cavity
defecation	(def-ek-KAY-shun)	The passage of fecal material through the rectum

deglutition	(**dee**-gloo-**TISH**-un)	The act of swallowing
eructation	(eh-ruck-**TAY**-shun)	The act of belching, or of ejecting gas or air from the stomach through the mouth
feces	(**FEE**-seez)	The solid waste remaining after digestion and absorption
flatulence	(**FLAT**-you-lens)	Excessive amounts of gas or air in the stomach or intestines
flatus	(**FLAY**-tus)	Expelling of gas, usually from the anus
gastroenterology	(**gas**-troh-**en**-ter-**OL**-oh-jee)	The branch of medicine concerned with the stomach and intestines and their diseases
halitosis	(hal-ih-**TOH**-sis)	Offensive or bad breath
hiccup, hiccough	(**HICK**-up)	An involuntary spasm of the diaphragm, ending with a characteristic sound; also called *singultus*
induration	(**in**-doo-**RAY**-shun)	The quality or the process of hardening; an abnormally hard spot or place on the body
inguinal	(**ING**-gwih-nal)	Pertaining to the groin
mastication	(**mass**-tih-**KAY**-shun)	The process of chewing food so it can be swallowed and digested
palpation	(pal-**PAY**-shun)	Examining by feeling with the hand or fingers
parenteral	(pah-**REN**-ter-ahl)	Referring to the introduction of substances into the body by some way other than by mouth or by rectum. For example, by injection into a muscle or an infusion into a vein
parotid	(pah-**ROT**-id)	Situated or occurring near the ear
regurgitation	(ree-**gur**-jih-**TAY**-shun)	A backward flow. For example, undigested food flowing from the stomach into the esophagus or

		blood flowing backward through the heart valves
singultus	(sing-**GUL**-tus)	Hiccup, hiccough
subcostal	(sub-**KOS**-tal)	Situated beneath a rib
sublingual	(sub-**LING**-gwal)	Located beneath the tongue
submandibular	(**sub**-man-**DIB**-you-lar)	Below the mandible (lower jaw)

Terms Related to Anatomy and Physiology

anus	**AY**-nus	The distal or terminal orifice (opening) of the alimentary canal
appendix	(ah-**PEN**-dicks)	An outgrowth. Pertaining to the digestive system, term refers to the *vermiform appendix*, a wormlike pocket or diverticulum of the cecum
bile	(byle)	A yellowish fluid secreted by the liver and stored in the gallbladder. Poured into the small intestine via the bile ducts, it helps digest fats
cardia	(**KAR**-dee-ah)	That part of the stomach surrounding the esophagogastric junction containing no acid-secreting or pepsin-secreting cells
cecum	(**SEE**-kum)	The first part of the large intestine; a dilated pouch into which the ileum, the colon, and the appendix vermiformis open
cementum	(see-**MEN**-tum)	The bonelike substance that covers the root of a tooth
chyme	(kym)	The semifluid, gruellike material resulting from the gastric digestion of food
colon	(**KOH**-lon)	The section of large intestine located between the cecum and the rectum
dentin	(**DEN**-tin)	The calcified tissue located beneath the enamel of a tooth

duodenum	(dew-oh-**DEE**-num)	The first part of the small intestine, extending from the pylorus to the jejunum
enzyme	(**EN**-zime)	A substance capable of initiating and accelerating chemical changes in living things. Usually a protein
esophagus	(eh-**SOPH**-ah-gus)	The tubular passage extending from the pharynx to the stomach
fundus	(**FUN**-dus)	A general term for the body, base, or larger part of an organ, or the part of a hollow organ farthest from its entrance
gallbladder	(**GAHL**-blad-der)	The pear-shaped reservoir for the storage and concentration of bile, located on the underside of the liver
gingivae	(**JIN**-jih-vee) (plural of *gingiva*)	The gums
ileum	(**ILL**-ee-um)	The distal portion of the small intestine, extending from the jejunum to the cecum
insulin	(**IN**-sew-lin)	A hormone secreted by cells in the islands (islets) of Langerhans in the pancreas. Important in the metabolism of carbohydrates and fat
islands of Langerhans, islets	(**LAHNG**-er-hanz)	Cells in the pancreas that secrete the hormone insulin. Important in the metabolism of carbohydrates and fat
jejunum	(jeh-**JOO**-num)	The middle portion of the small intestine, between the duodenum and the ileum
lingua	(**LING**-gwah)	The tongue
liver	(**LIHV**-er)	A large, dark-red gland situated in the upper part of the abdomen on the right side
mesentery	(**MESS**-en-**ter**-ee)	A membranous fold of peritoneum

attaching various organs to the body wall

mesocolon	(**mess**-oh-**KOH**-lon)	The fold of the peritoneum (mesentery), attaching the colon to the posterior abdominal wall
metabolism	(meh-**TAB**-oh-lizm)	The sum of the energy expended in the building up and breaking down of tissue
palate	(**PAL**-at)	The partition separating the nasal and oral cavities, divided into the hard palate and soft palate
peristalsis	(**per**-ih-**STALL**-sis)	A wavelike muscular contraction passing along the wall of a hollow tube or organ, for example, the esophagus and intestine propelling the contents forward
peritoneum	(**per**-ih-toh-**NEE**-um)	The thin membrane that lines the abdominal cavity and envelops the abdominal organs, helping keep them in position
pylorus	(pie-**LOR**-us)	The muscular outlet at the terminal end of the stomach that controls the passage of partially digested food into the duodenum
saliva	(sah-**LIE**-vah)	The clear, somewhat sticky secretion produced by the salivary glands
sigmoid	(**SIG**-moyd)	The term "sigmoid" means S-shaped and is frequently used to designate the *sigmoid colon*, the S-shaped portion of the colon immediately preceding the rectum.
stomach	(**STUM**-ack)	The large, upper-abdominal organ situated between the esophagus and the duodenum, where much of the digestion of food takes place

tongue	(tung)	The flexible, muscular organ on the floor of the mouth that manipulates food in chewing and swallowing and is important for speech and taste
uvula	(**YOU**-view-lah)	A small, soft structure hanging from the edge of the soft palate in the midline, above the root of the tongue
viscus	(**VIS**-kus)	Any one of the large internal organs situated within a body cavity (plural, *viscera*)

Terms Related to Pathology

achalasia	(ack-ah-**LAY**-zee-ah)	Failure of the smooth muscle fibers of the gastrointestinal tract to relax. For example, if the sphincter fails to relax, food cannot pass from the esophagus into the stomach.
achlorhydria	(**ah**-klor-**HIGH**-dree-ah)	The absence of hydrochloric acid
adenitis	(**add**-eh-**NIGH**-tis)	Inflammation of a gland
adhesion	(add-**HEE**-zhun)	A fibrous band or structure that abnormally holds two parts together
aerophagia	(**ay**-er-oh-**FAY**-jee-ah)	The spasmodic swallowing of air followed by belching
anorexia	(**an**-oh-**RECK**-see-ah)	Lack or loss of appetite for food. *Anorexia nervosa* is an eating disorder characterized by extreme weight loss.
aphagia	(ah-**FAY**-jee-ah)	Inability or refusal to swallow
ascites	(ah-**SIGH**-teez)	Escape of fluid from vessels and lymphatics, and accumulation of this serous fluid in the abdominal cavity
atresia	(ah-**TREE**-zee-ah)	An often congenital absence of a normal opening or closure of a normal body orifice or tubular organ; for example, *rectal atresia*

bulimia	(byou-**LIM**-ee-ah)	A neurotic eating disorder characterized by morbidly excessive appetite; current usage generally refers to bingeing and purging
cachexia	(kah-**KECK**-see-ah)	Profound ill health and malnutrition usually resulting from a chronic illness
cheilitis	(kye-**LIE**-tis)	Inflammation affecting the lips
cholecystitis	(koh-lee-sis-**TIE**-tis)	Inflammation of the gallbladder
cholelithiasis	(**koh**-lee-ligh-**THIGH**-ah-sis)	The presence or formation of gallstones
cirrhosis	(sir-**ROH**-sis)	Disease of an organ, particularly the liver, with the organ becoming nodular and scarred
cleft palate	(kleft **PAL**-et)	A congenital fissure in the midline of the roof of the mouth
colic	(**KOL**-ick)	Acute abdominal pain
constipation	(**kon**-stih-**PAY**-shun)	The infrequent or difficult evacuation of the feces, or waste matter, that is too hard to pass easily
debility	(deh-**BILL**-ih-tee)	A lack or loss of strength
diarrhea	(die-ah-**REE**-ah)	An abnormal, increased frequency and liquidity of the feces
diverticulitis	(**die**-ver-tick-you-**LIE**-tis)	Inflammation of a diverticulum, especially in the colon
diverticulum	(**die**-ver-**TICK**-you-lum)	An abnormal saclike pouch projecting from a weakness in the wall of a tube such as the colon or a cavity
dumping syndrome	(**SIN**-drome)	A set of symptoms in people who have had a gastrectomy. The symptoms include weakness, sweating, and dizziness and are caused by the too rapid passage of food into the small intestine.

dysentery	(**DIS**-en-**ter**-ee)	Inflammation of the intestinal mucosa, characterized by abdominal pain and frequent watery stools containing blood and mucus. There are several causes such as bacilli or amebas.
dyspepsia	(dis-**PEP**-see-ah)	The impairment of digestion characterized by epigastric discomfort following meals; indigestion
dysphagia	(dis-**FAY**-jee-ah)	Difficulty in swallowing
emesis	(**EM**-eh-sis)	Vomiting
enteritis	(**en**-ter-**EYE**-tis)	Inflammation of the intestine
esophagitis	(eh-**soph-ah-JYE**-tis)	Inflammation of the esophagus
fistula	(**FIS**-too-lah)	An abnormal passage or canal, connecting two internal organs, or leading from an internal organ to the surface of the body
gastritis	(gas-**TRY**-tis)	Inflammation of the stomach
gastrocele	(**GAS**-troh-seel)	A hernial protrusion of the stomach
gingivitis	(**jin**-jih-**VYE**-tis)	Inflammation of the gums
glossitis	(glos-**SIGH**-tis)	Inflammation of the tongue
harelip	(**HARE**-lip)	A congenital cleft or defect in the upper lip
hematemesis	(**hem**-ah-**TEM**-eh-sis)	The vomiting of blood
hemorrhoids	(**HEM**-oh-roydz)	Dilated varicose veins of the lower rectum or anus; sometimes called "piles"
hepatitis	(hep-ah-**TIE**-tis)	Inflammation of the liver
hernia	(**HER**-nee-ah)	The protrusion of a loop or knuckle of an organ or structure through the tissues that contain it
herpes simplex	(**HER**-peez)	An acute viral disease marked by groups of small blisters or vesicles on the skin, often on the borders of

		the lips or nostrils or on the genitals; cold sores, fever blisters
hiatal hernia	(high-AY-tal HER-nee-ah)	Protrusion of any structure, usually the stomach, through the esophageal hiatus of the diaphragm, where the esophagus passes through the diaphragm
ileus	(ILL-ee-us)	Obstruction of the intestines
icterus, jaundice	(ICK-ter-us, JAWN-dis)	Yellow discoloration of skin and mucous membranes due to excess bilirubin in the blood caused by obstruction of the bile ducts or liver dysfunction
ileitis	(ILL-ee-EYE-tis)	Inflammation of the ileum
incontinence	(in-KON-tih-nens)	The inability to control the excretory functions of defecation or urination
intussusception	(in-tus-sus-SEP-shun)	Telescoping of the intestine
jaundice	(JAWN-dis)	Icterus
melena	(meh-LEE-nah)	The passage of black, tarry stools, or black vomit (melenemesis), due to internal bleeding. The black color results from the action of intestinal juices on the blood.
nausea	(NAW-see-ah)	A vague, unpleasant sensation in the epigastrium and abdomen, and often followed by vomiting
pharyngitis	(far-in-JYE-tis)	Inflammation of the pharynx
polydipsia	(pol-ee-DIP-see-ah)	Excessive thirst resulting in frequent drinking
proctitis	(prock-TIE-tis)	Inflammation of the rectum
pruritus	(proo-RYE-tus)	Itching
pyloric stenosis	(pie-LOR-ick steh-NOH-sis)	A narrowing of the pylorus
pylorospasm	(PIE-LOH-roh-spazm)	A spasm of the pyloric portion of the stomach which may obstruct passage of food into the duodenum

pyorrhea	(pie-oh-**REE**-ah)	A discharge of pus
pyrexia	(pie-**RECK**-see-ah)	Abnormal elevation of the body temperature; fever
pyrosis	(pie-**ROH**-sis)	Heartburn
ulcer	(**UHL**-ser)	A defect in the skin or mucous membrane that causes an excavation of the underlying tissues. *Duodenal ulcer:* An ulcer that occurs in the duodenum, the first part of the small intentine. *Gastric ulcer:* An ulcer that occurs in the wall of the stomach, and may become malignant. *Peptic ulcer:* A general term that includes both duodenal and gastric ulcers.
vomiting	(**VOM**-it-ing)	The forcible and involuntary expelling of the contents of the stomach through the mouth

Terms Related to Surgery or Treatment

anastomosis	(ah-**nas**-toh-**MOH**-sis)	An opening created surgically between two normally distinct spaces or organs
appendectomy	(**ap**-en-**DECK**-toh-mee)	Surgical removal of the appendix
cheiloplasty	(**KYE**-loh-**plas**-tee)	Surgical repair of a defect of the lip
cholecystectomy	(**koh**-lee-sis-**TECK**-toh-mee)	Surgical removal of the gallbladder
colectomy	(koh-**LECK**-toh-mee)	Excision of a portion of the colon
colostomy	(koh-**LOS**-toh-mee)	The surgical creation of an opening between the colon and the surface of the body
exploratory laparotomy	(ecks-**PLOH**-roh-**toh**-ree lap-ah-**ROT**-oh-mee)	The surgical opening of the abdomen for diagnostic purposes
gastrectomy	(gas-**TRECK**-toh-mee)	Excision of all or part of the stomach

gastrostomy	(gas-**TROS**-toh-mee)	The surgical creation of an artificial opening into the stomach
hemorrhoidectomy	(**hem**-oh-roid-**ECK**-toh-mee)	Excision of hemorrhoids
herniorrhaphy	(her-nee-**OR**-ah-fee)	Surgical repair of a hernia
paracentesis	(**par**-ah-sen-**TEE**-sis)	The surgical puncture of a cavity for the purpose of withdrawing fluid
vagotomy	(vay-**GOT**-oh-mee)	The interruption of the impulses carried by the vagus nerve or nerves by surgery or by drugs. Results in decreased activity of the stomach

9.1 Review: System

DIRECTIONS: Cover the left column while you complete the statements on the right side.

internal medicine	The medical specialty that manages afflictions of the digestive system is _____ .
gastroenterology	The branch of medicine that deals with the stomach and intestines and their diseases is _____ .
digestion	The breaking down of complete foodstuffs into simpler substances that can be absorbed into the bloodstream is the process of _____ .
mouth	The buccal cavity is more commonly called the _____ .
tongue	The organ that is involved in taste, speech, swallowing, and chewing is the _____ .
behind	The soft palate is located _____ the hard palate.
pharynx	The _____ is what most of us call the throat.
air, food	Both _____ and _____ pass through the pharynx.
oropharynx	The _____ lies between the soft palate and the upper edge of the epiglottis.

laryngopharynx	The _____ lies below the upper edge of the epiglottis and opens into the larynx and esophagus.
esophagus	The _____ is about 10 to 12 inches long and extends from the pharynx to the stomach.
peristalsis	Rhythmic contractions, called _____ , help to move food through the digestive tract.
diaphragm	The musculomembranous partition that separates the thoracic and abdominal cavities is called the _____ .
three	The stomach has _____ distinctive parts.
fundus, body, pylorus	These parts are called: _____ _____
cardiac, pyloric	Food enters the stomach through the _____ sphincter, and leaves the stomach through the _____ sphincter.
duodenum, jejunum, ileum	The three major sections of the small intestine are: _____ , _____ , and _____ .
ileocecal	The small intestine opens via the _____ valve into the large intestine.
large intestine	The main function of the _____ is reabsorption of water into the body.
cecum, colon, rectum	The large intestine has three main parts which are: _____ , _____ , and _____ .
dentin	The bulk of a tooth consists of _____ .
cementum	The root portion of a tooth is covered with a bonelike material called _____ .
salivary	The parotid, submandibular, and sublingual glands are all _____ glands.
liver	The _____ is a vital organ that secretes bile.
gallbladder	The _____ is a small sac located on the inferior surface and under the right lobe of the liver.

Hepatic, cystic	_____ ducts carry bile from the liver to the _____ duct, which leads to the gallbladder.
common bile duct	Both of these ducts are connected with the _____ leading to the duodenum.
exocrine, endocrine	The pancreas serves as both a/an _____ gland and a/an _____ gland.
insulin	The islands of Langerhans secrete _____ .

9.2   Review: Building Blocks

DIRECTIONS: Write the meanings of the following building blocks.

1. cheil/o _____
2. gastr/o _____
3. nas/o _____
4. cec/o _____
5. –emesis _____
6. muc/o _____
7. chym/o _____
8. apo– _____
9. phag/o _____
10. gloss/o _____
11. enter/o _____
12. choledoch/o _____
13. –osmia _____
14. bucc/o _____
15. laryng/o _____

9.3   Review: Building Blocks

DIRECTIONS: Supply the combining form for the following words.

1. anus   _____
2. middle   _____
3. tongue   _____
4. anus/rectum   _____
5. large intestine   _____
6. gallbladder   _____
7. hernia   _____
8. lip   _____
9. speech   _____
10. saliva   _____
11. contraction   _____
12. bile; gall   _____
13. surgical repair   _____
14. liver   _____
15. gum   _____

9.4   Review: Word Building

DIRECTIONS: Fill in the blanks with the appropriate building block or medical term.

1. _____ is a root meaning *lip*.
   The suffix for *inflammation* is _____ .
   The term for inflammation affecting the lips is _____ .

2. The combining form for *stomach* is _____ .
   A suffix meaning *protrusion* or *hernia* is _____ .
   The term for *hernial protrusion of the stomach* is _____ .

3. The prefix for *bad* or *difficult* is _____ .
   The combining form for *swallow* is _____ .
   Difficulty with swallowing is called _____ .

4. The root for *liver* is _____ .
   The suffix for *inflammation* is _____ .
   Inflammation of the liver is called _____ .

5. The combining form for *gums* is _____ .
   The term for inflammation of the gums is _____ .

6. The root for *bile* or *gall* is _____ .
   The root for *stone* is _____ .
   _____ is a word ending that means presence or formation of.
   _____ is the presence or formation of gallstones.

7. A prefix meaning *many* or *excessive* is _____ .
   The combining form for *eat* is _____ .
   _____ means excessive or voracious eating.

8. A prefix meaning *not* or *without* is _____ .
   Abstention from eating (not eating) is called _____ .

9. _____ is a building block that means *vomiting*.
   A combining form for *blood* is _____ .
   _____ is the vomiting of blood.

10. _____ is the combining form for intestine.
    The suffix for *inflammation* is _____ .
    Inflammation of the intestine is called _____ .

9.5 Review: Structures

DIRECTIONS: Identify the numbered structures on the diagram.

1. _____
2. _____
3. _____
4. _____
5. _____
6. _____
7. _____
8. _____
9. _____
10. _____
11. _____
12. _____
13. _____
14. _____
15. _____
16. _____
17. _____
18. _____
19. _____
20. _____
21. _____
22. _____
23. _____
24. _____
25. _____
26. _____

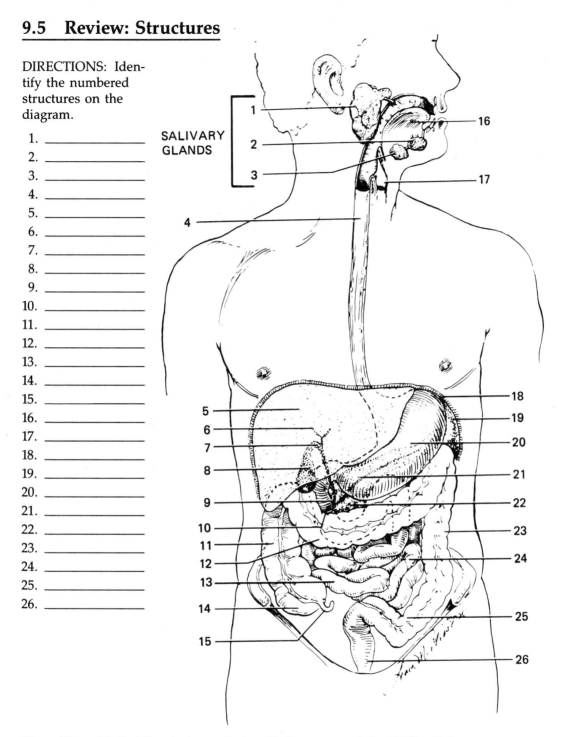

(From Kinn, *Medical Terminology—Review Challenge,* copyright 1987 by Delmar Publishers Inc.)

9.6   Review: Vocabulary

DIRECTIONS: Supply the corresponding medical terms for the following definitions.

1. _____ Absence of hydrochloric acid
2. _____ A fibrous band or structure by which parts abnormally stick together
3. _____ The act of swallowing
4. _____ Morbidly excessive appetite
5. _____ Protrusion of any structure through the esophageal hiatus of the diaphragm
6. _____ A membranous fold of peritoneum attaching various organs to the body wall
7. _____ Yellow discoloration of skin and mucous membranes
8. _____ Accumulation of fluid in the abdominal cavity
9. _____ Narrowing of the pylorus
10. _____ Inflammation of a gland

9.7   Review: Vocabulary

DIRECTIONS: Supply the terms for the following surgical procedures. Remember that spelling is important.

1. _____ Surgical creation of an artificial opening into the stomach
2. _____ Excision of a portion of the colon
3. _____ Creation of an opening between two normally distinct spaces or organs
4. _____ Surgical repair of a hernia
5. _____ Repair of a defect of the lip
6. _____ Interruption of the impulses carried by the vagus nerve(s)
7. _____ Surgical opening of the abdomen for diagnostic purposes
8. _____ Removal of the gallbladder
9. _____ Excision of all or part of the stomach
10. _____ Surgical creation of an opening between the colon and the surface of the body

Reading Comprehension 9.1

DIRECTIONS: Underline the medical terms as you go through the reading exercise. Then list and analyze the terms. Some will be completely new to you. Consult a medical dictionary for their meanings. Then re-read the material for better comprehension.

History and Review of Systems

Chief Complaint: Chest pain.

History of Present Illness:
The patient is a 78-year-old Caucasian male who gives a history of 4 days of anterior chest pain, heavy, severe, dull, radiating down to both elbows, waxing and waning, but increasing in intensity, unrelieved by breathing or position. The patient states that he has been short of breath at times during these 4 days and has had some sweating with it. The patient denies any previous history of myocardial infarctions, rheumatic fever, angina. The patient states that he sleeps well, has nocturia times 1, no edema, and no PND, but on further questioning states that on exertion for the past 3 months he has had a dull ache in the chest lasting approximately 10 minutes and relieved by rest.

Past History:
Includes hearing loss for the past several years, bilateral cataract surgeries, and a retinal detachment as well as an appendectomy and an exploratory for what was thought to be cholecystitis but which turned out to be pancreatitis about a year and a half ago.

> Medications: None
> Allergies: None

Social History:
The patient is married with 1 child. He quit smoking 25 years ago and drinks about 1 drink per day. He is a retired salesman.

Family History:
Father died at 75 of a heart attack. Mother died at 70 of a stroke. No siblings. No family history of diabetes, or cancer.

Review of Systems:
Skin: The patient has had several skin cancers in the past and presently has several on the right side of his face.

Eyes: See above.

Ears: See above.

Mouth, Nose, Throat: Dentures.

Endocrine: No history of thyroid disease or diabetes. Weight is stable.

Respiratory: No history of pneumonia, wheezing, asthma, emphysema, or cough.

G.I.: No history of jaundice, hepatitis, ulcers, change in bowel habits, black tarry stools, or constipation.

G.U.: No history of prostatitis, narrowing of the stream, hematuria, infections, or stones.

Musculoskeletal: No history of serious injuries.

Neurological: No history of strokes, seizures, epilepsy, or palsies.

Hematological: No extreme bleeding disorders.

Reading Comprehension 9.2

DIRECTIONS: Underline the medical terms as you go through the reading exercise. Then list and analyze the terms. Some will be completely new to you. Consult a medical dictionary for their meanings. Then re-read the material for better comprehension.

Physical Examination

The patient appears as an elderly male lying in bed in no real distress. Blood pressure—135/95. Pulse—70 with several ectopics. Respirations—12.

Some senile changes noted. The patient has 2 red angry lesions approximately 1/2 cm in the right forearm and right malar area.

Head:
Normocephalic.

Eyes:
Pupils are irregular with iris scarring noted. Status post cataract removal. Patient has contacts on. Fundi somewhat difficult to visualize but look pale bilaterally. Discs are discernible however. Sclera are clear. Extraocular movements within normal limits. Ears are clear. Hearing grossly decreased.

Nose, Mouth, Throat:
Soft palate has small ruddy like growth to the right of the uvula. Dentures in place.

Neck:
Supple, no neck vein distention. Carotids full bilaterally without bruits. Negative hepatojugular reflux.

Lungs:
Breath sounds heard throughout. Few rales heard in the base.

Chest:
Moves symmetrically; no CVA or spine tenderness elicited.

Heart:
Regular at 70. PMI not appreciated. S1, S2 audible. Grade I/VI systolic ejection murmur heard along the left sternal border. No gallops are heard.

Abdomen:
Well-healed gallbladder scar. No hepatosplenomegaly. No tenderness, no bruits heard. Bowel sounds are active. Femoral arteries strong bilaterally.

Genitalia:
Grossly normal.

Rectal:
Deferred.

Extremities:
Distal pulses strong in the feet; no clubbing, cyanosis, or edema noted.

Neurological:
Deep tendon reflexes are symmetrical. Toes downgoing. Cranial nerves II–XII grossly within normal limits, except for eyes as stated above.

Reading Comprehension 9.3

DIRECTIONS: Underline the medical terms as you go through the reading exercise. Then list and analyze the terms. Some will be completely new to you. Consult a medical dictionary for their meanings. Then re-read the material for better comprehension.

Operative Report

Preoperative Diagnosis:
Carcinoma of the left vocal cord

Postoperative Diagnosis:
Same.

Operation:
Laryngoscopy with excision of extensive left vocal cord tumor. Esophagoscopy. Bronchoscopy.

Procedure:

The patient was placed on the operating table in the supine position. General anesthesia was induced by an endotracheal tube. A round cross-section esophagoscope was then passed into the oral cavity over the dorsum of the tongue and base of the tongue into the right piriform sinus through the cricopharyngeal sphincter into the upper esophagus and then down approximately 2/3 of the way to the cardiac sphincter. The walls of the lumen were inspected carefully on antegrade and retrograde passage of the esophagoscope and no lesions were noted. A 7 mm ventilating bronchoscope was then introduced into the oral cavity and passed into the endolarynx anterior to the endotracheal tube. After passing the vocal cord level, the endotracheal tube balloon was encountered and this was deflated. The bronchoscope was continued down to the carina into the right mainstem bronchus and passed the upper and middle lobe orifices. The lumen was without mucosal lesions in all these areas. The bronchoscope was then passed retrograde into the carina and the left mainstem bronchus was entered. The bronchoscope was advanced into the division of the upper and lower lobe orifices and again these were all normal and no mucosal lesions were noted. The bronchoscope was passed retrograde to the level of the vocal cords and removed. The endotracheal tube balloon was then reinflated. A Hollinger laryngoscope was then passed into the oral cavity, and the piriform sinuses and post cricoid region as well as the vallecula were reinspected and again no lesions were found in these areas. The laryngoscope was passed into the laryngeal vestibule and the tumor of the left vocal cord was visualized. This tumor was biopsied extensively until almost complete excision of the tumor was noted. The laryngeal ventricle was palpated with a right-angle hook and appeared to be soft and free of tumor. The tumor appeared to be limited to the vocal cord. The anterior commissure was free and the tumor extended to the tip of the vocal process of the arytenoid but not into the posterior commissure. As noted above, the tumor was excised in multiple bites with the micro-biting forceps. When this was completed, the upper trachea was suctioned, and retained blood was removed. The patient was then awakened and extubated. He was returned to recovery room in satisfactory condition.

Reading Comprehension Vocabulary

Use the space below to list the terms for analysis and definition.

_____

_____

_____

_____

_____

_____

_____

_____

_____

CHAPTER 10

Male Reproductive System

OBJECTIVES

When you have successfully completed Chapter 10, you should be able to:

— Recall terms describing the anatomy and physiology of the male reproductive system.
— Define the building blocks introduced in this chapter.
— Define common terms related to the male reproductive system.
— Recall the medical terms for structures and functions defined in the chapter.
— Identify the structures of the male reproductive system in a familiar drawing.
— Build medical terms using the building blocks introduced in this and previous chapters.

KEY TERMS

ascend	(ah-**SEND**)	To go or move upward
bulbous	(**BUHL**-bus)	Bulb-shaped
cavernous	(**KAV**-er-nus)	Having hollow spaces
erectile tissue	(eh-**RECK**-tile **TISH**-you)	Vascular tissue that becomes erect or stiff
gonad	(**GOH**-nadd)	A primary sex gland, either male (testis) or female (ovary)
hormone	(**HOR**-mohn)	One of the many secretions of the ductless glands such as insulin from the pancreas that are absorbed by the body and control some of the body processes
motile	(**MOH**-till)	Able to move without conscious effort; moving
perpetuate	(per-**PETCH**-you-ate)	To ensure a lasting existence; for example, to *perpetuate* a species
propagation	(prop-ah-**GAY**-shun)	The act of reproducing or giving birth
puberty	(**POO**-ber-tee)	The period during which sexual maturity is reached, which occurs at about age 14 in the human male, age 12 in the female
reproduction	(**ree**-proh-**DUCK**-shun)	The act or process by which plants and animals create their young
vesicle	(**VEHS**-ih-kal)	A cavity or sac filled with fluid; a small blister

OVERVIEW

The principal function of the human reproductive system is to perpetuate our species. In very simple forms of life, reproduction is asexual; each half of the dividing cells becomes a new individual (a process called mitosis). In humans, as in all complex animals and plants, propagation requires both a male and a female of the species; that is, it is sexual.

Each of the two sexes has *gonads* that produce reproductive cells and sex hormones. The gonads, the ducts that transport the reproductive cells, and a number of accessory organs constitute the reproductive system. Each structure in the system has a special function, and the entire system must function properly for reproduction to take place. The male reproductive system consists of the gonads, called testes; the testicular ducts; and the external genitalia.

There is no medical specialty concerned exclusively with the male reproductive system as such. Most conditions related to this system are managed medically and surgically by urologists.

MALE GONADS

Testes

The male *gonads* are the paired *testes*. They are carried outside the abdominal cavity in the pouchlike *scrotum* (Figure 10.1). The testes have two functions: (1) to produce androgens, or male sex hormones, and (2) to produce *spermatozoa*, the male reproductive cells, which are transported in fluid called *semen*. The *chromosomes* within each sperm carry the entire hereditary pattern of the male parent.

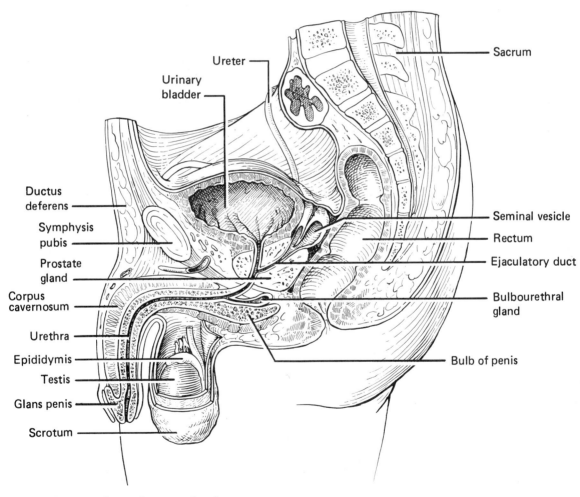

FIGURE 10.1 **The male reproductive system**

Seminiferous Tubules

Within the testes, cells lining structures called *seminiferous tubules* produce *spermatozoa*, or sperm from puberty onward. When reproduction occurs, the sex of the new individual is determined by the sperm, which contains both male (Y) and female (X) chromosomes. The production of spermatozoa by the seminiferous tubules is called *spermatogenesis*. In addition to their part in spermatogenesis, the seminiferous tubules produce androgens (male hormones), the most important of which is *testosterone*. Testosterone is necessary for normal male growth and development and for the normal functioning of the male reproductive organs. During puberty, this hormone stimulates the development of the male's *secondary sex characteristics* such as deepening of the voice, the growth of a beard and pubic and axillary hair, and a high proportion of lean muscle tissue. Testosterone also stimulates maturation of the male genitalia.

DUCT SYSTEM

The system of ducts that comprise a major part of the male reproductive system is very complex in structure and function (Figure 10.2).

Atop and behind each testis lies the *epididymis*, a coiled tube that is tiny in diameter but would be nearly 20 feet long if it were uncoiled. The seminiferous tubules of the testes empty into the epididymis, where the sperm are stored while they mature and become *motile*, that is, able to move by themselves. The tail of the epididymis straightens out to form the *ductus deferens*, also called the *vas deferens*, which ascends from the epididymis to the ejaculatory duct. En route it leaves the scrotum and passes through the inguinal rings and inguinal canal and into the abdominal cavity. As the duct ascends it is accompanied by blood vessels, lymphatics, and nerve fibers, and is enveloped by fascia (tissue wrappings). This entire structure is called the *spermatic cord*. After the vas deferens enters the abdominal cavity it loses its wrappings, extends posteriorly and medially into the pelvic cavity, and ends behind the urinary bladder. The function of the vas deferens is to store and carry sperm.

Near its end, the vas deferens and ducts from the seminal vesicles (see Glands) join to form the *ejaculatory duct*, which passes through the *prostate gland* before emptying into the first part of the *urethra*. The urethra, which transports both semen and urine extends from the urinary bladder and the ejaculatory duct through the penis. The male urethra is about 8 inches (20 cm) long.

GLANDS

Two glands called *seminal vesicles* lie, one on each side, just behind the urinary bladder. The seminal vesicles are blind pouches that secrete an alkaline fluid that contributes nutrients to semen.

The *prostate gland*, which is partly muscular and partly glandular, is cone-shaped and about the size of a chestnut. It lies beneath the urinary bladder and surrounds the urethra. The prostate gland also secretes alkaline fluids that enhance sperm motility and contract smooth muscle to assist in *ejaculation*, the rhythmic contraction of the penis by which semen is ejected during the peak of sexual excitement (orgasm).

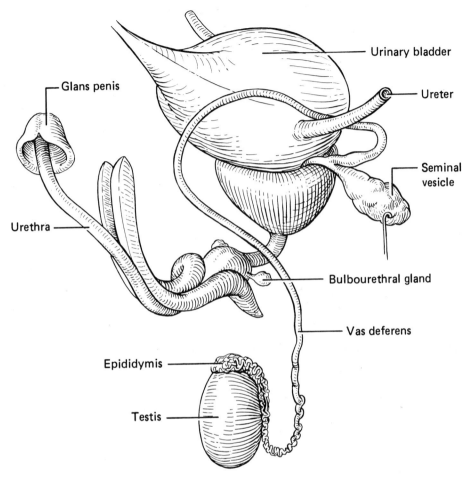

Glans penis

Urethra

Urinary bladder

Ureter

Seminal vesicle

Bulbourethral gland

Vas deferens

Epididymis

Testis

FIGURE 10.2 The male urogenital system

Two small, pea-sized *bulbourethral glands* called *Cowper's glands* lie on either side of the urethra and open into the urethra through ducts. These glands produce an alkaline fluid that mingles with the seminal fluid to help neutralize the acidity of the uretha, which would otherwise harm the sperm.

EXTERNAL GENITALIA

The male external genital organ, the *penis,* is suspended from the front and sides of the pubic arch (see Figure 10.1). The penis is formed of cavernous *erectile tissue* (the *corpus cavernosum*), which surrounds the urethra. The bulbous end of the penis, called the *glans penis,* is covered by the *prepuce,* or *foreskin.*

The *scrotum* is an external sac that develops from the layers of the abdominal wall. A midline septum divides the sac into two chambers, one for each testis. The scrotum contains muscle fibers that contract during exercise or exposure to cold temperatures, causing it to become smaller and wrinkled. Figure 10.3 shows the male perineum and the muscles of the perineum major.

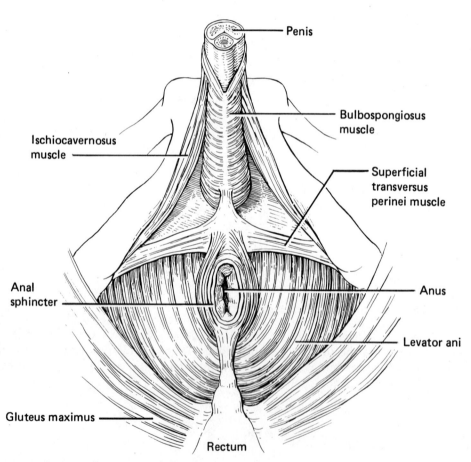

FIGURE 10.3   The male perineum

BUILDING BLOCKS

ROOTS AND COMBINING FORMS

Word Elements	Meaning
andr/o	male
balan/o	glans penis
chrom/o	color
crypt/o	hidden
gen/o	producing
genit/o	genital
gon/o	seed
gynec/o	woman, female
heter/o	other
hom/o	same
hydr/o	water
olig/o	little, scanty
orchi/o	testis
prostat/o	prostate gland
spermat/o	spermatozoa
urethr/o	urethra
vas	vessel, duct
vesicul/o	seminal vesicle

SUFFIXES

Word Elements	Meaning
–algia	pain
–cele	hernia
–cide	to kill
–ectomy	excision
–genesis	producing, forming
–mastia	breast
–megaly	large, enlargement
–pexy	fixation
–plasia	formation, development
–spermia	spermatozoa
–uria	urine

Word Elements	Meaning
a–	not, without
circum–	surrounding, around
inter–	between

VOCABULARY

General Terms

coitus	(KOH-ih-tus)	Sexual intercourse between male and female; penile/vaginal intercourse
condom	(KON-dum)	A thin, flexible sheath, usually made of rubber, worn over the penis during sexual intercourse to guard against conception and sexually transmitted disease
copulation	(kop-you-LAY-shun)	Sexual intercourse
ejaculation	(ee-jack-you-LAY-shun)	Ejection of the seminal fluid from the male urethra during sexual climax
eunuch	(YOU-nuck)	A castrated male; one whose testicles have been removed. If castration is accomplished before puberty, the male secondary sexual characteristics do not develop
heterosexual	(het-er-oh-SECKS-you-ahl)	Having to do with or directed to the opposite sex; being sexually oriented toward persons of the opposite sex
homosexual	(hoh-moh-SECKS-you-ahl)	A person who is sexually attracted to another of the same sex
orgasm	(OR-gazm)	The peak of sexual excitement during which, in the male, semen is expelled in a series of penile contractions (ejaculation)

puberty	(POO-ber-tee)	Period in life during which either the male or the female becomes functionally capable of reproduction
spermaturia	(sper-mah-TOO-ree-ah)	The condition of discharging semen with the urine
spermicide	(SPER-mih-side)	An agent that kills spermatozoa

Terms Related to Anatomy and Physiology

androgen	(AN-droh-jen)	Any substance that possesses masculinizing qualities, such as the testicular hormones
bulbourethral glands	(buhl-boh-you-REE-thal glanz)	Two small glands, one on each side of the prostate gland, that secrete a sticky, alkaline fluid forming part of the seminal fluid. Cowper's glands
chromosome	(KROH-moh-sohm)	A structure in the nucleus of a cell that contains the gene-carrying DNA
corpus cavernosum	(KOR-pus kav-er-NOH-sum)	The hollow, erectile tissue that forms the penile shaft
Cowper's glands		Bulbourethral glands. Correspond to the Bartholin glands in the female
ductus deferens	(DUCK-tus DEF-er-enz)	The testicular duct that carries sperm from the epididymis to the ejaculatory duct; vas deferens
epididymis	(ep-ih-DID-ih-miss)	Oblong coiled body on top of each testis that carries and stores the sperm cells before they enter the vas deferens
flagellum	(flah-JELL-un)	A hairlike, motile "tail" on the extremity of an organism. A flagellum attached to the spermatozoon gives it the power of self-propulsion
foreskin	(FOR-skin)	Loose skin covering the end of the penis or clitoris like a hood; prepuce

genitalia	(jen-ih-TAY-lee-ah)	The reproductive organs of male and female
glans penis	(glanz PEE-nis)	The cone-shaped head of the penis
penis	(PEE-nis)	The male organ of copulation and of urination
perineum	(per-ih-NEE-um)	The pelvic floor. In the male, the area between the scrotum and the anus; in the female, the area between the vulva and the anus
prepuce	(PREE-pyous)	The fold of skin over the glans penis in the male and the clitoris in the female
prostate	(PROS-tayt)	A fluid-secreting gland in the male that surrounds the neck of the bladder and the urethra
scrotum	(SKROH-tum)	The double pouch, found in most male mammals, that contains the testicles and part of the spermatic cord
semen	(SEE-men)	The thick, whitish secretion containing spermatozoa that is discharged from the male urethra at the climax of sexual excitement (orgasm)
seminal vesicle	(SEM-ih-nahl VEHS-ih-KAL)	One of two paired structures located at the base of the bladder in the male that produces the fluid portion of the semen
seminiferous tubules	(seh-mih-NIF-er-us TOO-buhlz)	Very small channels in the testes in which sperm develop and through which they leave the testes
spermatogenesis	(sper-mah-toh-JEN-ih-sis)	The formation of mature, functional spermatozoa
spermatozoa	(sper-mah-toh-ZOH-ah)	Plural of *spermatozoon*. The mature male sex cells or germ cells
testicle	(TES-tih-KAL)	The male gonad

testis	(**TES**-tis)	The testicle; plural, *testes*
testosterone	(tes-**TAHS**-ter-ohn)	The hormone, produced by the interstitial cells of the testes, that induces and maintains the male secondary sex characteristics
urethra	(you-**REE**-thra)	A canal through which urine is discharged, extending from the bladder to the outside of the body
vas deferens	(vass-**DEF**-er-enz)	The ductus deferens

Terms Related to Pathology

anorchism	(an-**OR**-kihzm)	Congenital absence of one or both testes
aspermatogenesis	(ah-**sper**-mah-toh-**JEN**-ih-sis)	Failure to develop spermatozoa
aspermia	(ah-**SPER**-mee-ah)	Failure of the formation or ejaculation of semen
azoospermia	(ay-**zoh**-oh-**SPER**-mee-ah)	Absence of spermatozoa in the semen
balanitis	(**bal**-ah-**NIGH**-tis)	Inflammation of the glans penis
benign prostatic hyperplasia (BPH)	(bee-**NINE** pros-**TAT**-ick high-per-**PLAY**-zee-ah)	Noncancerous overgrowth of the glandular tissue of the prostate
chancre	(**SHANG**-ker)	The primary sore of syphilis
cryptorchism	(krip-**TOR**-kizm)	Failure of the testicles to descend into scrotum. Cryptorchidism
epididymitis	(**ep**-ih-did-ih-**MY**-tis)	Inflammation of the epididymis
epispadias	(**ep**-ih-**SPAY**-dee-us)	A congenital opening of the urethra on the back of the penis. In the female, an opening formed by separation of the labia minora and a fissure of the clitoris
gynecomastia	(**jin**-eh-koh-**MASS**-tee-ah)	Abnormal enlargement of the male mammary glands
hydrocele	(**HIGH**-droh-seel)	The accumulation of serous fluid within the scrotum, especially in

the cavity of the tunica vaginalis testis

hypospadias	(**high**-poh-**SPAY**-dee-us)	A congenital abnormal opening of the male urethra on the underside of the penis
impotence	(**IHM**-poh-tens)	In general, lack of power. Lack of sexual power in the male
oligospermia	(**ol**-ih-goh-**SPER**-mee-ah)	Scanty spermatozoa in the semen
orchitis	(or-**KYE**-tis)	Inflammation of a testis. Orchiditis
paraphimosis	(**par**-ah-fih-**MOH**-sis)	The retraction (drawing back) of the prepuce behind the glans penis resulting in edema
phimosis	(fye-**MOH**-sis)	Stenosis or tightness of the prepuce, leading to the inability of the foreskin to be pushed back over the glans penis
prostatalgia	(**pros**-tah-**TAHL**-jee-ah)	Pain of the prostate gland
prostatitis	(**pros**-tah-**TIE**-tis)	Inflamed condition of the prostate gland
prostatomegaly	(**pros**-tah-toh-**MEG**-ah-lee)	Enlargement of the prostate gland
spermatocele	(**SPER**-mah-toh-**seel**)	A cystic tumor of the epididymis that contains spermatozoa
varicocele	(**VAR**-ih-koh-**seel**)	Enlargement of the veins of the spermatic cord
vesiculitis	(veh-**sick**-you-**LIE**-tis)	Inflammation of a vesicle, particularly the seminal vesicle

Terms Related to Sexually Transmitted Disease

A *sexually transmitted disease* (STD) is an infectious disease in which the infectious organism is transmitted to another during a sexual act such as vaginal or anal intercourse. Formerly called venereal disease. The list below is a partial list.

acquired immune deficiency syndrome (AIDS)	(aydz)	A syndrome involving the total collapse of the immune system, whereby the body loses all defense against infection, certain cancers, pneumonia, etc. It is believed to be

		due to the human immunodeficiency virus (HIV).
gonorrhea	(**gon**-oh-**REE**-ah)	Gonorrhea is the most common of the veneral diseases, and is caused by a one-celled organism. The first symptom in the male is usually an inflammation of the urethra. The female commonly has no symptoms.
herpes genitalis	(**HER**-peez **jen**-ih-**TAH**-lis)	Infection of the genital area with herpes virus type 2. Symptoms are itching and soreness followed by blisters. The infection can be spread to a fetus during delivery. It is usually spread by sexual contact. Genital herpes
syphilis	(**SIF**-ih-lis)	An infectious, sexually transmitted disease, characterized by a primary hard lesion (chancre), that may involve any organ or tissue and followed by a secondary skin eruption
trichomoniasis	(**trick**-oh-moh-**NIGH**-ah-sis)	An infection of the genitourinary tract caused by Trichomonas, a one-celled organism. May affect either sex, but symptoms are more commonly found in women. The male carrier may be asymptomatic but infectious to a sexual partner

Terms Related to Surgery or Treatment

circumcision	(**ser**-kum-**SIZH**-un)	The removal of all or part of the prepuce, or foreskin
epididymectomy	(**ep**-ih-**did**-ih-**MECK**-toh-mee)	Removal of the epididymis
orchiectomy	(**or**-kee-**ECK**-toh-mee)	Excision of one or both testes
orchiopexy	(**or**-kee-oh-**PECK**-see)	The surgical placement of an undescended testis into its normal position in the scrotum

prostatectomy	(**pros**-tak-**TECK**-toh-mee)	Excision of part or all of the prostate gland
sterilization	(**ster**-ih-lie-**ZAY**-shun)	The process of rendering a male or female incapable of reproduction, such as by vasectomy or tubal ligation
transurethral resection of the prostate, TUR, TURP		Excision of all or part of the prostate gland through the urethra
vasectomy	(vah-**SECK**-toh-mee)	Removal of all or a segment of the vas deferens

10.1   Review: System

DIRECTIONS: Cover the left column while you complete the statements on the right side.

gonad	The _____ of each sex produces the reproductive cell and hormones.
testes, scrotum	The male sex organs are the paired _____ , which lie in the _____ , external to the body.
androgen **testes**	The male sex hormone, _____ , is produced by the _____ .
semen	The reproductive fluid of the male is called _____ .
X and Y	Spermatozoa contain the _____ chromosome(s).
epididymis	The seminiferous tubules of the testes empty into the _____ .
sperm	The function of the vas deferens is to store and carry _____ .
prostate **urethra**	The ejaculatory duct passes through the _____ gland and empties into the _____ .

Cowper's glands	Two small, pea-sized glands called
	_____ lie on either side of the
	urethra.
scrotum	The _____ is an external sac that
	develops from the layers of the abdominal wall.

10.2 Review: Building Blocks

DIRECTIONS: Write the meanings of the following building blocks

1. hydr/o _____
2. gen/o _____
3. orchi/o _____
4. vesicul/o _____
5. –cele _____
6. gon/o _____
7. –plasia _____
8. andr/o _____
9. spermat/o _____
10. –cide _____
11. urethr/o _____
12. genit/o _____
13. chrom/o _____
14. olig/o _____
15. hom/o _____
16. balan/o _____
17. crypt/o _____
18. –genesis _____
19. heter/o _____
20. –megaly _____

10.3   Review: Word Building

DIRECTIONS: Fill in the blanks with the appropriate building block or medical term.

1. The combining form for *spermatozoa* is _____ .
   The suffix for *producing* or *forming* is _____ .
   The word _____ means *producing spermatozoa.*

2. A prefix meaning *not* or *without* is _____ .
   The word _____ means *not producing sperm.*

3. _____ is a prefix meaning *deficient* or *scanty.*
   _____ is a deficiency in the number of sperm in the semen.

4. The combining form for *prostate* is _____ .
   A suffix for *enlargement* is _____ .
   The medical term for enlargement of the prostate gland, affecting many men past middle age, is _____ .

5. A suffix meaning *pain* is _____ .
   _____ means pain of the prostate gland.

6. The combining form for *woman* is _____ .
   _____ is a word ending meaning *pertaining to the breast* or *mammary glands.*
   The condition of excessive development of the male mammary glands is called _____ .

7. The combining form for the *glans penis* is _____ .
   _____ is the suffix meaning *inflammation.*
   Inflammation of the glans penis is called _____ .

8. The combining form for *testis* is _____ .
   The term for *congenital absence of the testis* is _____ .

9. A prefix meaning *hidden* is _____ .
   The condition of having a *hidden or undescended testis* is called _____ .

10. A suffix meaning *surgical fixation* is _____ .
    _____ means surgical fixation in the scrotum of an undescended testis.

10.4   Review: Anatomy

DIRECTIONS: Identify the lettered structures of the male reproductive system in the diagram below.

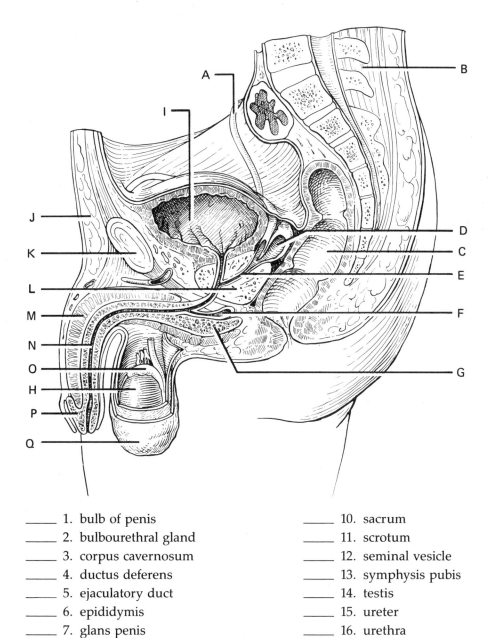

_____ 1. bulb of penis
_____ 2. bulbourethral gland
_____ 3. corpus cavernosum
_____ 4. ductus deferens
_____ 5. ejaculatory duct
_____ 6. epididymis
_____ 7. glans penis
_____ 8. prostate gland
_____ 9. rectum

_____ 10. sacrum
_____ 11. scrotum
_____ 12. seminal vesicle
_____ 13. symphysis pubis
_____ 14. testis
_____ 15. ureter
_____ 16. urethra
_____ 17. urinary bladder

10.5   Review: Vocabulary

DIRECTIONS: Match the terms in the first column with their definitions in the second column.

1. _____ heterosexual
2. _____ puberty
3. _____ androgen
4. _____ sterilization
5. _____ chancre
6. _____ spermatozoa
7. _____ varicocele
8. _____ eunuch
9. _____ impotence
10. _____ coitus

A. Any substance that possesses masculinizing properties
B. The primary sore of syphilis
C. Sexual intercourse between male and female
D. A castrated male
E. Pertaining to the opposite sex
F. Inability of the male to achieve or maintain erection
G. The period in life at which an individual of either sex becomes functionally capable of reproduction
H. The mature male sex cells formed within the seminiferous tubules of the testes
I. The process of rendering an individual incapable of reproduction
J. Enlargement of the vein of the spermatic cord

10.6   Review: Vocabulary

DIRECTIONS: Match the terms in the first column with their definitions in the second column.

1. _____ phimosis
2. _____ circumcision
3. _____ vasectomy
4. _____ benign prostatic hypertrophy
5. _____ spermatocele
6. _____ ejaculation
7. _____ homosexual
8. _____ transurethral resection of the prostate
9. _____ genitalia
10. _____ spermaturia

A. Overgrowth of the glandular tissue of the prostate
B. One sexually attracted to another of the same sex
C. Removal of all or part of the prepuce
D. Ejection of the seminal fluid from the male urethra
E. Condition in which the foreskin cannot be pushed back over the glans
F. A cystic tumor of the epididymis containing spermatozoa
G. Semen discharged with the urine
H. External reproductive organs
I. Removal of all or a segment of the vas deferens
J. Excision of part or all of the prostate gland through the urethra

10.7 Review: Vocabulary

DIRECTIONS: Write the medical or surgical term for the following definitions.

1. _____ Removal of all or a segment of the vas deferens
2. _____ Excision of all or a part of the prostate gland through the urethra
3. _____ The process of rendering a male or female incapable of reproduction
4. _____ The mature male sex cells formed within the seminiferous tubules of the testes
5. _____ A cystic tumor of the epididymis that contains spermatozoa
6. _____ The period in life at which either the male or female becomes functionally capable of reproduction
7. _____ Enlargement of the prostate gland
8. _____ Pain of the prostate gland
9. _____ Condition in which the foreskin cannot be pushed back over the glans penis
10. _____ Surgical placement of an undescended testis into its normal position in the scrotum
11. _____ Deficiency in the number of spermatozoa in the semen
12. _____ Inability of the male to achieve or maintain erection
13. _____ One who is sexually attracted to another of the same sex
14. _____ Ejection of the seminal fluid from the male urethra
15. _____ Removal of all or part of the prepuce
16. _____ Overgrowth of the glandular tissue of the prostate
17. _____ Absence of development of spermatozoa
18. _____ Any substance that possesses masculinizing qualities

Reading Comprehension 10.1

DIRECTIONS: Underline the medical terms as you go through the reading exercise. Then list and analyze the terms. Some will be completely new to you. Consult a medical dictionary for their meanings. Then re-read the material for better comprehension.

Return Examination

10 December 19—. Patient G.W. returned for complete exam. He has been feeling well. He has been exercising regularly and makes constant efforts at maintaining good health habits. He has minimal to no back discomfort. He has had nocturia at least once nightly in the last five of seven nights, but seems to have no hesitancy or difficulty with urination at other times.

On exam his weight is 181, BP 110/70, temp. 98, pulse rate 60. On exam of HEENT eyes and eyegrounds were normal. Ears showed no abnormalities. Mouth: Tongue was papillated. Neck was supple with no thyroid enlargement. Carotid pulses normal. There were no neck nodes or bruits. Chest was symmetrical. Lungs were resonant to percussion. No rales or rhonchi. Heart size was normal with no murmurs or third or fourth heart sound. No chest wall tenderness was noted. No axillary nodes palpable. Abdomen soft. No enlargement of liver or spleen. There was no abdominal mass. Testes were of normal size and consistency. Extremities showed no edema, clubbing, or cyanosis. Reflexes hypoactive. On rectal examination there was 1+ smooth symmetric prostatic enlargement. No rectal mass was noted. Stool negative for occult blood.

Hemoglobin 14.6, hematocrit 43, white count 4000, platelets 157,000. Blood chemistries, urinalysis, sed. rate and chest x-ray are to be done. EKG is within normal limits.

Blood was drawn for electrophoretic pattern.

Impression:
1. Multiple myeloma, in remission.

Advised he is doing well, continue on no treatment, return in two months for followup visit.

Marrow examination in March showed small numbers of plasma cells. Marrow examination should be repeated early in 19—.

Reading Comprehension 10.2

DIRECTIONS: Underline the medical terms as you go through the reading exercise. Then list and analyze the terms. Some will be completely new to you. Consult a medical dictionary for their meanings. Then re-read the material for better comprehension.

Pathology Report

Specimen: Left testicle

Preoperative Diagnosis: Tumor, left testicle

Gross:
The specimen received fresh from surgery is a left testicle, stated, and this weighs approximately 71 grams and shows overall measurements of about $8 \times 5 \times 3.3$ cm. When sectioned, the testicle shows a tan lobulated appearance and is firmer than usual. The cross sectional diameters of the testicle are approximately 4.0 and 3.0 cm. A rapid frozen section is reported as consistent with seminoma. Multiple sections are embedded for permanent section evaluation, while the material from rapid frozen section is labeled F.

Microscopic:
Multiple sections of left testicle show a cellular tumor characterized by sheets and aggregates and islands of cells separated from each other by a fibrocollaginous stroma. Reactive vessels are also present scattered throughout the tumor, but residual testicular tubules are not positively identified. The tumor cells show round, rather large, oval vesicular nuclei containing nucleoli. The cytoplasm is amphophilic and finely granular. Mitoses are not infrequent. Lymphocytes are scattered throughout many areas of the tumor itself. There are variable zones of fibrosis associated with the tumor in the multiple sections examined. Sections of epididymis show acidophilic amorphous material containing poorly preserved cells. The tumor does not involve the sections of spermatic cord. Areas of hemorrhage and necrosis are not a feature in the sections examined. The testicle appears totally replaced by pure seminoma.

Diagnosis:
Seminoma, left testicle (left orchiectomy)

Comment: Multiple sections show a pure seminoma which has apparently replaced the entire testicular parenchyma.

Reading Comprehension Vocabulary

Use the space below to list the medical terms for analysis and definition.

_____

_____

_____

_____

_____

_____

_____

_____

_____

_____

_____

_____

_____

_____

_____

_____

_____

_____

_____

_____

_____

_____

_____

_____

_____

_____

_____

_____

CHAPTER 11

Female Reproductive System

OBJECTIVES

When you have successfully completed Chapter 11, you should be able to:
— Recall terms describing the anatomy and physiology of the female reproductive system.
— Define the building blocks introduced in this chapter.
— Define common terms related to the female reproductive system.
— Recall the medical terms for structures and functions defined in the chapter.
— Identify the structures of the female reproductive system on a familiar drawing.
— Analyze surgical terms applied to the female reproductive system.
— Build medical terms using the building blocks introduced in this and previous chapters.

KEY TERMS

axilla	(ack-**SILL**-ah)	The armpit
deposition	(**dep**-oh-**ZIH**-shun)	The act or process of putting or laying something down
excretory organ	(**ECKS**-kreh-**toh**-ree)	An organ that serves to eliminate waste products from the body
follicle	(**FOL**-ih-kal)	A small cavity or depression
gynecology	(**guy**-neh-**KOL**-oh-jee)	The study of the female reproductive system, including the breasts
inhibit	(in-**HIB**-it)	Restrain; hold in check
junction	(**JUNGK**-shun)	The place or point of joining
laterally	(**LAT**-er-ahl-lee)	Directed toward the side
ligament	(**LIG**-ah-ment)	The tough band of tissue serving to connect the extremities of bones or to support an organ in place
longitudinal	(**lon**-jih-**TOO**-dih-nal)	Placed or running lengthwise, not crosswise
obstetrics	(ob-**STEH**-tricks)	The branch of medicine that manages the health care of women during pregnancy, childbirth, and immediately after delivery
pigment	(**PIG**-ment)	Coloring matter
prolapse	(pro-**LAPS**)	The falling downward of an internal part
sebaceous	(seh-**BAY**-shus)	Pertaining to fatty matter or sebum
secretory	(see-**KREE**-toh-ree)	Pertaining to promoting secretion, the process whereby cells of glandular organs produce certain materials from the blood
spiral	(**SPY**-rahl)	Circling round a center or pole
subcutaneous	(**sub**-kyou-**TAY**-nee-us)	Pertaining to beneath the skin
ventrally	(**VEN**-trah-lee)	Pertaining to or toward the abdominal surface of the body

OVERVIEW

The female reproductive system (Figure 11.1) includes not only the organs of reproduction but also the organs that contain and nourish the fertilized ovum (egg) through the period of prebirth development (gestation) and expel it from the mother's body during labor. The lactating (milk-producing) organs are considered a part of this system. The study of the female reproductive system, including the breasts, is called *gynecology* and is practiced by gynecologists. *Obstetrics* is a branch of medical practice concerned specifically with pregnancy and birth.

FEMALE GONADS (Ovaries)

The female reproductive organs or *gonads* are the paired *ovaries*, located near the lateral walls of the pelvic cavity. These almond-shaped glands, about 1.5 inches long, are connected by ligaments to the uterus, or womb. The function of the ovaries is to release

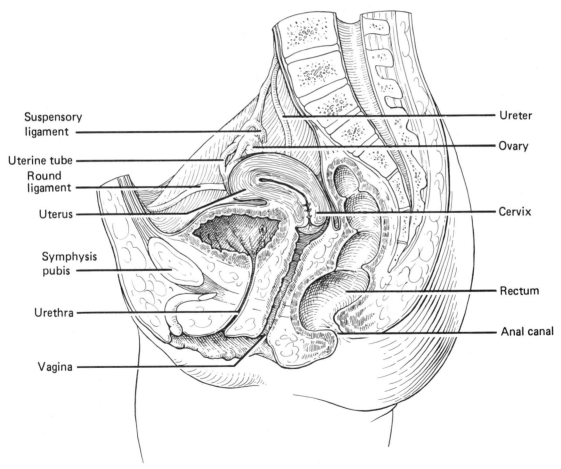

FIGURE 11.1 Female reproductive system

eggs (ova) which are present in the female at birth, from *puberty* to *menopause*, the end of the female's reproductive span. Each of the ova contains the entire genetic inheritance of the female parent, except that the ovum contains only a single sex chromosome, an X (female) chromosome. The X chromosome of the female combines with an X or Y chromosome from the male sperm, determining whether the offspring will be female (XX) or male (XY). The ovaries produce the female hormones *estrogen* and *progesterone*.

INTERNAL ORGANS

Uterus

The uterus lies between the urinary bladder and the rectum and is suspended in the pelvic cavity by ligaments. It receives the embryo resulting from a fertilized egg cell and sustains its life during development. In the nonpregnant female the uterus serves as the organ of menstruation.

The uterus is a hollow, pear-shaped organ, about 3 inches long and 2 inches wide (Figure 11.2). It has two main portions, the uterine body and the cervix. The *uterine body*, which forms the upper two-thirds of the uterus, is joined by the *uterine tubes* at its broadest part. The expanded portion above the entrance of the uterine tubes is called the *uterine fundus*. The inferior third of the uterus, its tubular *cervix*, or neck, extends distally into the upper portion of the vagina. The cervix is a very common site of cancer.

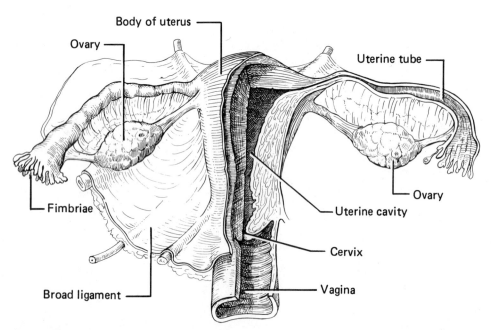

FIGURE 11.2 The uterus and ovaries

Uterine Walls

The walls of the uterus consist of three layers. The outer layer, or *perimetrium*, is a thin layer of serous-coat *peritoneum*. The middle *myometrium*, or muscle layer, is very thick. It is formed by three poorly defined layers of smooth muscle fibers arranged in longitudinal, circular, and spiral patterns. The *endometrium* is the inner layer of the uterine wall formed by mucous membrane that lines the fundus and cervix.

Normally the fundus is tipped ventrally. A condition called *uterine retroversion* is a tilting backward of the uterus with no change in the relationship of the body to the cervix. *Uterine prolapse* occurs when the uterine ligaments are stretched and the uterus descends to a lower than normal level.

Uterine Tubes

The *uterine tubes* receive ova as they are released from the ovary and convey the ovum to the uterus.

Paired uterine tubes, often called the *fallopian tubes* or *oviducts*, are approximately 4 inches long and 0.3 inches in diameter. They lie on either side of the uterus, joining the uterine body just below the fundus and extending laterally toward the ovaries. The narrow isthmus of each tube opens into the uterine cavity. The middle portion, or *ampulla*, arches over the ovary. Near the ovary the tube expands to form a funnel-shaped *infundibulum*, which partially encircles the ovary. The infundibulum ends in irregular fringed structures called *fimbriae*.

Vagina

The *vagina* is the organ of copulation. It also serves as a passage for the fetus during the birth process and is the excretory duct for the menses.

The vagina is a fibromuscular tube approximately 3.5 inches long, extending from the uterus to the *vestibule*. It is lined with mucous membrane arranged in folds called *rugae*. The vagina is located posterior to the urinary bladder and urethra and anterior to the rectum. A fold of mucous membrane, the *hymen*, partially covers the external opening.

EXTERNAL STRUCTURES

The external accessory structures of the female reproductive system consist mainly of those associated with copulation (Figure 11.3).

Vulva

The term *vulva* is used to refer to a group of external sexual structures of the female, including the labia majora, the labia minora and the vestibule, and the clitoris.

LABIA MAJORA. The *labia majora* are two large lips (labia) of fatty tissue that lie on either side of the vaginal opening (vaginal os). The labia majora form the lateral borders of the vulva and become covered with hair at puberty. They enclose and protect the other external reproductive organs, a function equivalent to the scrotum in the male.

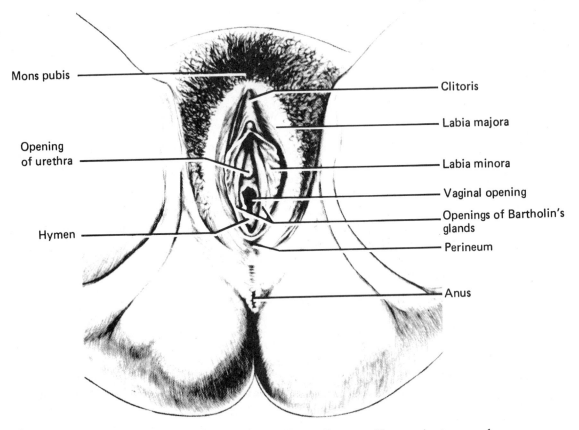

Mons pubis

Opening
of urethra

Hymen

Clitoris

Labia majora

Labia minora

Vaginal opening

Openings of Bartholin's
glands

Perineum

Anus

FIGURE 11.3   **The external female genitalia** (From Creager, *Human Anatomy and Physiology,* copyright 1983 by Wadsworth, Inc. Reprinted by permission of the publisher.)

LABIA MINORA. The *labia minora,* smaller lips, are located within the cleft between the labia majora. Composed of connective tissue richly supplied in blood vessels, they contain sebaceous glands but no fat. These hairless lips enclose the *vestibule.* The vestibule encloses the opening of the urethra, situated anteriorly, and the opening of the vagina, situated posteriorly.

CLITORIS. The *clitoris* is located just behind the juncture of the labia majora. It is partially covered by folds of skin called the *prepuce.* Like the penis of the male, the clitoris is composed of two columns of cavernous erectile tissue. These columns converge anteriorly to form a hoodlike covering. The anterior end of the clitoris contains a small mass of erectile tissue, the *glans,* which is abundantly supplied with sensory nerve fibers that respond to sexual stimulation.

VESTIBULAR GLANDS. A pair of *vestibular* glands called *Bartholin's* (**BAR**-toh-linz) *glands*, lie one on each side of the vagina. They produce mucus for lubrication and correspond to Cowper's glands in the male.

MONS PUBIS

The *mons pubis* is the skin-covered pad of fat located over the *symphysis pubis*, or pubic bone. The mons is covered with coarse hair after puberty.

PERINEUM

The *perineum* is the external floor of the pelvis extending from the pubic arch to the *coccyx*. It includes the underlying muscles and fascia. Figure 11.4 shows a section through the female perineum. During *parturition* (childbirth) the perineum is stretched and the tissues may become weakened. Sometimes an *episiotomy*, a cutting of the perineum, is done during delivery to prevent this stretching. Weakening of the perineum may lead to a protrusion of the urinary bladder (*cystocele*) or a herniation of the rectum (*rectocele*).

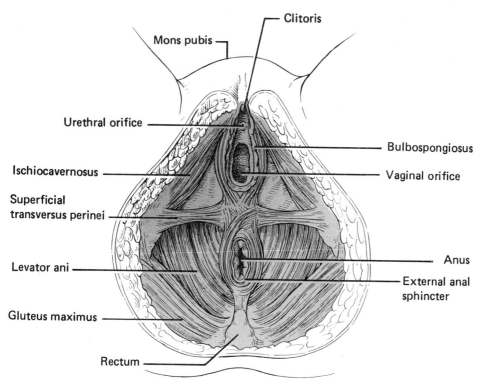

FIGURE 11.4   The female perineum

MAMMARY GLANDS (BREASTS)

The mammary glands are the organs of lactation. In structure (Figure 11.5) they are modified sweat glands. The breasts, which are composed of fatty tissue in addition to the glands, lie on the anterior surface of the thorax. They are supported by the pectoral muscles, which extend from the second to the sixth ribs and from the sternum to the axillae. Each gland is composed of 15 to 20 irregularly shaped lobes which are further subdivided into lobules. At the center of each breast is a *nipple* surrounded by a pigmented area called the *areola*. The areolae are usually pink but become brown during pregnancy. Each mammary lobe contains a *lactiferous duct* (milk duct) that leads to openings in the nipple.

HORMONES

The female hormones belong to two major groups, *estrogen* and *progesterone*. The primary source of estrogen is the ovaries. Estrogens induce *ovulation*, the monthly release of the ova. They also control maturation of the uterus, uterine tubes, vagina, ovaries, and mammary ducts. During puberty, estrogens stimulate development of secondary sex characteristics such as increased deposition of fat in the subcutaneous tissues, especially

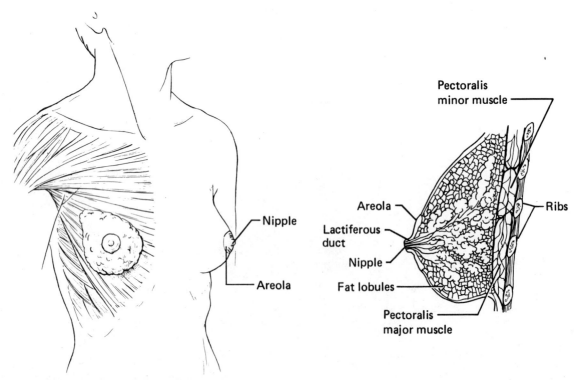

FIGURE 11.5   Mammary glands

in the breasts, thighs, and buttocks; the growth of pubic and axillary hair, and the development of a smoother, softer-textured skin than is found in males. Estrogens play a part in the cessation of growth through the closing of the epiphyseal plates in the long bones, which occurs sooner in females than in males.

Progesterone is the female hormone secreted by the *corpus luteum*, the name given to the mature ovarian follicle that has released its ovum. The most important function of progesterone is to prepare the lining of the uterus for implantation of a fertilized ovum. During pregnancy, the milk-producing glands enlarge and become secretory under the influence of progesterone, which also inhibits ovulation during this time.

MENSTRUATION

The *menstrual cycle* in the female reflects the cyclical changes that occur approximately monthly. The cycle includes both secretion of hormones and changes in the reproductive organs themselves. For example, when ovulation occurs, changes in the uterine lining prepare it to receive and nourish a fertilized ovum. If fertilization does not occur, these cells are sloughed off in the process known as the *menses*, or menstruation. The entire cycle is repeated about every 28 days from puberty through menopause, when it becomes irregular and eventually ceases.

MENOPAUSE

After about 35 years of menstrual cycling, the menses become irregular and eventually, after a few months or years, cease entirely. This period in the life of the female is called *menopause* and generally occurs in the late forties or early fifties.

≡ BUILDING BLOCKS

ROOTS AND COMBINING FORMS

Word Elements	Meaning
alb/o	white
amni/o	amnion
cervic/o	neck, cervix
colp/o	vagina
corpus	body
culd/o	cul de sac
cyst/o	urinary bladder, cyst
galact/o	milk
gynec/o	woman, female
hyster/o	uterus, womb
lact/o	milk

ROOTS AND COMBINING FORMS (continued)

Word Elements	Meaning
leuk/o	white
mamm/o	breast
mast/o	breast
men/o	month
metr/o	uterus, womb
nat/i	birth
oophor/o	ovary
ov/o	egg
perine/o	perineum
pseud/o	false
rect/o	rectum
salping/o	uterine tube
trachel/o	neck
uter/o	uterus, womb
vagin/o	vagina
version	turning

SUFFIXES

Word Elements	Meaning
–arche	beginning
–cele	hernia
–rhea	flow, discharge
–tocia	labor, birth

PREFIXES

Word Elements	Meaning
ante–	before, forward
eu–	good
neo–	new
nulli–	none
pan–	all
para–	near, beside, abnormal
primi–	first
retro–	behind, back
sym–	together, with
tri–	three
uni–	one

VOCABULARY

General Terms

ampulla	(am-**PULL**-lah)	A saclike dilatation of a tubular structure. The ampulla of the uterine tube is the dilated distal end of the tube resembling a funnel
anovular	(an-**AHV**-you-lar)	Not associated with, or without, ovulation, the discharge of an ovum
anteflexion	(an-tee-**FLECK**-shun)	The abnormal bending forward of part of an organ
antenatal	(an-teh-**NAY**-tal)	Occurring before birth
antepartum	(an-tee-**PAR**-tum)	Occurring before the onset of labor
bipara	(**BIP**-ah-rah)	A woman who has given birth for the second time to one or more infants
coitus	(**KOH**-ih-tus)	Sexual intercourse by insertion of the penis into the vagina
colposcope	(**KOL**-poh-skohp)	An instrument used for internal examination of the tissues of the vagina and cervix by means of a light and a magnifying lens
conception	(kon-**SEP**-shun)	The union of the male sperm and the female ovum resulting in fertilization
contraception	(**kon**-trah-**SEP**-shun)	The prevention of pregnancy
copulation	(**kop**-you-**LAY**-shun)	Sexual intercourse in humans or animals
dehiscence	(dee-**HISS**-ens)	A splitting open
fertilization	(**fer**-tih-lie-**ZAY**-shun)	The union of the female ovum with the male sperm
frigidity	(frih-**JID**-ih-tee)	In general, coldness. A term sometimes used to denote sexual unresponsiveness, especially in the female

gestation	(jes-TAY-shun)	The period from conception to birth. In humans, this normally ranges from 37 weeks to 39 weeks.
gravida	(**GRAV**-ih-dah)	A pregnant woman
gynecology	(**guy**-neh-**KOL**-oh-jee)	The study of the female reproductive system, including the breasts
intrauterine	(**in**-trah-**YOU**-ter-in)	Within the uterus
isthmus	(**IS**-mus)	A narrow passage between two cavities or two larger parts
lactation	(lack-**TAY**-shun)	The secretion of milk
lactiferous	(lack-**TIF**-er-us)	Yielding or conveying milk
menarche	(meh-**NAR**-kee)	The establishment or beginning of the menstrual function in the human female
menopause	(**MEN**-oh-pawz)	Cessation of menstruation in the human female, occurring in the late forties or early fifties
multipara	(mul-**TIP**-ah-rah)	A woman who has given birth to two or more infants of a defined minimum weight and period of gestation
neonatal	(**nee**-oh-**NAY**-tal)	Pertaining to the first four to six weeks after birth
nullipara	(nuh-**LIP**-ah-rah)	A woman who has never borne viable offspring
obstetrics	(ob-**STET**-ricks)	The medical specialty dealing with the care of women during pregnancy, labor, and the puerperium
orifice	(**OR**-ih-fis)	An opening such as the mouth. The entrance or outlet of any body cavity
parturient	(par-**TYOU**-ree-ent)	Giving birth, or concerning childbirth; a woman in labor

parturition	(**par**-tyou-**RISH**-un)	The act or process of giving birth; labor
postpartum	(post-**PAR**-tum)	Occurring after childbirth
prenatal	(pree-**NAY**-tal)	Existing or occurring before birth
primipara	(pry-**MIP**-ah-rah)	A woman who has given birth to one infant of 500 grams or 20 weeks' gestation, regardless of viability
puberty	(**POO**-ber-tee)	The period during which the capability of sexual reproduction is attained
puerpera	(pyou-**ER**-per-ah)	A woman who has just given birth
puerperium	(**pyou**-er-**PEE**-ree-um)	The period after childbirth during which the reproductive organs return to normal, generally about six weeks
retroflexion	(**ret**-roh-**FLECK**-shun)	Bending backward. Retroflexion of the uterus involves a bending backward of the body of the uterus toward the cervix, resulting in a sharp angle where the bend occurs
retroversion	(**ret**-roh-**VER**-zhun)	The tipping of an entire organ backward. *Uterine retroversion* is the turning backward of the entire uterus with the cervix pointing forward
sterility	(steh-**RILL**-ih-tee)	In general, the state of being free from microorganisms. Regarding the reproductive system, the inability to produce offspring
Trichomonas	(trick-oh-**MOH**-nas)	A genus of flagellate parasitic protozoa. *Trichomonas vaginalis* is the species found in the vagina that causes vaginal infection resulting in a whitish discharge. Frequently occurs during pregnancy, following vaginal surgery, and in diabetic women

trimester	(try-**MEHS**-ter)	A three-month period; used to describe the major stages of pregnancy, as in *first trimester*
unipara	(you-**NIP**-ah-rah)	A woman who has had one pregnancy of over 20 weeks gestation or has produced a fetus of at least 500 grams, whether viable or not
version	(**VER**-zhun)	A turning, or change of direction. Converting an abnormal position in the uterus to a more normal position

Terms Related to Anatomy and Physiology

adnexa	(ad-**NECK**-sah)	Accessory parts. *Adnexa uteri* are the ovaries and oviducts, parts of the uterus
alveolus	(al-**VEE**-oh-lus)	A small, saclike dilatation; plural, *alveoli*
amnion	(**AM**-nee-on)	The inner fetal membrane
areola	(ah-**REE**-oh-lah)	A circular area of different pigmentation, as around a wheal, around the nipple of the breast, or the part of the iris around the pupil
Bartholin's glands	(**BAR**-toh-linz)	Small, compound mucus glands, one situated in each of the two lateral walls of the vestibule of the vagina, near the vaginal opening at the base of the labia majora
cervix	(**SER**-vicks)	The neck or a necklike part of an organ. The *cervix uteri* is the neck of the uterus.
chorion	(**KOH**-ree-on)	The outermost membrane surrounding the developing embryo
clitoris	(**KLIT**-oh-ris)	A small elongated structure of erectile tissue located anterior to the vaginal orifice and in front of the

		urethral outlet; analogous to the penis in the male
coccyx	(**KOCK**-sicks)	A small bone at the lower (caudal) end base of the spinal column
corpus albicans	(**KOR**-pus **AHL**-bih-kanz)	A mass of fibrous tissue that replaces the regressing corpus luteum after an ovarian follicle has ruptured (released an ovum). A white scar forms that gradually shrinks and eventually disappears
corpus luteum	(**KOR**-pus **LOO**-tee-um)	A small yellow body that develops within a ruptured ovarian follicle
cul de sac	(**KUHL**-deh-sahk)	A blind pouch or cavity. In the female, an extension of the peritoneal cavity lying between the rectum and the posterior wall of the uterus
embryo	(**EM**-bree-oh)	The earliest developmental stage of an organism. In humans, this stage of development is from conception until the end of the second month of gestation.
endometrium	(**en**-doh-**MEE**-tree-um)	The mucous membrane lining the inner surface of the uterus
estradiol	(**es**-trah-**DIE**-ol) (es-**TRAY**-dee-ul)	An ovarian steroid possessing estrogenic properties
estrogen	(**ES**-troh-jen)	The estrogenic hormones estradiol, and estrone, produced by the ovary; or any natural or artificial substance that induces estrogenic activity
eutocia	(you-**TOH**-see-ah)	Normal or natural labor and childbirth
fallopian tubes	(fal-**LOH**-pee-an)	Paired tubes attached to and entering the uterus, which convey the ova from the ovaries to the uterus; uterine tubes

fetus	(FEE-tus)	In humans, the developing infant from the beginning of the third month to birth
fimbria	(FIM-bree-ah)	The outer fringelike end of each fallopian tube
follicle	(FOL-lih-KAL)	A small cavity or depression
follicle stimulating hormone (FSH)		A hormone secreted by the anterior lobe of the hypophysis; stimulates maturation of the ovarian follicles in the female and helps maintain spermatogenesis in the male
fundus	(FUN-dus)	The bottom or base of anything. The *fundus uteri* is the body of the uterus situated above the orifices of the uterine tubes.
gamete	(GAM-eet)	A mature male (spermatozoon) or female (ovum) reproductive cell
genitalia	(jen-ih-TAY-lee-ah)	The reproductive organs
gonad	(GOH-nadd)	An ovary or testis; the primary sex glands
graafian follicle	(GRAPH-ee-an)	The thin membranous structure surrounding and including each ovum before its escape from the ovary
human chorionic gonadotropin (HCG)	(koh-ree-ON-ick gon-ah-doh-TROH-pin)	A hormone produced by the placenta that helps sustain pregnancy
hymen	(HIGH-men)	The membranous fold that partially or wholly occludes the external orifice of the vagina
infundibulum	(in-fun-DIB-you-lum)	A funnellike tubular structure. The infundibulum of the uterine tube is located at the distal end of the tube.
labia	(LAY-bee-ah)	The folds of the female external genitalia, consisting of the labia majora, the outer folds, and the

		labia minora, the inner folds; singular, *labium*
lochia	(**LOH**-kee-ah)	The uterine discharge of blood-tinged mucus and tissue that takes place during the first week or two after childbirth
luteinizing hormone	(**loo**-tee-in-**EYE**-zing **HOR**-mohn)	A hormone secreted by the anterior lobe of the hypoplysis that promotes ovulation (LH)
mammary glands	(**MAM**-er-ee)	The milk-secreting glands of the female breast
meconium	(meh-**KOH**-nee-um)	The first feces of a newborn infant
menorrhea	(**men**-oh-**REE**-ah)	The normal discharge of the menses
menstruation	(men-stroo-**AY**-shun)	Cyclic, physiologic uterine bleeding that normally recurs at intervals of about four weeks during the reproductive span of the female, except during pregnancy; menses
mons pubis	(monz **PYOU**-bis)	The rounded prominence over the symphysis pubis that is covered with hair following puberty
myometrium	(my-oh-**MEE**-tree-um)	The muscular layer of the uterus that forms the main mass of the organ
oocyte	(**OH**-oh-sight)	A developing or immature ovum, which passes through two stages, primary and secondary
oogenesis	(**oh**-oh-**JEN**-eh-sis)	The process of formation of the female gametes (ova)
ovary	(**OH**-vah-ree)	The female gonad. A female has two ovaries, sexual glands in which the ova are formed
oviduct	(**OH**-vih-duckt)	A uterine tube; fallopian tube
ovulation	(**oh**-view-**LAY**-shun)	The release of an ovum from an ovarian follicle
ovum	(**OH**-vum)	The female reproductive cell, an egg

perimetrium	(per-ih-**MEE**-tree-um)	Serous layer of the uterus
perineum	(per-ih-**NEE**-um)	The structures comprising the pelvic floor, the area between the external genitalia and the anus
placenta	(plah-**SEN**-tah)	Vascular structure that develops in the uterine wall during pregnancy and serves as a link between the maternal and fetal bloodstreams
progesterone	(pro-**JES**-teh-rohn)	A steroid hormone produced in the corpus luteum and the placenta
pudendum	(pyou-**DEN**-deum)	The external genitalia; in the female, the vulva
rugae	(**ROO**-jee)	Rugae of the vagina are small transverse folds of the vaginal mucous membrane; singular, ruga
secundines	(seh-**KUN**-dines)	The placenta and membranes expelled following the birth of a child; the afterbirth
symphysis pubis	(**SIM**-fih-sis **PYOU**-bis)	The junction of the pubic bones on the anterior midline
umbilical cord	(um-**BIL**-ih-kal)	The cord that attaches the fetus to the placenta.
uterine tube	(**YOU**-ter-in)	Fallopian tube
uterus	(**YOU**-ter-us)	The female organ that carries and nourishes the embryo and fetus from conception to birth; the womb
vagina	(vah-**JYE**-nah)	The tubular passageway between the cervix uteri and the vulva
vernix caseosa	(**VER**-nicks kays-ee-**OH**-sah)	A protective substance covering the fetus during intrauterine life
vestibule	(**VES**-tih-byoul)	In general, a small space or cavity at the beginning of a canal. The vestibule of the vagina is an almond-shaped space between the labia minora containing the openings of the vagina and urethra

vulva	(**VUL**-vah)	The external genitalia of the female
zygote	(**ZYE**-goht)	The cell produced by two gametes; the fertilized ovum

Terms Related to Pathology

amenorrhea	(ah-**men**-oh-**REE**-ah)	Absence or abnormal stoppage of menstruation
azotemia	(**az**-oh-**TEE**-mee-ah)	Presence of nitrogenous compounds in the blood
bradytocia	(**brad**-ee-**TOH**-see-ah)	Slow parturition (birth)
cervicitis	(ser-vih-**SIGH**-tis)	Inflammation of the cervix uteri
condyloma	(**kon**-dih-**LOH**-mah)	A wartlike growth occurring on the external genitalia or near the anus
cystocele	(**SIS**-toh-seel)	Hernia of the urinary bladder protruding through the vaginal wall
dysmenorrhea	(**dis**-men-oh-**REE**-ah)	Pain associated with menstruation
dyspareunia	(**dis**-pah-**ROO**-nee-ah)	Pain or discomfort experienced by a woman during sexual intercourse
dystocia	(dis-**TOH**-see-ah)	Difficult or abnormal labor during childbirth
ectopic pregnancy	(eck-**TOP**-ick)	Pregnancy occurring outside of the uterine cavity
endocervicitis	(**en**-doh-**ser**-vih-**SIGH**-tis)	Inflammation of mucous lining of the cervix uteri
endometriosis	(**en**-doh-**mee**-tree-**OH**-sis)	A condition in which endometrial tissue is found in various places throughout the pelvis or in the abdominal wall
endometritis	(**en**-doh-mee-**TRY**-tis)	Inflammation of the endometrium
eutocia	(you-**TOH**-see-ah)	Normal or natural labor and childbirth
fibroma	(figh-**BROH**-mah)	A tumor composed of fibrous connective tissue; also called a fibroid tumor
galactorrhea	(gah-**LACK**-toh-**REE**-ah)	Excessive or spontaneous flow of

milk from the breasts; persistent secretion of milk after cessation of nursing

hematosalpinx	(**hem**-ah-toh-**SAL**-pincks)	An accumulation of blood or menstrual fluid in a uterine tube
hydrosalpinx	(**high**-droh-**SAL**-pincks)	An accumulation of watery fluid in a uterine tube
leukorrhea	(**loo**-koh-**REE**-ah)	A whitish, mucoid discharge from the vagina and uterine cavity
mastitis	(mass-**TIE**-tis)	Inflammation of the mammary gland, or breast
menorrhagia	(**men**-oh-**RAY**-jee-ah)	Excessive uterine bleeding occurring at the regular time of menstruation
menorrhea	(**men**-oh-**REE**-ah)	The normal discharge of the menses
metritis	(meh-**TRY**-tis)	Inflammation of the uterus
metrorrhagia	(**mee**-troh-**RAY**-jee-ah)	Uterine bleeding that occurs at completely irregular intervals in which the amount of bleeding is normal but the period of flow is prolonged
myometritis	(**my**-oh-meh-**TRY**-tis)	Inflammation of the muscular layer of the uterus (the myometrium)
oligomenorrhea	(ol-ih-goh-**men**-oh-**REE**-ah)	Markedly diminished menstrual flow
polyemia	(**pol**-ee-**EE**-mee-ah)	Excessive amount of blood in the body system
procidentia	(**pro**-sih-**DEN**-shee-ah)	A prolapse, or downward displacement, especially prolapse of the uterus to the extent that the cervix protrudes outside the vaginal outlet
prolapse	(proh-**LAPS**)	A falling down or sinking of an organ or internal part, such as the uterus or rectum; procidentia
pseudocyesis	(**soo**-doh-sigh-**EE**-sis)	False pregnancy; phantom pregnancy

pyosalpinx	(pie-oh-SAHL-pincks)	A collection of pus in a fallopian tube
rectocele	(RECK-toh-seel)	Bulging of part of the rectum through the posterior vaginal wall; proctocele
salpingitis	(sal-pin-JYE-tis)	Inflammation of the uterine tube
toxic shock syndrome (TSS)	(TOCK-sick shock SIN-drom)	A severe infection caused by the bacterium *staphylococcus aureus* that occurs mainly in young women who are using vaginal tampons during menstruation
vaginitis	(vaj-ih-NIGH-tis)	Inflammation of the vagina

Terms Related to Diagnostic Procedures

Culdoscopy	(kuhl-DAHS-koh-pee)	Visual examination of the female pelvic viscera by means of an endoscope introduced into the pelvic cavity through the posterior vaginal fornix
mammography	(mam-AHG-rah-fee)	Radiologic (x-ray) study of the breast, used in the diagnosis of cancer
Papanicolaou test	(pap-ah-nick-oh-LAY-oo)	A study for early detection of cancer cells; pap smear
Rubin's test (ROO-bins test)		Instillation of carbon dioxide into the fallopian tubes by way of the uterus (transuterine insufflation) to determine whether the tubes are open (patent); may cause pain in one or both shoulders of the patient

Terms Related to Surgery or Treatment

amniocentesis	(am-nee-oh-sen-TEE-sis)	Transabdominal puncture of the amniotic sac and withdrawal of fluid for purposes of testing
cauterization	(kaw-ter-eye-ZAY-shun)	The destruction of tissue for therapeutic purposes. May be accomplished with a caustic agent, a

hot iron, or an electric current; cautery. If done with cold, is called cryocautery.

cesarean section	(seh-**SAY**-ree-an)	Delivery of a fetus by way of an incision through the abdominal and uterine walls
colpocleisis	(**kol**-poh-**KLIGH**-sis)	Surgical closure of the vaginal canal
colpohysterectomy	(**kol**-poh-**hihs**-ter-**ECK**-toh-mee)	Vaginal hysterectomy
colporrhaphy	(kol-**POHR**-ah-fee)	Suturing (stitching or closing) of the vagina
colpotomy	(kol-**POT**-oh-mee)	Incision of the vagina for entry into the cul de sac
culdocentesis	(**kul**-doh-sen-**TEE**-sis)	Obtaining fluid from the posterior vaginal cul de sac through a puncture or surgical incision of the vaginal wall
curettage	(**kyou**-reh-**TAHZH**)	Scraping of a cavity with a curet, a circular instrument with sharp edges, for the removal of growths or for obtaining a specimen for diagnosis. Also called *curettement*.
dilatation	(dill-ah-**TAY**-shun)	Expansion of an organ, opening, or vessel with a dilator
dilation and curettage (D & C)	(die-**LAY**-shun **kyou**-reh-**TAHZH**)	A surgical procedure during which the cervical canal is dilated and the lining of the uterine wall is scraped (curetted)
episioplasty	(eh-**piz**-ee-oh-**PLAS**-tee)	A plastic operation to repair the vulva
episiotomy	(eh-**piz**-ee-aht-oh-mee)	Surgical incision of the perineum to aid in delivery of a fetus and to avoid accidental laceration
fibroidectomy	(**figh**-broyd-**ECK**-toh-mee)	Excision of a fibroid tumor (fibroma) of the uterus
hysterectomy	(**his**-teh-**RECK**-toh-mee)	Surgical removal of the uterus

hysterosalpin-gectomy	(his-teh-roh-**SAL**-pin-**JECK**-toh-mee)	Excision of the uterus and uterine tubes
hysterosalpingo-oophorectomy	(**his**-teh-roh-sal-**ping**-goh-**oh**-awf-oh-**RECK**-toh-mee)	Surgical removal of the uterus, uterine tubes and ovaries
hysterotomy	(**his**-ter-**AHT**-oh-mee)	Incision of the uterus
lumpectomy	(lum-**PECK**-toh-mee)	Surgical removal of a tumor from the breast, without extension to other tissue or lymph nodes
mammoplasty	(**MAM**-oh-**plas**-tee)	Surgical reconstruction of the breasts which may include augmentation or reduction
mastectomy	(mass-**TECK**-toh-mee)	Surgical excision of a breast
oophorectomy	(**oh**-awf-oh-**RECK**-toh-me)	The surgical removal of an ovary or ovaries
panhysterectomy	(**pan**-his-teh-**RECK**-toh-me)	Total hysterectomy, including the uterus and cervix
radical mastectomy	(**RAD**-ih-kal mass-**TECK**-toh-mee)	Surgical procedure in the treatment of cancer to remove the breast, lymph nodes, and adjacent chest wall muscles
salpingectomy	(**sal**-pin-**JECK**-toh-mee)	Surgical removal of the uterine tube
salpingo-oophorectomy	(**sal**-ping-goh-**oh**-awf-oh-**RECK**-toh-mee)	Surgical removal of a uterine tube and ovary
tracheloplasty	(**TRAY**-keh-loh-**plas**-tee)	Surgical procedure to repair defects of the neck of the uterus
vaginoperineotomy	(**vaj**-ih-noh-**per**-ih-nee-**AHT**-oh-mee)	Surgical incision of the vagina and perineum to facilitate childbirth

11.1   Review: System

DIRECTIONS: Cover the left column while you complete the statements on the right side.

gynecology
The study of the female reproductive system is called _____ .

ovaries
The paired _____ are the female sex organs.

fallopian, oviducts
Joined to either side of the uterus, and extending laterally toward the ovaries are two tubes called _____ tubes, or _____ .

infundibulum
fimbriae
The funnel-shaped expansion of the tube near the ovary is the _____ , which is edged by irregular fringed processes called _____ .

body
cervix
The upper main portion of the uterus is the _____ , and the lower portion is the _____ .

perimetrium
myometrium
endometrium
Three separate layers together make up the wall of the uterus. The outer layer is the _____ ; the middle layer is the _____ ; and the inner layer is the _____ .

vagina
A fibromuscular tube, the _____ , extends from the uterus to the vestibule.

vulva
The _____ is a composite of the external genital structures of the female.

clitoris
The female counterpart of the male penis is the _____ .

perineum
The external floor of the pelvis, extending from the pubic arch to the coccyx, is the _____ .

ovaries
The primary source of estrogen is the _____ .

corpus luteum
Progesterone is secreted by the _____ and the placenta.

11.2   Review: Building Blocks

DIRECTIONS: Write the meanings of the following building blocks.

1. uni–   _____
2. pseudo–   _____
3. oophor/o   _____
4. leuk/o   _____
5. culd/o   _____
6. mast/o   _____
7. lact/o   _____
8. sym–   _____
9. tri–   _____
10. –cele   _____

Write the building blocks for the following terms:

11. amnion   _____
12. before, forward _____
13. neck, cervix _____
14. body   _____
15. urinary bladder _____
16. egg   _____
17. perineum   _____
18. rectum   _____
19. womb, uterus _____
20. vagina   _____

11.3 Review: Building Blocks

DIRECTIONS: Match the words in the right column with the building blocks in the left column. Write the letter in the space provided.

1. _____ alb/o	A. birth
2. _____ –arche	B. neck
3. _____ colp/o	C. first
4. _____ eu–	D. white
5. _____ galact/o	E. month
6. _____ gynec/o	F. all
7. _____ hyster/o	G. beginning
8. _____ men/o	H. labor, birth
9. _____ metr/o	I. good
10. _____ nat/i	J. none
11. _____ neo–	K. vagina
12. _____ nulli–	L. uterine tube
13. _____ pan–	M. near, beside
14. _____ para–	N. flow, discharge
15. _____ primi–	O. uterus, womb
16. _____ retro–	P. milk
17. _____ –rrhea	Q. uterus, womb
18. _____ salping/o	R. behind, back
19. _____ –tocia	S. new
20. _____ trachel/o	T. woman, female

11.4   Word Building

DIRECTIONS: Fill in the blanks with the appropriate building block or medical term.

1. The combining form for *birth* is _____ .
   A prefix meaning *before* is _____ .
   The word _____ means *before birth*.
   A prefix meaning *new* is _____ .
   The term for *newborn* is _____ .
2. The word _____ means *the process of giving birth.*
   A prefix indicating *after* or *following* is _____ .
   The word _____ means *after giving birth*.
   The word _____ means *before* giving birth.

3. The word ending _____ means *labor* or *birth*.
   A prefix for *slow* is _____ .
   _____ means *slow birth*.
   The prefix _____ means *difficult* or *painful*.
   _____ means *difficult* or abnormal labor.
   The prefix _____ means *good* or *normal*.
   Normal or natural labor and childbirth is called _____ .

4. The combining form for *vagina* is _____ .
   The suffix that means *suturing* is _____ .
   Suturing of the vagina is called _____ .
   The suffix for *incision* or *cutting* is _____ .
   Incision of the vagina is called _____ .

5. The combining form _____ means *month*.
   The suffix that means *flow* or *discharge* is _____ .
   The *normal discharge of the menses* is called _____ .
   _____ is the term for *scanty menstrual flow.*
   Painful menstruation is called _____ .

6. The combining form for *vulva* is _____ .
   A suffix for *surgical repair* is _____ .
   Surgical repair of the vulva is _____ .
   The suffix for *incision* or *cutting* is _____ .
   _____ is a surgical incision of the vulvar orifice.

7. _____ is a combining form for *uterus* or *womb*.
   The suffix for *inflammation* is _____ .
   The term for inflammation of the uterus is _____ .

8. A suffix meaning *excessive flow* or *hemorrhage* is _____ .
   _____ means prolonged uterine bleeding.
   _____ means excessive bleeding during the regular menstrual
   period.

9. The prefix for *false* is _____ .
   A word ending that means *pregnancy* is _____ .
   The term for *false pregnancy* is _____ .

10. The combining form for *uterine tube* is _____ .
    _____ means inflammation of the uterine tube.
    The prefix meaning *pus* is _____ .
    _____ means a collection of pus in a uterine tube.
    The prefix meaning *water* is _____ .
    A collection of watery fluid in a uterine tube is called _____ .

11. A prefix meaning *first* is _____ .

A woman who has produced one infant is a _____ .

A prefix meaning *two* or *twice* is _____ .

A woman who has given birth the second time is a _____ .

A prefix meaning *none* is _____ .

A woman who has borne no children is a _____ .

A prefix meaning *many* or *several* is _____ .

A _____ is a woman who has had two or more pregnancies resulting in viable fetuses.

12. The word _____ means a *turning.*

A prefix for *behind* or *back* is _____ .

_____ means the tipping of an entire organ backward.

13. Two combining forms meaning *breast* are _____ and

_____ .

_____ is a suffix meaning the *process of recording.*

The process of X-ray study of the breast is called _____ .

Inflammation of the breast is called _____ .

14. The suffix _____ means *beginning.*

The beginning of the menstrual function is _____ .

The end or cessation of the menstrual function is known as _____ .

15. A prefix for *white* is _____ .

A suffix meaning *flow* or *discharge* is _____ .

The word _____ means a whitish discharge from the vagina and uterine cavity.

11.5   Review: Vocabulary

DIRECTIONS: Match the terms in the first column with their definitions in the second column.

1. _____ adnexa
2. _____ areola
3. _____ cesarean section
4. _____ copulation
5. _____ corpus luteum
6. _____ curettage
7. _____ ectopic pregnancy
8. _____ fertilization
9. _____ fundus
10. _____ gamete

A. Removal of the fetus through the abdominal wall
B. A small yellow body that develops within a ruptured ovarian follicle
C. Mature reproductive cell
D. The union of an ovum with the spermatozoon of the male
E. Accessory parts of a structure
F. The bottom or base of anything
G. Sexual intercourse
H. A circular area of pigmentation around the nipple of the breast
I. Implantation of the fertilized ovum outside of the uterine cavity
J. Removal of growths from the wall of a cavity with a small instrument

11.6   Review: Vocabulary

DIRECTIONS: Match the terms in the first column with their definitions in the second column.

1. _____ gravida
2. _____ isthmus
3. _____ lactation
4. _____ orifice
5. _____ parturition
6. _____ perineum
7. _____ puerpera
8. _____ puerperium
9. _____ trimester
10. _____ zygote

A. The entrance or outlet of any cavity
B. The pelvic floor and the associated structures occupying the pelvic outlet
C. The act or process of giving birth to a child
D. A three-month period
E. A woman who has just given birth
F. A narrow passage connecting two cavities or two larger parts
G. The period or state of confinement after labor
H. A pregnant woman
I. The cell produced by gametes; the fertilized ovum
J. The secretion of milk

11.7 Review: Vocabulary

DIRECTIONS: Analyze the following surgical terms.

1. colpocleisis

   _____

2. hysterectomy

   _____

3. hysterolaparotomy

   _____

4. hysterosalpingo-oophorectomy

   _____

5. mammoplasty

   _____

6. mastectomy

   _____

7. oophorectomy

   _____

8. panhysterectomy

   _____

9. radical mastectomy

   _____

10. salpingo-oophorectomy

    _____

11. tracheloplasty

    _____

12. vaginoperineotomy

    _____

11.8   Review: Anatomy

DIRECTIONS: Identify the lettered structures of the female reproductive system in the diagram below.

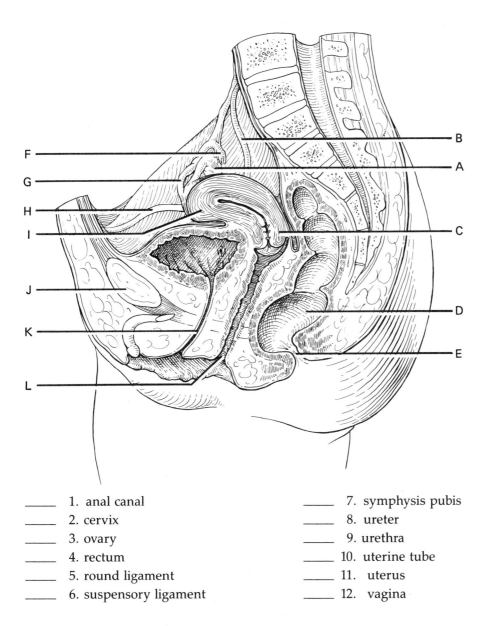

_____	1. anal canal
_____	2. cervix
_____	3. ovary
_____	4. rectum
_____	5. round ligament
_____	6. suspensory ligament

_____	7. symphysis pubis
_____	8. ureter
_____	9. urethra
_____	10. uterine tube
_____	11. uterus
_____	12. vagina

Reading Comprehension 11.1

DIRECTIONS: Underline the medical terms as you go through the reading exercise. Then list and analyze the terms. Some will be completely new to you. Consult a medical dictionary for their meanings. Then re-read the material for better comprehension.

Operation Record

Preoperative Diagnosis: Tumor of rt breast, probable carcinoma, rt breast

Postoperative Diagnosis: Carcinoma of right breast

Operation: Right radical mastectomy

Procedure:

This patient presented with a deep tumor in the upper outer quadrant of the right breast. At the time of biopsy this was grossly typical of a malignancy and this was confirmed by frozen section.

Initially a small transverse incision was made over the lesion and a portion of it excised for frozen section. The defect was packed with a Merthiolate silk sponge, and the wound sewn tight. The area was then reprepped and redraped and using new gauze, gowns, and instruments, the breast was circumscribed with the transverse elliptical incision; this was used because of the rather lateral position of the breast tumor with this incision providing wider encompassment. Flaps of skin and subcutaneous tissue were dissected superiorly up to the clavicle and inferiorly down over the rectus muscle following which the lower half of the pectoralis major muscle was outlined and separated from the upper half, and the lower portion was transected at its insertion into the humerus.

The pectoralis major muscle was reflected medially, the pectoralis minor muscle was transected at its insertion and reflected inferiorly. An axillary dissection was then performed, all fatty adventitious and lymphatic tissue being excised from the axillary space en masse, being left attached to the operative specimen. During the course of the axillary dissection, the long thoracic and thoracodorsal nerves were visualized and preserved. Following completion of the axillary dissection, the pectoral musculature was removed from the chest wall along with the overlying breast and the attached axillary contents en masse.

All suture material used was both silk and cotton and the wound was dry at the closure of the procedure. Because of the vascularity of the area in this particular patient, blood loss was more than usual, approximating 700 ml. Following completion of the procedure, the wound was irrigated with sterile saline. The HemoVac drains were then placed into the axillary space and under the lower skin flap and let out through stab wounds. The skin incision was then closed with moderate tension using interrupted silk.

The patient's condition throughout surgery was satisfactory and she left the operating room in good condition. Tissue as above to laboratory.

Reading Comprehension 11.2

DIRECTIONS: Underline the medical terms as you go through the reading exercise. Then list and analyze the terms. Some will be completely new to you. Consult a medical dictionary for their meanings. Then re-read the material for better comprehension.

Operation Record

Preoperative Diagnosis:

1. Pelvic pain of undetermined etiology
2. Dysfunctional uterine bleeding

Posteroperative Diagnosis:

1. Ectopic pregnancy, left fallopian tube, aborting in progress
2. Bilateral ovarian adhesions

What Was Done:

1. Laparoscopy
2. D&C
3. Pelvic exploratory laparotomy
4. Left salpingectomy

Procedure:
After satisfactory induction of assisted-inhalation cuffed endotracheal anesthesia, the patient was placed in the dorsolithotomy position in stirrups in 15 degree Trendelenburg position. The abdomen and perineum were prepped and draped in the usual fashion for pelvic surgery. The Veress needle was introduced through the umbilicus, and pneumoperitoneum was inducted utilizing carbon dioxide. Approximately 4.5 liters of carbon dioxide were used; the maximum filling pressure was 14 mm Hg. The rate of flow of carbon dioxide did not exceed 1 liter/min.

While pneumoperitoneum was being induced, attention was directed to the perineum. The anterior lip of the cervix was grasped with a Lahey tenaculum. The uterus was sounded to a depth of 10 cm. The lower endometrial cavity was nearly obliterated. It was very difficult to get the sound into the endometrial cavity.

The cervix was then dilated with a Goodell dilator. The endometrial cavity was explored and very abnormal-appearing prune-juice looking blood and histologic material was obtained. The endometrium was sharply curetted and a further amount of similar abnormal-appearing endometrial tissue was obtained. The Hulka sound cervical tenaculum instrument was applied. A #18 Foley with a 5 ml bag was placed in the urinary bladder.

Attention was next directed to the abdomen. A short, infraumbilical vertical incision was made through which the 11 mm ACMI laparoscopic trocar was introduced in Z-fashion. It could be immediately seen that the left fallopian tube was distended and appeared blue at its distal two-thirds; there was a large blood clot dropping out of the left fallopian tube from its fimbriated extremity. There were also numerous adhesions around the left ovary and also around the right ovary. In light of these circumstances, the laparoscope was removed after carbon dioxide was permitted to escape, and the infraumbilical incision was closed with Steristrips.

A pelvic exploratory operation was then performed utilizing a Pfannenstiel incision. The fascia was incised transversely, the recti were separated in the midline; the peritoneum was entered vertically. There was a small amount of dark blood in the cul-de-sac; there was also a large clot at the fimbriated extremity at the left fallopian tube and the distal two-thirds of the left fallopian tube was distended with what appeared to be blood. There were also numerous adhesions around the left ovary and around the right ovary. These were subsequently released. The uterus itself was somewhat larger than normal and seemed rather firm. A 00 suture was placed through the uterine fundus for traction and the left fallopian tube was then excised at the cornua by clamping the mesosalpinx in series, dividing and ligating with 00 chromic catgut stick ligatures. The fallopian tube was thus removed from its cornual insertion.

Peritonealization of the area was accomplished by bringing the round ligament over the area sutured on the mesosalpinx. The round ligament was attached to the uterine fundus with a series of interrupted 00 chromic catgut sutures. The appendix was inspected; it was grossly normal in appearance. The gallbladder was felt to be normal; there were no stones palpated. First sponge, instrument, needle count said to be correct by the circulating nurse, therefore closure of the abdominal wall in anatomic layers follows: Peritoneum running Vicryl 00 which was continued through the pyramidalis to the pubis; recti interrupted 00 Vicryl; fascia running 00 Vicryl with several interrupted left angle; 3–0 Vicryl interrupted subcutaneous, 1/4" Steristrips for the skin.

The patient withstood the operative procedure well, left the operating room for the recovery room with normal vital signs and crystal clear urine.

Reading Comprehension Vocabulary

Use the space below to list the medical terms for analysis and definition.

_____

_____

_____

_____

_____

_____

_____

_____

_____

_____

_____

_____

_____

_____

_____

_____

_____

_____

_____

_____

_____

_____

_____

_____

_____

_____

_____

_____

CHAPTER 12

Urinary System

OBJECTIVES

When you have successfully completed Chapter 12, you should be able to:
— Recall terms describing the anatomy and physiology of the urinary tract.
— Define the building blocks introduced in this chapter.
— Define common terms referring to the urinary system.
— Recall the medical terms for words defined in this chapter.
— Identify the structures of the urinary system in a familiar drawing.
— Build medical terms using the building blocks introduced in this and previous chapters.

KEY TERMS

concave	(KON-kayv)	Curved or rounded in an inward direction
conical	(KON-ih-kal)	Cone-shaped
convex	(KON-vecks)	Curved or rounded in an outward direction
filtrate	(FILL-trayt)	Fluid that has passed through a filter
granular	(GRAN-you-lar)	Roughened by grainy, raised areas
lateral	(LAT-er-al)	At or having to do with the side
medial	(MEE-dee-al)	At or occurring in the middle
parietal	(pah-RYE-eh-tal)	Related to the walls of an organ or cavity; for example, the parietal cells of the kidney
peristalsis	(per-ih-STAL-sis)	Involuntary, rhythmic wavelike movement in tubular body structures such as the ureters
peritoneum	(per-ih-toh-NEE-um)	The serous membrane that lines the abdominal cavity and envelops the abdominal organs, helping to keep them in position
reservoir	(REZ-er-vwar)	A place in which a liquid is stored

OVERVIEW

The *urinary system* (Figure 12.1) has three major functions:

- The production of urine by removal of wastes such as *urea* from the tissues and organs by way of the bloodstream
- Removal from the bloodstream of excess useful materials, such as excess sugar or protein
- Assisting in the maintenance of *homeostasis* (1) by regulating the balance of chemicals known as electrolytes, especially sodium (salt) and potassium in the blood and tissues; (2) by regulating the amount of fluid (water) in the blood and tissues; and (3) by regulating the acidity of the blood

Kidneys that are functioning well also conserve substances that the body needs. These substances, such as electrolytes, are reabsorbed from the filtered fluid produced

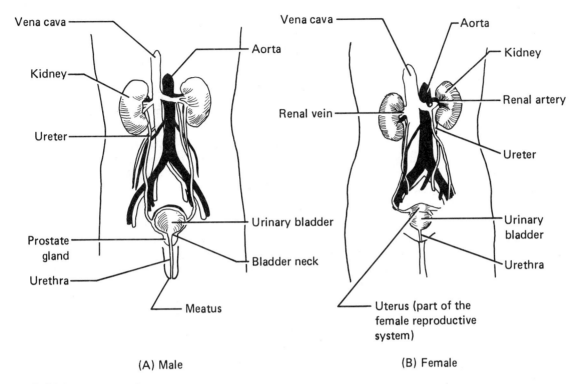

Vena cava

Kidney

Ureter

Prostate
gland

Urethra

Aorta

Urinary bladder

Bladder neck

Meatus

(A) Male

Vena cava

Renal vein

Uterus (part of the
female reproductive
system)

Aorta

Kidney

Renal artery

Ureter

Urinary
bladder

Urethra

(B) Female

FIGURE 12.1   Urinary system

by the renal tubules (tubular filtrate). Harmful substances, such as urea, are rejected by the kidney and excreted. The amount of such substances in the urine is an indicator of health or disease.

The foregoing functions are all related in some way to the production and excretion of urine. In addition, the kidneys play a role in the formation of red blood cells by secreting the hormone *erythropoietin*. They help regulate blood pressure in a complex process that involves the enzyme renin, which the kidneys produce; and they affect the body's absorption of calcium by activating vitamin D.

The urinary system consists of two kidneys, which produce urine; two ureters, which carry the urine from the kidneys to the urinary bladder; the urinary bladder, which stores the urine until a sufficient amount has accumulated to trigger the nerve signals for discharge, or voiding, and the *urethra*, through which the urine is discharged. These organs are referred to by their names; however, certain structures of the kidney are more commonly described by the adjective *renal* (for example, the renal pelvis), and certain structures of the bladder are referred to by the adjective *vesical* (for example, the *vesical trigone*). You may also, however, find "kidney" and "bladder" used as adjectives. Both forms are given here.

Urology is the branch of medicine concerned with the urinary tract in men, women, and children and the genital tract in the male. Physicians who specialize in this branch of medicine are called urologists.

KIDNEYS

The kidneys (Figure 12.2) are the principal functional organs of the urinary system; the other organs serve mainly in transporting and excretion of urine. They lie behind the peritoneum on either side of the vertebral column, extending from the twelfth thoracic vertebra (T_{12}) downward to the level of the third lumbar vertebra (L_3). The right kidney lies just below the liver. These bean-shaped organs are about 4 to 6 inches long and 2 inches wide. Anatomically, the kidney is divided into two distinct regions or zones (Figure 12.3). The outer region, the *renal cortex*, encloses the *renal medulla*, which is composed of conical masses of tissue called *renal pyramids*.

The lateral surface of each kidney is convex; the medial side is concave. The medial depression leads into a hollow chamber, the *renal sinus*, by way of the *hilum*. The hilum contains the major blood vessels and nerves that supply the kidney, as well as the continuation of the upper end of the ureter. This funnel-shaped structure is called the *renal pelvis* or the pelvis of the kidney.

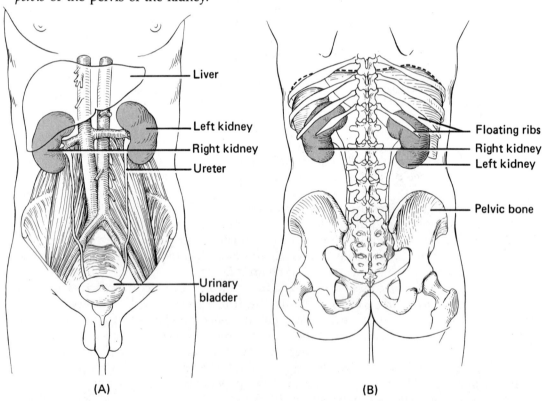

(A)   (B)

Position of kidneys anteriorly   **Position of kidneys posteriorly**

FIGURE 12.2   Locations of the kidneys

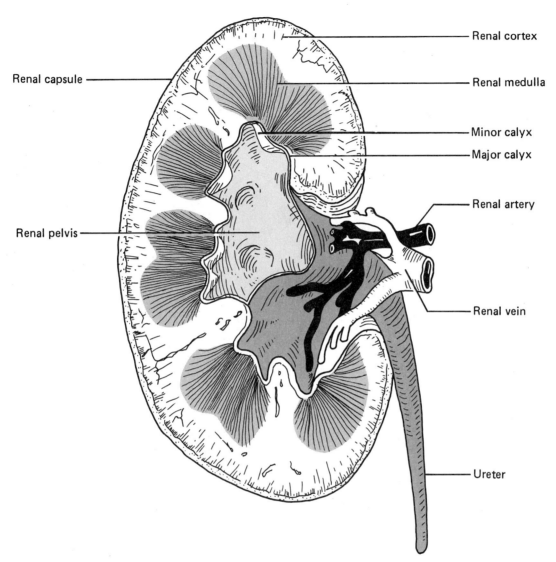

Renal capsule

Renal pelvis

Renal cortex

Renal medulla

Minor calyx

Major calyx

Renal artery

Renal vein

Ureter

FIGURE 12.3   Longitudinal section through kidney

The renal pelvis divides into two, sometimes three, large branches called *major calices* (sometimes spelled *calyces*), and each renal calyx (the singular) divides again into short branches named *minor calices*. Numerous nipplelike elevations on the wall of the renal sinus, *renal papillae,* have tiny openings into the minor calices.

The calices, in turn, are composed of *nephrons* (Figure 12.4), the structural and functional unit of the kidney. These structures are so tiny that each kidney contains about one million of them, yet their structure is extremely complex. Each nephron consists of a *renal corpuscle* and a *renal tubule*. The actual filtration of impurities and exchange of elec-

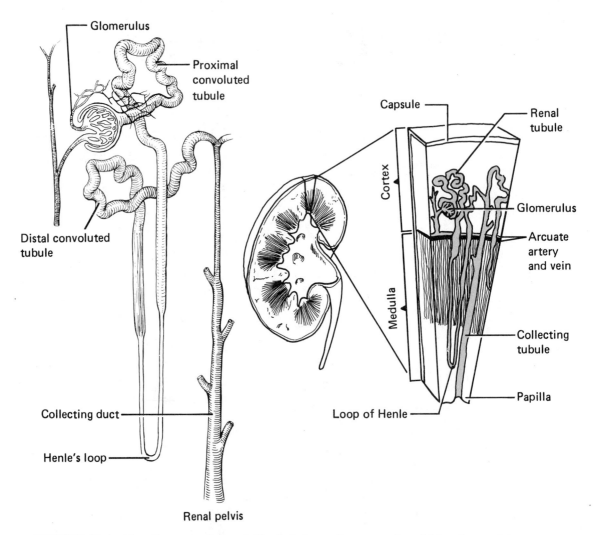

FIGURE 12.4   Renal corpuscles and Henle's loop (less associated blood supply)

trolytes takes place in the tangled clusters of blood capillaries, called a *glomeruli* (singular, *glomerulus*) of which the renal corpuscles are formed. The functional structures of the nephron are surrounded by a thin-walled, saclike structure called *Bowman's capsule.*

URETERS

Each kidney is drained by a *ureter,* which conducts urine to the urinary bladder. The ureters are 10 to 12 inches long. They lie behind the parietal peritoneum and extend from the hilum of the kidney to the urinary bladder, entering the bladder through its posterior surface. Urine collects in the renal pelvis, the expanded upper end of the ureter lying inside the kidney, before it passes by peristaltic contractions through the ureter to the bladder.

URINARY BLADDER

The urinary bladder is a flexible reservoir for urine. Its capacity ranges from about 1 to 3 cups of liquid. The *vesical trigone* is a triangular area formed by the two ureteral openings and the single urethral opening.

URETHRA

The function of the *urethra* is to transport urine to the outside of the body. The urinary sphincter holds urine until the signal for excretion is received from the nervous system.

Female Urethra

The female urethra is a tubular structure extending about 1.5 inches from the bladder to the outside orifice. This opening is called the *urinary meatus* and is located anterior to the opening of the vagina. Urethral glands open at the side of the orifice. The short length of the female urethra makes it easy for external bacteria to reach the bladder and cause infection.

Male Urethra

The male urethra is about 8 inches (20 cm) long, and is smaller in diameter than the female urethra. It transports both urine and male reproductive fluid (semen). Because of this dual function, the male reproductive and urinary system are often called the *genitourinary* system. The reproductive system of the male is discussed in Chapter 10.

URINE

The process of passing urine is called *voiding, micturition,* or *urination.* Laboratory examination of the urine, called *urinalysis,* is a routine part of most medical examinations because examination of the urine, like examination of the blood, yields clues to a vast number of health problems.

Normal Urine

About 95 percent of normal urine consists of water. The remainder is composed of metabolic wastes such as urea and *uric acid,* mineral salts such as sodium and potassium, and a pigment called *urochrome,* which gives the urine its color.

Abnormal Urine

A number of substances indicate a disease condition if they appear in the urine. The presence in the urine of blood (*hematuria*), sugar (*glycosuria*), or pus (*pyuria*) is a danger signal. If urination is painful (*dysuria*) or if an unusually great amount of urine (*polyuria*) or an unusually small amount of urine (*oliguria*) is passed, there is cause for further investigation. The complete absence of urination (*anuria*) may indicate a very dangerous situation.

BUILDING BLOCKS

ROOTS AND COMBINING FORMS

Word Elements	Meaning
cyst/o	urinary bladder, cyst, sac
flux	flow
glyc/o	sweet; pertaining to glucose
hemat/o	blood
home/o	same, similar
hydr/o	water
keton	ketone, acetone
lith/o	stone
lytos	soluble
meat/o	meatus
nephr/o	kidney
noct	night
olig/o	scanty
pyel/o	renal pelvis
ren/o	kidney
scler/o	hardening
ureter/o	ureter

SUFFIXES

Word Elements	Meaning
–itis	inflammation
–lysis	breakdown, separation
–oma	tumor
–pexy	fixation, putting in place
–poiesis	making
–ptosis	dropping, prolapse
–stasis	standing
–tripsy	crushing
–uria	urination, urine

Word Elements	Meaning
an–	no, not, without
dia–	through
pyo–	pus
re–	back
uro–	urine, urinary tract

VOCABULARY

General Terms

antidiuretic	(**AN**-tih-die-you-**RET**-ick)	Reducing urine output, or a drug that does so
calculus	(**KAL**-kyou-lus)	Commonly called stone; any abnormal concretion within the animal body
catheter	(**KATH**-eh-ter)	A tubular instrument passed into the body through a vessel or natural orifice for the purpose of withdrawing fluid from or injecting fluid into a body cavity.
cystoscope	(**SIS**-toh-skohp)	An instrument that is passed through the urethra for interior examination of the bladder and ureters
diuretic	(**die**-you-**RET**-ick)	Increasing production and output of urine, or, a drug that does so
electrolyte	(ee-**LECK**-troh-light)	Any solution that conducts electricity; in the human body, mainly salts of sodium, potassium, and chlorine in the blood and tissues
erythropoietin	(eh-**rith**-roh-**POY**-eh-tin)	A hormone that stimulates red blood cell production
filtration	(fill-**TRAY**-shun)	Natural or artificial removal of particles from a solution (such as

		blood) by passing it through a membrane; a kind of sieving
homeostasis	(hoh-mee-oh-STAY-sis)	Maintaining a state of equilibrium of the internal environment of the body
hyaline cast	(high-ah-line)	The commonest form of cast found in the urine
micturition	(MICK-too-RISH-un)	The voiding of urine; urination
nitrogenous waste	(nigh-TRAHJ-eh-nus)	Wastes that contain nitrogen (wastes from protein)
pH		The degree of acidity or alkalinity of a substance expressed as a potential of hydrogen
reflux	(REE-flucks)	A return or backward flow
residual urine	(reh-ZIJ-you-al)	Urine left in the bladder after urination; occurs if flow is blocked
urologist	(you-ROL-oh-jist)	A physician who specializes in diseases of the urinary tract
urology	(you-ROL-oh-jee)	The branch of medicine concerned with the urinary tract in both sexes and the genital tract in the male
vesical	(VES-ih-kal)	Pertaining to or shaped like a bladder
vesicle	(VES-ih-kal)	A small sac or bladder containing fluid
void	(voyd)	To evacuate the bowels or bladder; most often used to refer to urination

Terms Related to Anatomy and Physiology

Bowman's capsule		The renal structure that serves as a filter when urine is formed
calyx (calix)	(KAH-licks)	Any cuplike organ or cavity. Plural, *calyces* or *calices*
glomerulus	(glow-MER-you-lus)	One of the tiny urine-forming structures of the kidney

hilum, hilus	(**HIGH**-lum, **HIGH**-lus)	The large opening at the medial edge of the kidney through which blood vessels enter and leave the kidney
meatus	(mee-**AY**-tus)	A passage or opening in soft tissue; for example, the urethral meatus
medulla	(meh-**DULL**-ah)	Inner or central portion of an organ in contrast to the outer portion or cortex
nephron	(**NEF**-ron)	The structural and functional unit of the kidney
papilla	(pah-**PILL**-ah)	A small, nipplelike protuberance or elevation
parenchyma	(pah-**RENG**-kih-mah)	The essential parts of an organ that are concerned with its function; for example, the renal parenchyma
renal corpuscle	(**KOR**-pus-ul)	The renal corpuscle is made up of a tuft of blood vessels (the glomerulus) contained within a capsule; found at the proximal end of each renal tubule
renal cortex	(**KOR**-tecks)	The outer covering of the kidney, surrounding the medulla
renal pelvis	(**PEL**-vis)	A funnel-shaped expansion at the proximal end of the ureter that receives the urine through the major calyces.
renal pyramids	(**PEER**-ah-midz)	The cone-shaped structures that compose the medulla of the kidney
renal sinus	(**SIGH**-nus)	The area in the kidney composed of the renal pelvis, renal calyces, vessels, nerves, and fatty tissues
renal tubules	(**TOO**-byoulz)	The tubules that connect the glomeruli to the renal pelvis
renal veins		Short thick venous trunks that pass from the kidneys to the inferior vena cava.

renin	(REE-nin)	An enzyme produced by the kidney and involved in maintaining blood pressure by regulating excretion or conservation of fluid
Skene's glands	(SKEENZ glanz)	Paired glands that lie just inside of and on the posterior of the female urethra
trigone	(TRY-gohn)	A triangular area at the base of the bladder
urea	(you-REE-ah)	The chief nitrogenous constituent of urine
ureters	(you-REE-terz)	The paired tubes that carry urine from the kidneys to the bladder
urethra	(you-REE-thrah)	A passage for the discharge of urine extending from the bladder to the exterior of the body
uric acid	(YOU-rick AS-sid)	A crystalline acid often found in urinary and renal calculi
urinary bladder		Temporary reservoir for urine formed and excreted by the kidneys

Terms Related to Pathology and Laboratory Procedures

acetonuria	(ass-eh-toh-NEW-ree-ah)	An excess of acetone bodies in the urine; ketonuria
albuminuria	(AL-byou-mih-NEW-ree-ah)	Presence in the urine of serum albumin; proteinuria
anuria	(ah-NEW-ree-ah)	Absence of urine formation
cystitis	(sis-TIE-tis)	Inflammation of the bladder, acute or chronic
diabetes insipidus	(die-ah-BEE-teez in-SIP-ih-dus)	A disease characterized by excessive urination and excessive thirst caused by inadequte secretion of vasopressin, the antidiuretic hormone
diabetes mellitus	(die-ah-BEE-teez MELL-ih-tus, mell-LIE-tus)	A metabolic disorder caused by inadequate production or utilization of insulin, and characterized by

		elevated levels of blood sugar and glucose in the urine
diuresis	(**die**-you-**REE**-sis)	The secretion and passage of excessive amounts of urine; may be an early symptom of diabetes mellitus
dysuria	(dis-**YOU**-ree-ah)	Painful or difficult urination
enuresis	(**en**-you-**REE**-sis)	Involuntary urination; often used specifically to indicate bedwetting
glomerulonephritis	(glow-**mer**-you-loh-neh-**FRY**-tis)	Inflammation of the kidney involving primarily the glomeruli
glycosuria	(**glie**-koh-**SOO**-ree-ah)	The presence of glucose in the urine
hematuria	(**hem**-ah-**TOO**-ree-ah)	Blood in the urine
hydronephrosis	(**high**-droh-nah-**FROH**-sis)	Abnormal collection of urine in the renal pelvis due to obstruction
hypernephroma	(**high**-per-neh-**FROH**-mah)	A malignant tumor of the kidney
incontinence	(in-**KON**-tih-nens)	Inability to retain urine, semen, or feces
ketonuria	(**kee**-toh-**NEW**-ree-ah)	Acetone bodies in the urine
nephritis	(neh-**FRY**-tis)	Inflammation of the kidney
nephrolithiasis	(**nef**-row-lih-**THIGH**-ah-sis)	The presence of stones in the kidney
nephropathy	(neh-**FROP**-ah-thee)	Kidney disease
nephroptosis	(**nef**-rop-**TOH**-sis)	Prolapse or downward displacement of the kidney
nephrosclerosis	(**nef**-roh-sklee-**ROH**-sis)	Sclerosis (hardening) of renal tissues
nocturia	(nock-**TOO**-ree-ah)	Excessive urination during the night
oliguria	(ol-ih-**GOO**-ree-ah)	Scanty formation or discharge of urine
phenylketonuria	(**fen**-ill-**key**-toh-**NEW**-ree-ah)	An inborn disorder of phenylalanine metabolism that may be fatal early in life unless treated early by a diet low in the amino acid, phenylalanine (used in the

sweetener *Equal* and found in many foods). Some states require a test for this condition at birth.

polyuria	(POL-ee-YOU-ree-ah)	Excessive secretion and discharge of urine
pyelitis	(pie-eh-LIE-tis)	Inflammation of the pelvis of the kidney and its calyces
pyelonephritis	(pie-eh-loh-neh-FRY-tis)	Inflammation of the body and pelvis of the kidney
pyuria	(pie-YOU-ree-ah)	Pus in the urine, evidence of renal disease
uremia	(you-REE-mee-ah)	Toxic condition caused by retention in the blood of nitrogenous substances that are normally excreted by the kidney
ureterocele	(you-REE-ter-oh-seel)	An abnormal dilatation and protrusion of the end of the ureter into the bladder
urethritis	(you-ree-THRIGH-tis)	Inflammation of the urethra
urinary stress incontinence		Inability to prevent urination during stressful conditions such as lifting, sudden movement, laughing, coughing, or sneezing
urinary retention		Inability to expel urine
uropathy	(you-ROP-ah-thee)	Any disease affecting the urinary tract
Wilms' tumor	(vilmz TOO-mer)	Named for Marx Wilms, German surgeon, 1867–1918. Rapidly developing malignant tumor of the kidney that usually occurs in children

Terms Related to Diagnostic Procedures

cystogram	(SIS-toh-gram)	X-ray of the bladder
pyelogram	(PIE-eh-loh-gram)	X-ray of the ureter and renal pelvis. An *intravenous pyelogram* (IVP)

| | | involves injection of dye; also called an *excretory* urogram. |
| urinalysis | (**you**-rih-**NAHL**-ih-sis) | Physical, chemical, and/or microscopic analysis or examination of the urine |

Terms Related to Function Replacement Procedures

| dialysis | (**die-AHL**-ih-sis) | Basically the passage of a solute through a membrane. The general term *renal dialysis* refers to artificial removal by dialysis of substances normally removed by the kidneys. The two techniques of renal dialysis are *hemodialysis,* in which the blood is pumped through a kidney machine, and *peritoneal dialysis,* in which liquid is instilled into the peritoneal (abdominal) cavity, for removal by fluid exchange through the peritoneal membrane. |

Terms Related to Surgery

lithotripsy	(**LITH**-oh-**trip**-see)	Crushing of a calculus
meatotomy	(**mee**-ah-**TOT**-oh-me)	Incision of the urinary meatus to enlarge the opening
nephrectomy	(neh-**FRECK**-toh-mee)	Removal of a kidney
nephropexy	(**NEF**-roh-**peck**-see)	Surgical attachment of a floating or dropped kidney to improve its drainage
pyelolithotomy	(**pie**-eh-loh-lih-**THOT**-oh-mee)	Removal of stone from the renal pelvis through an incision
pyeloplasty	(**PIE**-eh-loh-**plas**-tee)	Reparative surgery on the renal pelvis of the kidney
renal transplantation	(**REE**-nal **trans**-plan-**TAY**-shun)	Surgical implantation of a donor kidney after removing the patient's kidney

12.1   Review: System

DIRECTIONS: Cover the left column while you complete the statements on the right side.

urinary tract   Urology is concerned with the _____
genital tract   in men, women, and children, and the
                           _____ in the male.

kidneys, ureters   The organs of the urinary system are:
bladder, urethra   _____
                           _____

peritoneum   The kidneys lie behind the _____
vertebral column   on either side of the _____
thoracic   extending from the 12th _____
lumbar   vertebra to the level of the 3rd _____
                           vertebra.

renal cortex   The outer region of the kidney is called the
                           _____ .

medulla   The inner region of the kidney is called the
                           _____ .

nephron   The structural and functional unit of the kidney is
                           the _____ .

ureter   The _____ conducts urine from
                           the kidney to the urinary bladder.

1 to 3   The urinary bladder has a holding capacity of about
                           _____ cups of liquid.

urethra   The function of the _____ is to
                           transport urine to the outside of the body.

12.2 Review: Building Blocks

DIRECTIONS: Match the words in the second column with their medical equivalents in the first column.

_____ 1. flux		A.	acetone
_____ 2. home/o		B.	crushing
_____ 3. hydr/o		C.	fixation
_____ 4. ketone		D.	flow
_____ 5. –pexy		E.	making
_____ 6. lith/o		F.	meatus
_____ 7. lytos		G.	night
_____ 8. met/o		H.	same
_____ 9. noct–		I.	soluble
_____ 10. –poiesis		J.	standing
_____ 11. –stasis		K.	stone
_____ 12. –tripsy		L.	water

12.3 Review: Building Blocks

DIRECTIONS: Write the meanings of the following building blocks.

1. an–	_____	11. –pexy	_____
2. cyst/o	_____	12. –ptosis	_____
3. dia–	_____	13. pyel/o	_____
4. glyc/o	_____	14. pyo–	_____
5. hemat/o	_____	15. re–	_____
6. –itis	_____	16. ren/o	_____
7. –lysis	_____	17. sclerosis	_____
8. nephr/o	_____	18. ureter/o	_____
9. olig/o	_____	19. –uria	_____
10. –oma	_____	20. uro–	_____

12.4   Review: Word Building

DIRECTIONS: Write the appropriate building blocks and terms in the blanks.

1. The word ending _____ means *urination* or *urine*.
   The prefix _____ means painful or difficult.
   _____ is painful or difficult urination.
   The prefix _____ means *not* or *without*.
   _____ is absence of urine formation.
   The combining form _____ means *glucose*.
   _____ is the presence of glucose in the urine.

2. A combining form for *blood* is _____ .
   The condition of blood in the urine is called _____ .
   The prefix for *scanty* or *diminished* is _____ .
   _____ is a diminished amount of urine formation.
   The prefix _____ means *excessive*.
   _____ means excessive secretion and discharge of urine.

3. The prefix that means *pus* is _____ .
   Pus in the urine is called _____ .
   The combining form for *night* is _____ .
   _____ means excessive urination at night.

4. The combining form for *bladder* is _____ .
   _____ is a suffix meaning *a record*.
   An X-ray of the bladder is called a/an _____ .
   The suffix _____ describes an instrument for viewing.
   An instrument for viewing the bladder is a _____ .

5. The combining form for *kidney* is _____ .
   _____ means the presence of stones.
   Presence of stones in a kidney is called _____ .

6. The combining form for *urine* is _____ .
   The suffix _____ indicates a *disease process*.
   _____ is any disease affecting the urinary tract.

7. The combining form _____ means *same* or *similar*.
   _____ is a suffix that means *standing*.
   A state of equilibrium of the internal environment of the body is referred to as
   _____ .

8. The combining form for *stone* is _____ .
   The suffix _____ describes *crushing*.
   Crushing of a stone in the bladder or urethra is _____ .

9. The combining form for *kidney pelvis* is _____ .

   The suffix _____ indicates *surgical repair.*

   _____ means surgical repair of the kidney pelvis.

   A suffix meaning *a record* is _____ .

   An X-ray of the ureter and kidney pelvis is called a _____ .

10. The combining form for *ureter* is _____ .

    The suffix _____ indicates *dilatation* or *hernia.*

    A cystlike dilatation of the ureter near its opening into the bladder is called a/an

    _____ .

12.5   Review: Vocabulary

Match the terms in the first column with their definitions in the second column.

1. _____ antidiuretic
2. _____ calyx
3. _____ dialysis
4. _____ enuresis
5. _____ incontinence
6. _____ micturition
7. _____ nephron
8. _____ reflux
9. _____ renal cortex
10. _____ renin
11. _____ trigone
12. _____ urinalysis
13. _____ vesical
14. _____ vesicle

A. The inability to retain urine
B. An enzyme produced by the kidney
C. Structural and functional unit of the kidney
D. Pertaining to or shaped like a bladder
E. A return or backward flow
F. The outer covering of the kidney
G. Physical, chemical, or microscopic analysis or examination of the urine
H. The passage of a solute through a membrane
I. Small sac or blader containing fluid
J. Any cuplike organ or cavity
K. A hormone or drug that decreases urine secretion
L. Voiding of urine
M. Triangular space at base of bladder
N. Involuntary urination, especially at night

12.6   Review Anatomy

DIRECTIONS: Identify the numbered structures in the figures below.

A. Male

1. _____
2. _____
3. _____
4. _____
5. _____
6. _____
7. _____
8. _____
9. _____

B. Female

1. _____
2. _____
3. _____
4. _____
5. _____
6. _____
7. _____
8. _____
9. _____

(A) Male

(B) Female

Reading Comprehension 12.1

DIRECTIONS: Underline the medical terms as you go through the reading exercise. Then list and analyze the terms. Some will be completely new to you. Consult a medical dictionary for their meanings. Then re-read the material for better comprehension.

Operation Record

Preoperative Diagnosis: Renal failure

Postoperative Diagnosis: Same

Operation: Insertion of Scribner shunt for hemodialysis

Procedure:

The patient was placed in the supine position on the operating table and an axillary block was performed by the anesthesiologist. The entire upper extremity was then thoroughly prepared with Betadine and appropriately draped. A vertical incision was made directly over the radial artery at the wrist and dissection carried down through the subcutaneous tissue to expose a segment of the radial artery. A pledget of cotton containing Regitine was placed on this structure and attention was then directed to search for a large vein. On the radial aspect of the arm the cephalic vein was encountered and was found to be of satisfactory size. A portion of this vein was freed and mobilized for the venous side of the shunt. At this point the distal vein was ligated with a 3–0 silk suture. A bulldog clamp was placed on the proximal vein and incision made on this structure. The distal exit wound was then made in the wrist and a Scribner shunt tube brought through this distal wound into the primary field. An appropriate vessel tip was inserted into the tube, which was then filled with heparinized saline. The vessel tip was then inserted into the vein and secured with a 3–0 silk suture. Heparinized saline was then used to irrigate into the vein and flow appeared without difficulty. Attention was then directed to the artery. The distal artery was ligated and the vascular clamp applied to the proximal portion of the vessel. An incision was made in the artery and using the lacrimal duct probes the vessel was adequately dilated for insertion of the vessel tip. Another distal puncture incision was made in line with the artery and a Silastic tube brought through this wound into the primary field. The vessel tip was then inserted into the artery and secured with a 3–0 silk. Flow was permitted and found to be excellent. The excess shunt tubing was then cut off and a bridge connector used to connect the two sides of the shunt. An excellent flow was noted. The wound was then closed in layers using 3–0 chromic in the subcutaneous tissue and 4–0 polyethylene in the skin. A dry sterile dressing was applied. A plaster splint was also applied and held in place with bias stockinette.

The patient appeared to have tolerated the procedure well and was taken to recovery room in satisfactory condition.

Reading Comprehension 12.2

DIRECTIONS: Underline the medical terms as you go through the reading exercise. Then list and analyze the terms. Some will be completely new to you. Consult a medical dictionary for their meanings. Then re-read the material for better comprehension.

Discharge Summary

Date Admitted: _____   Date Discharged: _____

Admitting Diagnosis:

1. Incapacitating interstitial cystitis
2. Elevated liver enzymes
3. Restrictive lung disease
4. Aortic insufficiency
5. Mitral regurgitation
6. Sclerosing mediastinitis

Discharge Diagnosis:

1. Incapacitating interstitial cystitis
2. Elevated liver enzymes
3. Restrictive lung disease
4. Aortic insufficiency
5. Mitral regurgitation
6. Sclerosing mediastinitis

Operations Performed:
12/01/— Anterior exenteration with ureteroileal cutaneous urinary diversion via a continent Kock ileostomy, appendectomy, temporary gastrostomy tube, liver biopsy. Placement of right subclavian line on 12/05/—.

History of Present Illness:
This 73-year-old white female has biopsy-proven incapacitating interstitial cystitis with frequency and nocturia. She is essentially a bladder cripple. Previously, she had undergone bladder biopsy which revealed no cancer, tuberculosis or fungal elements. She had failed essentially every treatment possible, including experimental parenteral Elmiron, as well as laser treatment.

Past Medical History:
Significant primarily for superior vena cava syndrome, secondary to sclerosing mediastinitis. Aortic insufficiency. Elevated liver enzymes. Restrictive pulmonary disease.

Allergies:
See admission history and physical.

Review of Systems:
Please refer to admission history and physical.

Physical Examination:
Please refer to admission history and physical for pertinent findings.

Hospital Course:
The patient was brought in and the patient underwent the standard neomycin/Neoloid bowel prep. It was modified because of her erythromycin allergy and Keflex was used instead. She was evaluated by Dr. A. and subsequent pulmonary function studies revealed a mild restrictive ventilatory defect which responded to bronchodilators. She was evaluated by Dr. B., who followed her closely through the hospitalization. On 12/01/—, she underwent the above surgical procedure, which was remarkably uneventful. She received her autologous blood in addition to blood captured and retrieved by the Cell Saver. She did not require any other blood products. Postoperatively, she was kept in the intensive care unit and did quite well. Initially, her sugars were elevated to the 300 range, but rapidly fell to normal. During her hospitalization, careful attention was paid to her potassium level and digoxin level, which remained therapeutic. She had mild fever postoperatively, which was attributed to atelectasis, and her intake and output were satisfactory with an expected positive balance that was later stabilized. Her ureteral stents were removed by about her 8th postoperative day and she had rapid return of bowel function. By discharge she was tolerating a regular diet with minimal need for analgesics and had assumed care of her Medena tube, which she was irrigating.

On her fourth postoperative day, because of poor intravenous access, a right subclavian line was placed, which was subsequently removed when she was able to tolerate regular diet. She met with the enterostomal therapist during her hospitalization for her pouch training.

Discharge Medications:
Premarin 0.625 mg per day, Duricef b.i.d, Tylenol #3 p.r.n, and she was continued on her digoxin 0.25 alternating with 0.125 mg per day.

Condition on Discharge:
Pathology showed significant interstitial cystitis in the bladder, small leiomyoma and chronic cervicitis in the uterus, cystic follicles in the fallopian tubes, a normal appendix, a liver biopsy that showed moderate fatty change with nonspecific triaditis, and an inactive granuloma. On 12/11/— her GGT was 80 and her AST was 42 with an ALT of 72 and bilirubin of 0.2 and LDH of 183. Alkaline phosphatase was 96. That same day, potassium was 4.3, BUN 18, creatinine 1.2. Histoplasmosis serology showed a yeast phase titer of 1:8 and a mycelial titer of less than 1:8. Histoplasmosis serology, ID on the first specimen was negative. Cocci routine serology, CF titer was less than 1:2, and the cocci serology ID specimen was negative. The cocci serology, LA, was negative. Total iron was 18 and

hematocrit on 12/11/— was 36.6 with a WBC of 9.9 and a normal differential. Postoperative chest x-rays were unremarkable except atelectasis in the right lung base.

Discharge Activity:
Discussed with patient. Office follow-up in one week.

_____ M.D.
Signature

Reading Comprehension Vocabulary

Use the space below to list the medical terms for analysis and definition.

_____
_____
_____
_____
_____
_____
_____
_____
_____
_____
_____
_____
_____
_____
_____
_____
_____
_____
_____
_____
_____
_____
_____
_____
_____

CHAPTER 13

Endocrine System

OBJECTIVES

When you have successfully completed Chapter 13, you should be able to:

— Recall terms relating to the structure and function of the endocrine glands.
— Write the meanings of building blocks introduced in this chapter.
— Name the five major glands of the endocrine system.
— Recall the regulatory functions of the thyroid gland
— Build medical terms using the building blocks introduced in this and previous chapters
— Identify endocrine glands on a familiar drawing

KEY TERMS

acceleration	(ack-**sell**-er-**AY**-shun)	Increasing speed
adolescence	(**add**-oh-**LES**-ens)	The period of life between the onset of puberty and maturity
anterior	(an-**TEE**-ree-er)	Before, in front of
asthmatic	(as-**MAT**-ick)	Pertaining to or having asthma
atrophy	(**AT**-roh-fee)	A wasting away from lack of nourishment or from disuse
carbohydrate	(**kar**-boh-**HIGH**-drayt)	One of the three classes of food; includes sugars, glycogen, starches, dextrins, and cellulose
endocrine gland	(**EN**-doh-krin)	Ductless gland that produces an internal secretion
exocrine glands	(**ECK**-soh-krin)	Glands that secrete their products into ducts that open onto some internal or external surface of the body
fat		One of the three classes of foods. Fats serve as a source of energy.
hormone	(**HOR**-mohn)	A substance produced by ductless glands that exerts control over many of the body processes
hyperactivity	(**high**-per-ack-**TIV**-ih-tee)	Increased or excessive activity of organism or any organ, part, or system
hyperthyroidism	(**high**-per-**THIGH**-royd-izm)	Condition caused by excessive secretion of the thyroid gland
hypoactivity	(**high**-poh-ack-**TIV**-ih-tee)	Decreased activity
lipid	(**LIP**-id)	Any one of a group of fats or fatlike substances
protein	(**PRO**-tee-in)	One of the three classes of food. Proteins provide the amino acids essential for the growth and repair of animal tissue
steroid hormone	(**STEE**-royd **HOR**-mohn)	The sex hormones and the hormones secreted by adrenal cortex
stimulant	(**STIM**-you-lant)	Any agent that temporarily increases functional activity

OVERVIEW

Recall that in Chapter 3, a body system was described as a group of organs that are closely allied anatomically and are involved in the same function. The exceptions to this definition are the organs known as glands. They form a system only in the functional sense.

The body has two types of glands, both of which manufacture and secrete (distribute) special kinds of substances. *Exocrine* (exo-outside) *glands* secrete such materials as saliva (the salivary glands) digestive enzymes (the pancreatic glands), or milk (the breasts, or mammary glands) through tubes or ducts. In contrast, the *endocrine* (endo-within), or *ductless, glands* secrete organic substances called hormones, which they release directly into the blood flowing through them. A *hormone* is a chemical substance secreted by a cell that affects the metabolic (energy-producing) activity of another cell or tissue. Some organs, such as the pancreas, contain both endocrine and exocrine glands.

STRUCTURE AND FUNCTION

The *endocrine system* consists of the ductless glands (Figure 13.1) Its general function is the regulation of major body processes under the overall direction of the brain. The major glands of the endocrine system are the:

- pituitary gland (hypophysis)
- thyroid gland
- parathyroid glands
- pancreatic islet cells (islets of Langerhans)
- adrenal glands

The pineal gland and the gonads (testes and ovaries) also have endocrine functions.

The medical discipline concerned with the study and treatment of the endocrine system is called *endocrinology,* and physicians who practice this specialty are called *endocrinologists.*

Pituitary Gland (Hypophysis)

The *pituitary gland* or *hypophysis* in considered to be the master gland because its secretions affect the activity of other glands. It is located at the base portion of the brain called the hypothalamus. Its anterior lobe, the *adenohypophysis,* produces growth hormone (GH); insufficient GH in a youth results in *dwarfism,* while excessive production of GH in youth results in *gigantism.* In later life, after growth has ceased, an overproduction of GH will produce a condition called *acromegaly,* in which the bones of the face, hands, and feet, are abnormally enlarged. The adenohypophysis also secretes a wide variety of other hormones including some that affect reproduction and others that affect lactation and healing. The neurohypophysis apparently serves as a reservoir for hormones before release into the blood stream.

Thyroid Gland

The *thyroid gland* is located in the anterior aspect of the pharynx, or neck, just below the larynx on either side and in front of the trachea. It has two lateral lobes connected by

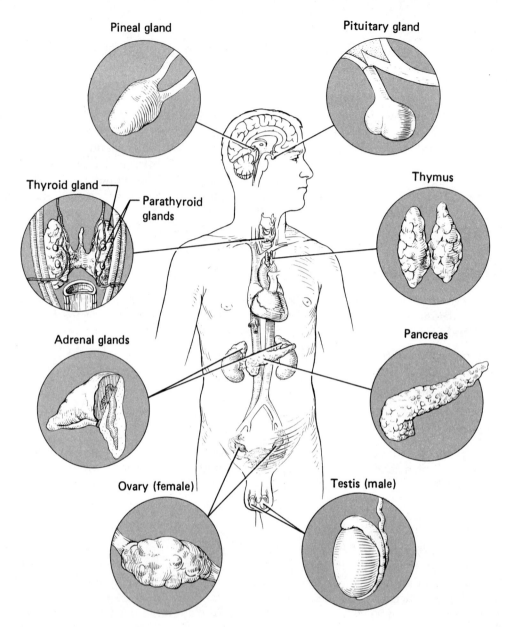

FIGURE 13.1   Glands of the endocrine system

a central isthmus. The principal hormones of the thyroid are *thyroxine* (T4) and *triiodothyronine* (T3), which regulate the speed at which carbohydrates, fats, and proteins are metabolized. Thyroid hormones are needed for normal growth and development. Either an excess (hyperthyroidism) or a deficiency (hypothyroidism) of thyroid hormone can lead to various health problems.

A congenital condition of hypothyroidism is associated with *cretinism*, a condition characterized by mental and physical abnormalities. In an adult, hypothyroidism leads to problems such as myxedema or goiter. Hyperactivity of the thyroid is sometimes called Graves' disease. The symptoms include *exophthalmos*, enlargement of the thyroid gland, acceleration of the pulse, increased basal metabolic rate (BMR), and nervous manifestations. Individuals with hyperthyroidism sometimes have white patches on the skin of the hands and feet called *vitiligo*.

Parathyroid Glands

The *parathyroid glands* are located on the dorsal surface of the thyroid gland, usually two on each lobe. They secrete *parathormone* (PTH), which regulates the levels of calcium and phosphorus in the blood. An excess of PTH causes softening of the bones (*osteomalacia*), whereas a deficiency leads to spasmodic twitching and contraction of the muscles (*tetany.*)

Pancreas

As already mentioned, the pancreas contains both endocrine and exocrine cells. The exocrine portion of the gland is attached to the duodenum by a duct through which its digestive juices are released to the small intestine (see Chapter 9). The endocrine portion of the gland consists of clusters of cells called the *islets of Langerhans* or simply pancreatic islets. These islets produce the hormone *insulin* which is involved in the utilization of carbohydrates by the body cells. The islet cells also secrete the hormone glucagon, which has several complex functions.

Insufficient secretion of insulin by the islet cells (*hypoinsulinism*) leads to a severe form of the disease *diabetes mellitus*. Excess sugar in the blood (*hyperglycemia*) causes damage to blood vessels and organs, especially the kidneys and delicate vessels such as those of the eye.

Excessive levels of insulin (*hyperinsulinism*) may bring on a condition known as insulin shock. The blood sugar may drop low enough (*hypoglycemia*) to cause fainting, coma, or convulsions. This condition may be caused by a tumor of the pancreas but more often occurs in diabetics who are taking insulin injections or other medications that lower the blood sugar.

Adrenal Glands

The paired *adrenals*, or adrenal glands, situated above each kidney, are sometimes called the *suprarenal glands*. Each has an outer cortex and an inner medulla. The adrenal cortex and the adrenal medulla function as separate glands.

Adrenal Cortex The *adrenal cortex* is essential for life. The hormones it secretes are called *corticosteroids* and include:

- The *glucocorticoids*, for example, hydrocortisone
- The *mineralocorticoids*, for example, aldosterone
- The *androgenic hormones*, for example, androsterone

The pituitary gland stimulates the adrenal cortex to produce these hormones by releasing *adrenocorticotropic hormone* (ACTH). The function of these hormones is too complex for discussion here.

Adrenal Medulla The *adrenal medulla* secretes two vitally important hormones, *epinephrine* (adrenaline) and *norepinephrine* (noradrenaline), also called *catecholamines*. The catecholamines act in combination to stimulate and inhibit a wide variety of organs including the heart, the respiratory centers, and others. The well-known "fight or flight response" is a function of these hormones acting in concert with the nervous system.

Pineal Gland

The *pineal gland* is a small cone-shaped structure located deep between the hemispheres (halves) of the brain. It secretes the hormone *melatonin*, which is thought to affect some aspects of reproduction. Its function in the human body is still being studied.

Gonads

The male and female gonads secrete important hormones; consequently, the gonads are considered a part of the endocrine system. The ovaries produce *estrogens* and *progesterone;* the testes produce *testosterone*. These hormones are discussed more fully in Chapters 10 and 11.

BUILDING BLOCKS

ROOTS AND COMBINING FORMS

Word Elements	Meaning
aden/o	gland
andr/o	male
cortex	outer layer, bark
crine	secrete
dips/o	thirst
edema	swelling
geros	old age
glyc/o	sweet
gynec/o	woman
hexis	condition
kal	potassium
renal	pertaining to kidney

SUFFIXES

Word Elements	Meaning
–emia	blood
–megaly	enlargement
–phagia	eat

Word Elements	Meaning
acro–	extremity
endo–	within
epi–	upon
eu–	healthy, normal
exo–	outside
myx–	mucus
neo–	new
supra–	above

VOCABULARY

General Terms

cretinism	(KREE-tin-izm)	Congenital condition due to lack of thyroid secretion, generally accompanied by dwarfism and mental retardation
dwarfism	(DWORF-izm)	The condition of being abnormally short or undersized, sometimes because of glandular dysfunction
endocrinologist	(en-doh-krin-OL-oh-jist)	A specialist in the diagnosis and treatment of disorders of the endocrine glands
endocrinology	(en-doh-krin-OL-oh-jee)	The science of the endocrine, or ductless, glands and their functions
euthyroid	(you-THIGH-royd)	Normal thyroid gland function
exocrine	(ECK-soh-krin)	The external secretion of a gland. Opposed to endocrine
hirsutism	(HER-soot-izm)	Abnormal hairiness or the growth of hair in unusual places, especially in women
homeostasis	(hoh-mee-oh-STAY-sis)	A relatively stable state of equilibrium of the internal environment of a cell or organism

Terms Related to Hormones

adrenaline	(ah-**DREN**-ah-len)	Alternative name for epinephrine, mostly in British usage; *Adrenalin* (upper-case *A*, no *e*) is the trade name for manufactured rather than secreted epinephrine
adrenocorticotropic hormone	(add-**ree**-noh-**kor**-tee-koh-**TROP**-ick)	A secretion of the anterior lobe of the pituitary that stimulates the growth, development, and continued function of the adrenal cortex
aldosterone	(**ALE**-doh-ster-**ohn**, al-**DOS**-ter-ohn)	A mineralocorticoid hormone secreted by the adrenal cortex; helps regulate use and excretion of sodium, chloride, and potassium
androsterone	(an-**DROS**-ter-ohn)	A masculinizing steriod found in the urine; thought to be a metabolite of testosterone
antidiuretic hormone (ADH)	(**an**-tih-**die**-you-**RET**-ick)	A hormone formed in the hypothalamus; reduces the secretion of urine when the body needs to conserve sodium or water. Also called vasopressin.
calcitonin	(**kal**-sih-**TOH**-nin)	A hormone from the thyroid gland, important in bone and calcium metabolism
catecholamines	(**kat**-eh-**KOL**-ah-meenz, **kat**-eh-**KOL**-ah-minz)	Epinephrine (adrenaline) and norepinephrine (noradrenaline); these hormones affect the nervous and cardiovascular systems, metabolic rate, temperature, and smooth muscle. Involved in so-called fight-flight responses.
corticosteroid	(**kor**-tih-koh-**STEE**-roid)	Any of several hormonal steroid substances secreted by the adrenal cortex
cortisol	(**KOR**-tih-sol)	An adrenocortical hormone (hydrocortisone)

cortisone	(**KOR**-tih-sohn)	A hormone from the adrenal cortex and also prepared synthetically
epinephrine	(ep-ih-**NEF**-rin)	A hormone secreted by the adrenal medulla; adrenaline
glucagon	(**GLOO**-kah-gon)	A polypeptide hormone secreted by the pancreas to increase the concentration of glucose in the blood
glucocorticoid	(**gloo**-koh-**KOR**-tih-koyd)	Adrenal cortical hormones that are active mainly in protecting against stress and in enabling protein and carbohydrate metabolism
gonadotrophic hormones	(**gon**-ah-doh-**TROHP**-ick)	Hormones that stimulate the gonads
hormone	(**HOR**-mohn)	A substance produced by ductless glands which regulates body processes under the direction of the brain
hydrocortisone	(**high**-droh-**KOR**-tih-sohn)	The corticosteriod hormone produced by the adrenal cortex; cortisol
insulin	(**IN**-sul-in)	A natural hormone secreted by the beta cells of the islets of Langerhans of the pancreas, involved in the metabolism of sugar in the body, and therefore with the presence and treatment of diabetes. Also produced commercially
melatonin	(**mel**-ah-**TOH**-nin)	Hormone produced by the pineal gland in mammals. Its function in humans is not known
norepinephrine	(nor-**eh**-pih-**NEF**-rin)	One of the catecholamines produced by the adrenal medulla; noradrenaline
oxytocin	(**ock**-seh-**TOH**-sin)	A pituitary hormone that induces labor by stimulating the uterus to contract

parathormone	(par-ah-**THOR**-mohn)	Hormone secreted by the parathyroid glands that regulates the metabolism of calcium and phosphorus
somatotropin	(**so**-mah-toh-**TROH**-pin)	Growth hormone; in humans, also called *human growth hormone*(HGH)
steroid hormones	(**STEE**-royd)	The sex hormones and the hormones of the adrenal cortex
thyroxine	(**thigh-ROCK**-sin)	A hormone produced by the thyroid gland; also manufactured and used in the treatment of hypothyroidism
triiodothyronine	(**tri**-eye-**oh**-doh-**THIGH**-roh-neen)	One of the principal thyroid hormones
vasopressin	(**vas**-oh-**PRESS**-in)	An antidiuretic hormone formed in the hypothalamus; also has a constrictive (pressor) effect on the blood vessels and thereby elevates blood pressure. See antidiuretic hormone.

Terms Related to Anatomy and Physiology

adenohypophysis	(**ad**-eh-noh-high-**POFF**-ih-sis)	The anterior lobe of the pituitary gland
adrenal gland	(ah-**DREE**-nal)	A triangular body on the superior surface of each kidney. Also called *suprarenal gland*.
cortex	(**KOR**-tecks)	The outer layer of an organ as distinguished from the inner portion or medulla, as in adrenal cortex
deoxyribonucleic acid (DNA)	(dee-**OCK**-seh-**rye**-boh-new-**KLEE**-ick)	The chemical basis of heredity and the carrier of genetic information found within each chromosome
electrolyte	(ee-**LECK**-troh-light)	In general, a solution that conducts electricity. In medicine, the term refers to salts found in blood, tissue fluids, and cells including salts of

		sodium, potassium, calcium, and chlorine
endocrine gland	(**EN**-doh-krin)	A ductless gland that produces an internal secretion
glycogenesis	(**glie**-koh-**JEN**-eh-sis)	The formation of glycogen from carbohydrate sources
glyconeogenesis	(**glie**-koh-nee-oh-**JEN**-eh-sis)	The formation of glycogen from noncarbohydrate sources
glycogen	(**GLIE**-koh-jen)	Animal starch.
hypophysis	(high-**POFF**-ih-sis)	The pituitary body or gland
islets of Langerhans	(**EYE**-letz of **LAHNG**-er-hahnz)	The endocrine portion of the pancreas consisting of cells arranged in groups that include three distinct types of hormone-secreting cells. The *alpha cells* secrete glucagon, the *beta cells* secrete insulin, and the *delta cells* secrete somatostatin.
lipid	(**LIP**-id)	Any one of a group of fats or fatlike substances. Lipids are not soluble in water but are soluble in fat solvents such as alcohol, ether, and chloroform
medulla	(meh-**DULL**-ah)	The inner or central portion of an organ
neurohypophysis	(**new**-roh-high-**POFF**-ih-sis)	Posterior portion of the pituitary gland
pancreas	(**PAN**-kree-as)	A large, elongated gland situated behind the stomach that produces insulin and a digestive juice
parathyroid gland	(**par**-ah-**THIGH**-royd)	One of four small endocrine glands that lie posterior to and at the lower edge of the thyroid gland or embedded within its substance
pineal body	(**PIN**-ee-al)	A glandlike structure situated in the brain. Named because of its resemblance to a pine cone.

Appears to be associated with the formation of melatonin.

pituitary gland	(pih-**TOO**-ih-tair-ee)	A gland situated beneath and attached to the base of the brain; has major regulatory functions including effects on other endocrine glands
renin	(**REH**-nin)	An enzyme produced by the kidney and active in regulating urine production; elevated in some forms of hypertension
sella turcica	(**SELL**-ah-**TUR**-sih-kah)	A concave area atop the sphenoid bone that houses the hypophysis (pituitary gland). Literal translation: Turkish saddle

Terms Related to Pathology

acromegaly	(ack-roh-**MEG**-ah-lee)	A disorder of adults caused by overproduction of the growth hormone; it results in enlargement of the bones of the extremities and certain bones of the head
Addison's disease		Disease caused by deficient secretion of adrenocortical hormones. Named for Thomas Addison, a 19th-century British physician.
adrenomegaly	(add-**ren**-oh-**MEG**-ah-lee)	Enlargement of the adrenal gland(s)
cachexia	(kah-**KECK**-see-ah)	A state of severe ill health, malnutrition, and wasting often associated with such diseases as cancer
coma	(**KOH**-mah)	An abnormal deep stupor from which the patient cannot be roused; unconsciousness
Conn's syndrome		A condition of excess production of aldosterone; associated with muscle weakness, polyuria, hypertension,

		hypokalemia, and alkalosis. Named for J. W. Conn, U.S. physician
Cushing's syndrome		A disease caused by hypersecretion of the adrenal cortex with excessive production of glucocorticoids. Symptoms include protein loss, fatigue, osteoporosis, amenorrhea, impotence, edema, diabetes mellitus, skin discoloration, and striae (striping) of the skin. (Named for Harvey Cushing, a U.S. surgeon)
diabetes insipidus	(**die**-ah-**BEE**-teez in-**SIP**-ih-dus)	A disease characterized by polyuria and polydipsia caused by inadequate secretion of vasopressin, the antidiuretic hormone
diabetes mellitus	(**die**-ah-**BEE**-teez mell-**LIE**-tus)	A metabolic disorder of carbohydrate metabolism caused by inadequate production or utilization of insulin; characterized by hyperglycemia and glycosuria
exophthalmos	(**eck**-sof-**THAL**-mos)	Abnormal protrusion of the eyeball
gigantism	(jye-**GAN**-tizm, **JYE**-gan-tism)	Excessive development of the body or of a body part
goiter	(**GOY**-ter)	An enlargement of the thyroid gland
gout	(gowt)	A hereditary metabolic disease actually a form of acute arthritis, marked by inflammation of the joints. Gout usually begins in the knee or foot, but affected joints may be at any location.
gynecomastia	(**jin**-neh-koh-**MAS**-tee-ah)	Abnormally large mammary glands in the male
hyperglycemia	(**high**-per-glie-**SEE**-mee-ah)	Abnormal increase of blood sugar such as occurs in diabetes mellitus
hypergonadism	(**high**-per-**GOH**-nadd-izm)	Excessive secretion of the sex glands

hyperinsulinism	(**high**-per-**IN**-soo-lin-**izm**)	An excessive amount of insulin in the blood
hyperkalemia	(**high**-per-kal-**EE**-mee-ah)	Excessive amount of potassium in the blood
hypernatremia	(**high**-per-nah-**TREE**-mee-ah)	Excessive sodium in the blood
hyperthyroidism	(**high**-per-**THIGH**-royd-izm)	A condition caused by excessive secretion of the thyroid glands; goiter and protruding eyeballs are prominent symptoms
hypocalcemia	(**high**-poh-kal-**SEE**-mee-ah)	Abnormally low blood calcium
hypoglycemia	(**high**-poh-glie-**SEE**-mee-ah)	Deficiency of sugar in the blood
hypoinsulinism	(**high**-poh-**IN**-soo-lin-izm)	Insufficient secretion of insulin
myxedema	(**mick**-seh-**DEE**-mah)	A condition caused by decreased function of the thyroid gland.
pheochromocytoma	(fee-oh-**kroh**-moh-sigh-**TOH**-mah)	A vascular tumor of the adrenal medulla that causes an excessive production of the catecholamines norepinephrine and epinephrine, resulting in hypertension
polydipsia	(**pol**-ee-**DIP**-see-ah)	Excessive thirst leading to excessive consumption of fluids
polyphagia	(**pol**-ee-**FAY**-jee-ah)	Eating excessive amounts of food at a meal
Simmond's disease	(**SIM**-onz)	A condition caused by complete atrophy of the pituitary body resulting in loss of function of the thyroid, adrenals, and gonads. Signs and symptoms include premature senility and cachexia.
tetany	(**TET**-ah-nee)	A condition of the nervous system in which the muscles twitch or contract violently, usually involving the muscles of the extremities

thyroiditis	(thigh-roy-**DIE**-tis)	Inflammation of the thyroid gland
thyrotoxicosis	(**thigh**-roh-**tock**-sih-**KOH**-sis)	Toxic condition due to hyperactivity of the thyroid gland; exophthalmic goiter
virilism	(**VIR**-ih-lizm)	Presence or development in the female of male secondary sexual characteristics

Terms Related to Surgery or Treatment

hypophysectomy	(high-**poff**-ih-**SECK**-toh-mee)	Excision of the hypophysis cerebri
parathyroidectomy	(**par**-ah-**thigh**-roy-**DECK**-to-me)	Excision of one or more of the parathyroid glands
thymectomy	(thigh-**MECK**-toh-mee)	Surgical removal of the thymus
thyroidectomy	(**thigh**-roy-**DECK**-toh-mee)	Excision of the thyroid gland

13.1 Review: System

DIRECTIONS: Cover the left column while you complete the statements on the right side.

exocrine
endocrine
The body has both _____ glands and _____ glands.

exocrine
The secretions from _____ glands are carried by tubes or ducts.

endocrine
hormones
The _____ glands secrete organic substances called _____ that are released directly into the bloodstream.

metabolic
The general function of ductless glands is to regulate_____processes.

adenohypophysis
neurohypophysis
The hypophysis has an anterior lobe called the _____ and a posterior lobe called the _____ .

dorsal
The parathyroids are located on the _____ surface of the thyroid.

calcium	They regulate the levels of _____
phosphorus	and _____ in the blood.
insulin, glucagon	The endocrine portion of the pancreas produces
	_____ and _____ .
ACTH	The pituitary stimulus for secretion of hormones from
	the adrenal cortex is _____ .
corticosteroids	The hormones secreted by the adrenal cortex are
	called _____ .

13.2 Review: System

DIRECTIONS: Complete the following statements by filling in the blanks.

1. The five major glands of the endocrine system are:

    a. _____

    b. _____

    c. _____

    d. _____

    e. _____

2. The thyroid hormones regulate the metabolism of:

    a. _____

    b. _____

    c. _____

13.3 Review: Building Blocks

DIRECTIONS: Write the meanings of the following building blocks.

1. acro–   _____

2. aden/o   _____

3. adrenal   _____

4. cortex   _____

5. crine   _____

6. dipsa   _____

7. edema   _____

8. geros   _____

9. glyc/o   _____

10. hexis   _____

11. andr/o   _____

12. kal _____
13. myx– _____
14. –phagia _____
15. renal _____

13.4   Review: Structures

Identify the glands in the figure below:

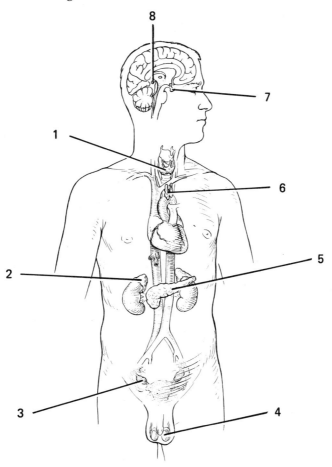

1. _____   5. _____
2. _____   6. _____
3. _____   7. _____
4. _____   8. _____

13.5   Review: Word Building

DIRECTIONS: Fill in the blanks with the appropriate building blocks and medical terms.

1. The root that means *secrete* is _____ .
   The prefix for *within* is _____ .
   The prefix for *outside* is _____ .
   The suffix _____ means the *study or science of.*
   The word for internal secretion is _____ .
   The word for external secretion is _____ .
   _____ is a study of the ductless glands and their functions.

2. The suffix _____ means *enlargement.*
   The combining form for *extremity* is _____ .
   Enlargement of the extremities is called _____ .

3. The combining form for *adrenal glands* is _____ .
   A condition of enlarged adrenal glands is _____ .

4. The combining form for *eye* is _____ .
   _____ is a prefix meaning *outside.*
   _____ is an abnormal protrusion of the eyeball.

5. The combining form for *thymus gland* is _____ .
   The suffix _____ means surgical excision.
   _____ is surgical removal of the thymus gland.

6. The prefix _____ means *above* or *excessive.*
   The combining form for *sweet* or *sugar* is _____ .
   _____ is a suffix meaning *blood.*
   _____ is an increase of blood sugar.
   The prefix _____ means *below* or *decrease.*
   _____ is a deficiency of sugar in the blood.

7. The word _____ means *sex gland.*
   _____ is a word ending meaning *condition.*
   _____ is the condition of excessive secretion of the sex glands.
   _____ is the building block for *potassium.*
   _____ is excessive potassium in the blood.

8. The prefix _____ means *excessive.*
   _____ is the combining form for *thirst.*
   The word _____ means excessive thirst.

9. _____ is the combining form for *eat.*
   The word _____ means eating abnormally large amounts of food at a meal.

326   Body Systems

10. The combining form for *thyroid* is _____ .

_____ is the combining form that means *poison*.

The suffix _____ means *abnormal condition* or *increase*.

_____ is a condition due to hyperactivity of the thyroid gland.

13.6 Review: Vocabulary

DIRECTIONS: Match the terms in the first column with their definitions in the second column.

1. _____ cretinism
2. _____ hirsutism
3. _____ insulin
4. _____ electrolyte
5. _____ glycogen
6. _____ hypophysis
7. _____ lipid
8. _____ cachexia
9. _____ coma
10. _____ edema
11. _____ goiter
12. _____ virilism

A. Animal starch
B. An enlargement of the thyroid gland
C. Any one of a group of fats or fatlike substances
D. Excessive growth of hair or the presence of hair in unusual places
E. The presence or development of male secondary characteristics in a woman
F. An abnormal, deep stupor occurring in illness or injury
G. A solution that is a conductor of electricity
H. Swelling due to collection of fluid in body tissues
I. Congenital condition due to lack of thyroid secretion
J. The pituitary body or gland
K. A natural hormone secreted by the beta cells of the islets of Langerhans
L. A state of ill health, malnutrition, and wasting

Reading Comprehension 13.1

DIRECTIONS: Underline the medical terms as you go through the reading exercise. Then list and analyze the terms. Some will be completely new to you. Consult a medical dictionary for their meanings. Then re-read the material for better comprehension.

Operation Record

Preoperative Diagnosis: Nontoxic nodular goiter

Postoperative Diagnosis: Adenoma of the thyroid

Operation: Thyroidectomy

Procedure:
This patient presented a hard, solitary large adenoma occupying most of the right lobe of the thyroid gland. The remainder of the gland was slightly diffusely enlarged without palpable nodularity or abnormal consistency.

A classical transverse thyroid incision was made with elevation of inferior and superior flaps of skin and platysma. The straps were incised in the midline and their underside separated from the surface of the gland. The right lobe was gently elevated from its bed, the inferior thyroid vessels being transected between clamps, and with gradual mobilization the majority of the lobe was excised; some normal thyroid was left at the superior pole and a posterior shell of thyroid along the capsule was left in situ.

The isthmus was dissected free from the trachea and was removed in continuity with the portion of the right lobe described containing the adenoma. Frozen sections were obtained and were reported by the pathologist to represent a fetal adenoma without evidence of malignancy. A small anterior portion of the left lobe was excised in order to entirely bury the trachea and tear the gland down to normal size. All bleeders were controlled with cotton ties and the wound was thoroughly dry at the time of closure. One inferior parathyroid gland was identified on the right side and preserved. The recurrent nerves were not visualized but dissection was carried out in the plane above their course. The strap muscles were reapproximated in the midline using interrupted cotton and skin and the platysma closed with clips. Vocal cords were checked at the end of the procedure and found to move normally.

The patient's condition throughout surgery was satisfactory and she left the operating room in good condition. Thyroid as above to laboratory.

Reading Comprehension 13.2

DIRECTIONS: Underline the medical terms as you go through the reading exercise. Then list and analyze the terms. Some will be completely new to you. Consult a medical dictionary for their meanings. Then re-read the material for better comprehension.

Pathology Report

Preoperative Diagnosis: Nontoxic nodular goiter

Tissue Removed: Nodule L. lobe thyroid

Gross:
The specimen consists of a mass of tissue from the left lobe of the thyroid gland presented in two masses a total weight of which is 12 grams. In the larger mass there is an encapsulated adenomatous nodule measuring 1.5 cm in diameter and at the time of surgery a frozen section was done on this tumor.

Frozen Section Impression:
Sections taken of the nodule showed a benign adenoma with no evidence of malignant change.

Additional material from the nodule will be taken for further study. Parathyroid tissue is not observed upon the specimen.

Microscopic:
Sections taken of the adenomatous nodule confirm the diagnosis made by frozen section of a benign process. The acini vary somewhat in size but all are lined with a single layer of low cuboidal cells and are filled with pink-staining colloid. The epithelium is perfectly normal throughout. Parathyroid tissue is not observed.

Diagnosis:
Adenoma of the thyroid.

Reading Comprehension Vocabulary

Use the space below to list the medical terms for analysis and definition.

_____
_____
_____
_____
_____
_____
_____
_____
_____
_____
_____
_____
_____
_____
_____
_____
_____
_____
_____
_____
_____
_____
_____
_____
_____
_____

CHAPTER 14

Nervous System

OBJECTIVES

When you have successfully completed Chapter 14, you should be able to:
— Recall terms relating to the structure and function of the nervous system.
— Write the meanings of building blocks introduced in this chapter.
— Name the two main divisions of the nervous system.
— Name the basic structural and functional units of the nervous system.
— Identify the anatomic structures of the nervous system on a familiar drawing.
— Build medical terms using the building blocks introduced in this and previous chapters.

331

antagonist	(an-**TAG**-on-nist)	A substance or process that counteracts the action of something else
congenital malformation	(kon-**JEN**-ih-tal mal-for-**MAY**-shun)	An abnormal shape or structure present at birth
functional	(**FUNGK**-shun-al)	In medicine, pertaining to the action performed by a structure, organ, or system
hemisphere	(**HEM**-ih-sfeer)	Half of a spherical body; the *cerebral hemisphere* consists of half of either the cerebrum or the cerebellum
impulse	(**IHM**-puhls)	A nerve impulse is an electrochemical process transmitted through nerve fibers and muscles that results in physical change or activity
innervate	(in-**ER**-vayt)	To stimulate a part or provide the pathway for the stimulation, as the nerve supply of an organ
sheath	(sheeth)	A covering structure
shock		A condition of circulatory failure marked by hypotension, coldness of the skin, and other symptoms; can have a number of causes and can lead to death if not reversed
structural	(**STRUCK**-shur-al)	Pertaining to the arrangement of component parts of an organism

OVERVIEW

The nervous system is the body's communication network; working closely with the endocrine system (Chapter 13), it unifies and coordinates all functions of the human body. The nervous system has two major divisions and several structural and functional subdivisions (Figure 14.1). The *central nervous system* (CNS), consists of the brain and the spinal cord. The *peripheral nervous system* (PNS) includes all the individual nerves, both cranial and spinal that connect the central nervous system with other parts of the body.

NEURONS AND NERVES

The basic structural and functional component of the nervous system is called the *neuron*, or nerve cell. Neurons are the most complex and varied of body cells (Figure

14.2), but each consists of the cell body, with its nucleus, and nerve fibers called axons and dendrites. The structures we call *nerves* are actually bundles of nerve fibers much like many-stranded electrical cables. Other cells of the nervous system that are not involved in impulse transmission are called *glial cells*.

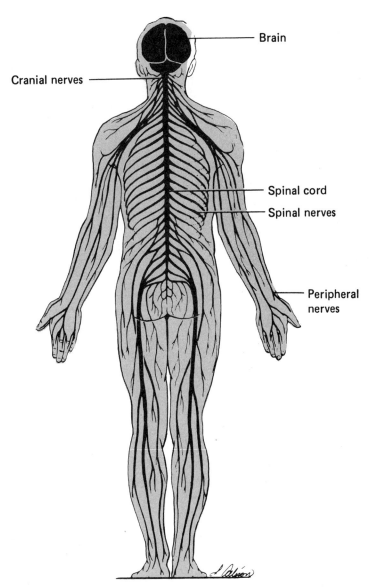

Cranial nerves

Brain

Spinal cord

Spinal nerves

Peripheral nerves

FIGURE 14.1   Nerve cells (neurons) (From Kinn, *Medical Terminology—Review Challenge,* copyright 1987 by Delmar Publishers Inc.)

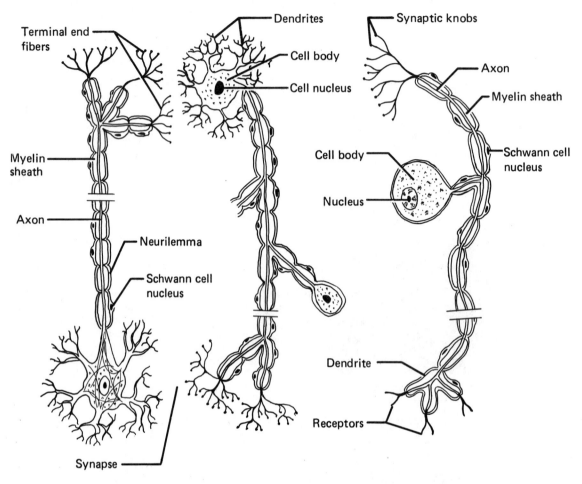

Terminal end fibers

Dendrites

Synaptic knobs

Cell body

Axon

Cell nucleus

Myelin sheath

Myelin sheath

Cell body

Schwann cell nucleus

Axon

Nucleus

Neurilemma

Schwann cell nucleus

Dendrite

Receptors

Synapse

Motor (efferent) neuron

Sensory (afferent) neuron

FIGURE 14.2   The nervous system

Types of Neurons

There are two major types of neurons: *sensory*, or *afferent* neurons and *motor*, or *efferent neurons*, plus connector neurons which carry messages between the two major types. Neurons communicate by means of electrical charges and chemical reactions called *nerve impulses*.

- Sensory (afferent) neurons transmit impulses *toward* the central nervous system.
- Motor (efferent) neurons transmit impulses *from* the CNS to body structures.

Structure of the Neuron

The three main parts of the neuron consist of:

- A *cell body*, the main part of the cell, containing the *cell nucleus*.
- One or more *dendrites*, the nerve fibers, or processes, that conduct impulses *toward* the cell body. Motor neurons have more than one dendrite; sensory neurons have only one.
- One *axon*, the nerve fiber, or process that conducts impulses *away from* the cell body.

Larger axons are covered with an insulating layer called the *myelin sheath*. A second covering, outside the myelin, is called the *neurilemma*. Axons that have a myelin sheath are called *myelinated* or *medullated nerve fibers*. Those axons that have no myelin sheath are called *unmyelinated nerve fibers*.

Function of the Neuron

Each neuron is a separate and distinct unit whose axons communicate with the dendrites of other neurons. The nerve fibers do not actually touch; the microscopic space through which neurons communicate is called a *synapse*. The nerve impulse is transmitted across the synapse through the action of chemicals called neurotransmitters, including acetylcholine, epinephrine, dopamine and others. The activities of these chemicals has only recently been identified, and additional neurotransmitters are still being discovered.

CENTRAL NERVOUS SYSTEM

The brain is enclosed within the protective covering of the skull. The spinal cord, which is named separately but is actually continuous with the brain, occupies a canal within the vertebral column (see Chapter 5). In addition to these bony coverings, the brain and spinal cord are further protected by three-layered membranes called *meninges*. Structures within the brain called *ventricles* manufacture a watery, *cerebrospinal fluid* which is similar to plasma or lymph which cushions and protects the brain and spinal cord from shock.

Brain and Associated Structures

The brain is the largest and most complex part of the nervous system. It is composed of billions of neurons and countless nerve fibers arranged in intricate networks. The brain has many regions which have distinct functions but nonetheless interact (Figure 14.3).

CEREBRUM The largest part of the brain is the *cerebrum*, which is divided into two hemispheres (halves). The cerebrum controls the higher brain functions.

CEREBELLUM The cerebellum, the second-largest part of the brain, is located below the occipital lobe of the cerebrum. It is a reflex center for the control of skeletal muscles (see Chapter 6).

BRAIN STEM The brain stem which connects the cerebrum to the spinal cord, consists of the *diencephalon*, the *midbrain*, the *pons*, and the *medulla oblongata*. The functions of these areas are complex and not entirely understood.

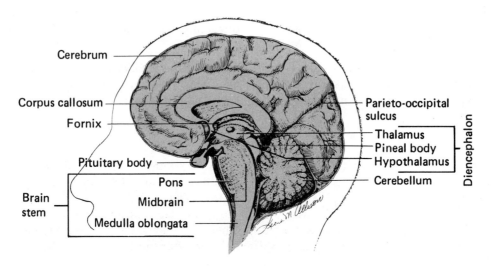

FIGURE 14.3 **The brain** (From Kinn, *Medical Terminology—Review Challenge*, copyright 1987 by Delmar Publishers Inc.)

CRANIAL NERVES There are 12 paired cranial nerves (Table 14.1). One pair originates in the cerebrum. The other 11 pairs originate in the brain stem. They lead to various parts of the head, neck, and trunk. Each cranial nerve has a name but is often referred to by number.

Spinal Cord

In adults, the spinal cord extends from the base of the brain to about the level of the first lumbar vertebra (L_1). It has 31 segments, each of which has a pair of *spinal nerves* that branch out to various body parts and connect those parts with the central nervous system. Major nerve pathways called *nerve tracts* exist within the spinal cord.

The spinal cord has two major functions:

• to conduct nerve impulses and
• to serve as a center for spinal reflexes.

An incoming nerve impulse (*stimulus*) is received from *afferent* nerves. Outgoing responses are carried to muscles and visceral organs via *efferent* nerves to effect a response. Between stimulus and response, the spinal cord may communicate with the brain if a considered response is required; however the spinal cord may itself process a *reflex response* without involving the brain. Common reflex pathways include the knee jerk reflex, the withdrawal reflex, and the ankle jerk reflex.

TABLE 14.1. The Cranial Nerves

Number	Name	Type	Function
I	Olfactory	Sensory	Sense of smell
II	Optic	Sensory	Vision
III	Oculomotor	Primarily motor	Reflex adjustment of the eyes to light and accommodation
IV	Trochlear	Primarily Motor	Voluntary movements of the eyeballs
V	Trigeminal	Mixed	Sensations of face, scalp, and teeth; chewing
VI	Abducens	Primarily Motor	Coordinates contraction of extrinsic muscles of the eyes
VII	Facial	Mixed	Sensations of face, scalp, and muscles of facial expression
VIII	Vestibulocochlear	Sensory	Hearing and sense of balance
IX	Glossopharyngeal	Mixed	Sense of taste
X	Vagus	Mixed	Sensations of throat, swallowing, peristalsis, heart contraction; stimulates production of gastric juices
XI	Accessory	Motor	Stimulates muscles of larynx and pharynx
XII	Hypoglossal	Motor	Stimulates movement of the tongue

The Meninges

Both the brain and the spinal cord have outer coverings of membranes called *meninges* (Singular, *menix*). The outer membrane is the *dura mater,* the middle layer the *arachnoid,* and the innermost the *pia mater.* The dura mater is separated from the bony-walls of the skull by an *epidural space* containing blood vessels and protective tissues. The *subdural* space lies between the dura mater and the arachnoid. Between the arachnoid and pia mater is the *subarachnoid space,* which contains cerebrospinal fluid. The very thin pia mater, which closely covers the brain and spinal cord, contains many nerves as well as blood vessels from which the underlying cells of these organs receive nourishment.

PERIPHERAL NERVOUS SYSTEM

Functionally, the *peripheral nervous system* (PNS) is divided into two systems:

- the voluntary nervous system and
- the autonomic nervous system (ANS).

Voluntary Nerves

The *voluntary nervous system* regulates functions that are under conscious control. For example, the neural connections that innervate the musculoskeletal system for the purpose of walking.

Autonomic Nerves

The *autonomic nervous system* regulates body activities that occur without conscious control. For example, the autonomic system controls ongoing functions such as the heartbeat, breathing, digestion, and so forth. It does so by a complex series of stimulating and inhibiting effects regulated by *sympathetic* and *parasympathetic* nerves.

The two act as antagonists to balance each other's effect. The parasympathetic impulses utilize neurotransmitters to induce glandular secretion, increase the tone of smooth muscles, and dilate blood vessels. Sympathetic nerve impulses utilize epinephrine and other neurotransmitters to depress some secretions, relax smooth muscle, and contract blood vessels. These intricate interrelationships are too complex to discuss here.

MEDICAL CARE AND THE NERVOUS SYSTEM

Three specialities are specifically concerned with the nervous system and its disorders.

Neurology is the branch of medicine that deals with the nonsurgical aspects of neurologic diseases. Generally, the neurologist will study and manage infectious, metabolic, degenerative, and systemic involvements of the nervous system.

Psychiatry is more concerned with functional disorders involving the nervous system, especially those that affect behavior. No organic cause may be apparent, or the psychiatrist may work with the neurologist or neurosurgeon on managing the behavioral aspects of organic nerve disease.

Tumors, trauma, and congenital malformations of the nervous system are more likely to be treated definitively by a neurosurgeon. Postoperative care may be coordinated with the neurologist and in some cases with a psychiatrist also.

BUILDING BLOCKS

ROOTS AND COMBINING FORMS

Word Elements	Meaning
agor/a	marketplace, open area
astr/o	star
cephal/o	head
crani/o	skull
cyt/o	cell
encephal/o	brain
erg/o	work
kinesis	motion
men/o	mind
mening/o	membrane
narc/o	numbness, sleep
neur/o	nerve
paresis	slight paralysis, weakness
phobia	fear
praxis	action
psych/o	relationship to mind
radicle	little root
rhiz/o	root
soma	body
spondyl/o	vertebra
thalam/o	chamber
ventr/o	belly, cavity

SUFFIXES

Word Elements	Meaning
–algia	pain
–asthenia	weakness
–cele	hernia
–esthesia	sensation
–glia	glue
–ism	condition
–lepsis	seizure
–lexia	diction
–lysis	destruction

SUFFIXES (continued)

Word Elements	Meaning
–malacia	softening
–oma	tumor
–phasia	speaking
–plegia	stroke, paralysis
–sthenia	Strength

PREFIXES

Word Elements	Meaning
atel–	incomplete, imperfect
auto–	self
brady–	slow
macro–	large
micro–	small
mono–	single
para–	beside
quadri–	four

VOCABULARY

General Terms

afferent	(**AFF**-er-ent)	Carrying impulses toward a center; in neurology, referring to the direction of an impulse proceeding *toward* the cell body of the neuron or toward the central nervous system
anergic	(an-**ER**-jick)	Abnormal lack of energy; sluggishness
anesthesia	(an-es-**THEE**-zee-ah)	Partial or complete loss of sensation
arachnoid	(ah-**RACK**-noyd)	Resembling a web; for example, the arachnoid membrane
cranial	(**KRAY**-nee-al)	Pertaining to the cranium
efferent	(**EF**-fer-ent)	In neurology, referring to the direction of an impulse proceeding

		away from the cell body of the neuron or away from the central nervous system
hypnology	(hip-**NOL**-oh-jee)	Scientific study of sleep
inertia	(in-**ER**-she-ah)	Disinclination to engage in normal activities
inversion	(in-**VER**-zhun)	Turning inside out of an organ; for example, inversion of the uterus
neurologist	(new-**ROL**-oh-jist)	A specialist in the structure, function, and diseases of the nervous system
parasympathetic	(pair-ah-**sim**-pah-**THET**-ick)	Relating to the craniosacral division of the autonomic nervous system
psychosomatic	(**sigh**-koh-so-**MAT**-ick)	Pertaining to the relationship of the mind and the body
reflex	(**REE**-flecks)	An involuntary movement or action in response to a stimulus
sciatic	(sigh-**AT**-ick)	Pertaining to the hip or ischium
spinal	(**SPY**-nal)	Pertaining to the spine or spinal cord
sympathetic	(**sim**-pah-**THET**-ick)	Pertaining to the sympathetic nervous system; caused by or pertaining to sympathetic activity

Terms Related to Anatomy and Physiology

astrocyte	(**ASS**-troh-sight)	A star-shaped neuroglial cell that supports and binds nerve tissue together
autonomic nervous system	(aw-toh-**NOM**-ick)	The part of the nervous system that controls involuntary bodily functions
axon	(**ACK**-son)	The nerve fiber, or process, that conducts impulses away from the cell body
cell body		The main part of the neuron, containing the nucleus

central nervous system (CNS)		The brain and spinal cord
cerebellum	(sehr-eh-**BELL**-um)	The portion of the brain, near its base, that controls coordination and equilibrium
cerebrospinal fluid (CSF)	(sehr-eh-broh-**SPY**-nal)	A watery fluid produced in the ventricles of the brain to cushion the brain and spinal cord from physical impact
cerebrum	(seh-**REE**-brum, **SEHR**-eh-brum)	The largest part of the brain which consists of two hemispheres, and is the main seat of conscious mental processes and sensation
dendrites	(**DEN**-drights)	The nerve fibers, or processes, that conduct impulses toward the cell body
diencephalon	(die-en-**SEHF**-ah-lon)	The diencephalon is the second portion of the brain; it consists of the thalamus, the hypothalamus, and the pineal body.
dura mater	(**DOO**-rah **MAY**-ter)	The outermost of the three membranes (meninges) covering the brain and spinal cord
epidural space	(ep-ih-**DOO**-ral)	The space outside of or upon the dura mater
foramen magnum	(foh-**RAY**-men **MAG**-num)	Opening of the occipital bone through which the spinal cord exits the brain
frontal lobe	(**FRUN**-tal lowb)	The anterior portion of each cerebral hemisphere
ganglion	(**GANG**-glee-on)	A collection of nerve cells outside the brain or spinal cord that initiates or reinforces nerve impulses; plural, *ganglia*
hypothalamus	(high-poh-**THAL**-ah-mus)	A portion of the brain that plays a large part in maintaining homeostasis. It serves as a link

		between the nervous and endocrine systems.
medulla oblongata	(meh-**DULL**-ah **ob**-long-**GAH**-tah)	Enlarged continuation of the spinal cord within cranium extending from the foramen magnum to the pons; the lower portion of the brain stem
meninges	(meh-**NIN**-jeez)	The three membranes surrounding the spinal cord and brain; the dura mater, arachnoid, and pia mater. Singular, *menix*
microcephalus	(**my**-kroh-**SEF**-ah-lus)	Condition of having an exceptionally small head
motor neuron		A neuron that transmits signals to muscle tissue
nerve tract		A bundle of myelinated nerve fibers within the spinal cord or brain that constitutes a major nerve pathway
neuroglia	(new-**ROG**-lee-ah)	The tissue composed of neuroglial cells that forms the supporting elements of the brain and spinal cord
neuron	(**NEW**-ron)	The structural and functional unit of the nervous system consisting of a cell body and its processes
neurotransmitter	(**new**-roh-**TRANZ**-mit-er)	One of several chemicals including acetylcholine and the catecholamines that play a part in the transmission of nerve impulses across the synaptic junction
occipital lobe	(ock-**SIP**-ih-tal)	Posterior portion of the cerebral hemisphere that is shaped like a three-sided pyramid and separated from the cerebellum by an extension of the dura mater
parietal lobe	(pah-**RYE**-eh-tal)	The division of each side of the brain lying posterior to the frontal lobe and beneath each parietal bone

peripheral nervous system (PNS)	(peh-**RIFF** -er-al)	That part of the nervous system outside the central nervous system
pia mater	(**PIE**-ah **MAY**-ter)	The innermost of the three meninges
pons	(ponz)	A bridge; with reference to the nervous system, the pons is the bridge between the medulla oblongata and the midbrain.
sensorium	(sen-**SO**-ree-um)	The center of sensations in the brain
sensory neuron	(**SEN**-so-ree)	An afferent neuron that carries sensory impulses from peripheral body parts to the brain or spinal cord
spinal cord		A slender column of nerve tissue within the spinal canal and extending from the brain to the second lumbar vertebra (L_2)
subarachnoid space	(sub-ah-**RACK**-noyd)	Space between the arachnoid membrane and the pia mater
subdural space	(sub-**DOO**-ral)	Space between the arachnoid and dura mater
synapse	(**SIN**-ahps)	The microscopic space between dendrite and axon through which neurons communicate
temporal lobe	(**TEM**-poor-al)	The portion of the cerebrum that is located laterally and below the frontal lobe; it contains auditory receptive areas
thalamus	(**THAL**-ah-mus)	The brain center that relays sensory impulses from other parts of the nervous system to the cerebrum
ventricle	(**VEN**-trih-kul)	A small cavity. One of the cavities of the brain

Terms Related to Psychiatry

acrophobia	(ack-roh-**FOH**-bee-ah)	Great fear of high places

agoraphobia	(**ag**-oh-rah-**FOH**-bee-ah)	Great fear of being alone or of being in open spaces
autism	(**AW**-tizm)	A condition in which the patient withdraws from reality and displays self-centered activity
delusion	(dee-**LOO**-zhun)	A false belief that persists without explanation; for example, delusions of grandeur, delusions of persecution
disorientation	(**dis**-oh-ree-en-**TAY**-shun)	The state of being confused regarding one's position in space, time, or personal relationships
hallucination	(hah-**loo**-sih-**NAY**-shun)	A false perception regarding occurring events that has no relation to reality and that is not induced by any external stimuli
neurasthenia	(**new**-ras-**THEE**-nee-ah)	A neurotic illness marked by such symptoms as chronic abnormal fatigability, weakness, and lack of energy
obsession	(ob-**SEH**-shun)	An uncontrollable desire to dwell on an idea, an emotion, or an activity
paranoia	(pair-ah-**NOY**-ah)	A psychotic disorder in which suspicions develop in a logical order into delusions of persecution and grandeur
phobia	(**FOH**-bee-ah)	A persistent and unrealistic fear of a specific object or situation
psychosis	(sigh-**KOH**-sis)	A severe mental disorder in which the patient departs from the normal pattern of behavior and loses contact with reality
psychosomatic	(**sigh**-koh-so-**MAT**-ick)	Pertaining to the interaction of the mind (psyche) and the body (soma)

Terms Related to Pathology

akinesia	(ah-kih-NEE-zee-ah)	Loss of muscle movement, complete or partial. Also spelled *acinesia*.
Alzheimer's disease	(ALTZ-high-merz)	A presenile degenerative organic brain disease that results in complete loss of intellectual function
amentia	(ah-MEN-she-ah)	Congenital lack of mental ability; mental retardation
amnesia	(am-NEE-zee-ah)	A pathological loss of memory
anencephaly	(an-en-SEF-ah-lee)	Congenital absence of the brain and spinal cord
anorexia nervosa	(an-oh-RECK-see-ah ner-VOH-sah)	A serious psychosomatic condition in which the patient loses appetite, has an exaggerated fear of being overweight and systematically limits food intake, resulting in emaciation
apathy	(APP-ah-thee)	Indifference; lack of emotion
aphasia	(ah-FAY-zee-ah)	Loss of language comprehension
apraxia	(ah-PRACK-see-ah)	Loss of ability to perform skilled motor movements although there is no sensory or motor impairment
arachnitis	(ar-ack-NIGH-tis)	Inflammation of the arachnoid membrane
asthenia	(as-THEE-nee-ah)	Lack or loss of strength
ataxia	(ah-TACK-see-ah)	Loss of muscular coordination
atelencephalia	(ah-tell-en-seh-FAY-lee-ah)	Congenital imperfect development of the brain
bradykinesia	(brad-ee-kih-NEE-see-ah)	Extreme slowness of all motor activity
bulimia	(byou-LIM-ee-ah)	Excessive appetite. More recently used to describe a neurotic disorder characterized by bouts of extreme overeating followed by fasting, induced vomiting, or induced diarrhea (bingeing and purging)

cephalalgia	(**sef**-ah-**LAL**-jee-ah)	Headache, pain in the head
cerebral palsy	(**sehr**-eh-bral, seh-**REE**-bral **PAWL**-zee)	A motor disorder characterized by paralysis and lack of coordination due to trauma at birth or brain pathology occurring during infancy
cerebral hemorrhage	(seh-**REE**-bral **HEM**-or-idj)	Escape of blood into tissues of the brain
cerebromalacia	(sehr-eh-broh-mah-**LAY**-she-ah)	Softening of brain tissue, especially of the cerebrum
chorea	(koh-**REE**-ah)	A nervous disorder characterized by a variety of involuntary, highly complex, jerky movements
diplegia	(die-**PLEE**-jee-ah)	Paralysis of similar parts on both sides of the body
dyslexia	(dis-**LECK**-see-ah)	A condition in which an individual with normal vision cannot interpret or misinterprets written language
dysphasia	(dis-**FAY**-jee-ah)	Impairment of speech resulting in failure to arrange words in their proper order
encephalitis	(en-**sef**-ah-**LIE**-tis)	Inflammation of the brain
epilepsv	(**EP**-ih-**lep**-see)	A central nervous system disorder caused by temporary disturbances in normal brain impulses that results in convulsive seizures and loss of consciousness
hemiparesis	(**hem**-ee-**PAR**-ee-sis)	Incomplete paralysis; muscular weakness affecting one side of the body
hemiplegia	(**hem**-ee-**PLEE**-jee-ah)	Paralysis of only one half of the body
Huntington's chorea		A rare hereditary brain disorder characterized by chronic progressive chorea and mental deterioration. Named for G. Huntington, a U.S. physician.

hydrocephalus	(high-droh-**SEF**-ah-lus)	Abnormal accumulations of cerebrospinal fluid within the ventricles of the brain. In infants it results in enlargement of the head.
hyperesthesia	(**high**-per-es-**THEE**-zee-ah)	Increased sensitivity of the skin
hyperkinesis	(**high**-per-kih-**NEE**-sis)	Abnormally increased motor function and physical activity
macrocephalia	(**mack**-roh-seh-**FAY**-lee-ah)	Abnormal largeness of the head
meningioma	(meh-**nin**-jee-**OH**-mah)	A slow-growing tumor of the meninges that originates in the arachnoidal tissue
meningitis	(men-in-**JIGH**-tis)	Inflammation of the membranes of the spinal cord or brain
meningocele	(meh-**NING**-goh-seel)	Congenital hernia of the meninges through an opening of the skull or spinal column
monoplegia	(**mon**-oh-**PLEE**-jee-ah)	Paralysis of a single limb or a body part
multiple sclerosis		A chronic, generally progressive, incurable disease of the spinal cord. Symptoms include weakness, incoordination, nystagmus and tremor. There may be remissions and exacerbations.
myasthenia gravis	(**my**-as-**THEE**-nee-ah **GRAH**-vis)	A chronic neuromuscular disease characterized by muscular weakness of increasing severity. Symptoms may fluctuate.
myelitis	(**my**-eh-**LIE**-tis)	Inflammation of the spinal cord; also, inflammation of bone marrow
narcolepsy	(**NAR**-koh-**lep**-see)	A chronic ailment consisting of recurrent brief episodes of sleep which the patient is unable to control
neuralgia	(new-**RAL**-jee-ah)	Severe sharp pain along the course of a nerve

neuritis	(new-**RYE**-tis)	Inflammation of a nerve or nerves
neurosis	(new-**ROH**-sis)	An emotional disorder related to unresolved conflicts
palsy	(**PAWL**-zee)	Paralysis; may be temporary or permanent. There are many specific types of palsy; for example, Bell's palsy, cerebral palsy.
papilledema	(**pap**-ill-eh-**DEE**-mah)	Swelling of the optic nerve. Sometimes called choked disk.
paralysis	(pah-**RAL**-ih-sis)	Temporary or permanent loss of motor function, especially voluntary motion
paraplegia	(pair-ah-**PLEE**-jee-ah)	Paralysis involving the lower portion of the body and both legs
paresis	(pah-**REE**-sis, **PAR**-eh-sis)	Partial or incomplete paralysis
paresthesia	(pair-es-**THEE**-zee-ah)	The sensation of numbness, prickling, or tingling in a body part; the "pins and needles" sensation
poliomyelitis	(**poh**-lee-oh-**my**-eh-**LIE**-tis)	Often referred to simply as "polio." A viral disease affecting the nervous system. It may result in paralysis or atrophy of groups of muscles. *Bulbar poliomyelitis* causes respiratory paralysis.
quadriplegia	(**kwad**-rih-**PLEE**-jee-ah)	Paralysis of all four extremities and usually of the trunk
radiculitis	(rah-**dick**-you-**LIE**-tis)	Inflammation of spinal-nerve roots
Reye's syndrome	(rize **SIN**-drohm)	A disease occurring mainly in children, characterized by acute degeneration of brain tissue and tissue changes in the liver and other visceral organs; occurs following certain viral diseases
sciatica	(sigh-**AT**-ih-kah)	Severe pain along the course of the sciatic nerve beginning in the hip and progressing down the thigh, leg and foot

syncope	(SIN-koh-pee)	A fainting spell caused by inadequate blood flow to the brain

Terms Related to Diagnostic Procedures

electroencephalogram (EEG)	(ee-**leck**-troh-en-**SEF**-ah-loh-gram)	A tracing of the electrical activity of the brain
electromyography (EMG)	(ee-**leck**-troh-my-**AHG**-rah-fee)	Testing the innervation of muscle tissue and its contraction through the application of electrical current at selected locations
myelography	(**my**-eh-**LOG**-rah-fee)	Visualization of the spinal cord by X-ray after the injection of a radiopaque medium
pneumoencephalography	(**new**-moh-en-**sef**-ah-**LOG**-rah-fee)	Examination of the cerebral ventricles by x-ray after removing CSF and injecting air or gas

Terms Related to Surgery or Treatment

chordotomy, cordotomy	(kor-**DOT**-oh-mee)	Section (cutting) of lateral pathways of the spinal cord to relieve pain
craniectomy	(kray-nee-**ECK**-toh-me)	Surgical removal of a portion of the skull
craniotomy	(kray-nee-**OTT**-oh-mee)	An incision through the cranium; also, crushing of the skull of the fetus that has died in utero to facilitate delivery in difficult parturition
ganglionectomy	(**gang**-glee-oh-**NECK**-toh-mee)	Excision of a ganglion
laminectomy	(**lam**-ih-**NECK**-toh-mee)	The excision of a vertebral posterior arch in order to reach and remove a disk
lobotomy	(loh-**BOT**-oh-mee)	Incision into the frontal lobe of the brain to sever connecting nerve fibers between certain areas. It is done to relieve intractable pain or to promote changes in mood or behavior

neurectomy	(new-**RECK**-toh-mee)	Partial or total excision of a nerve
neurolysis	(new-**ROL**-ih-sis)	Freeing of adhesions surrounding a nerve. Relief of tension of a nerve by stretching
rhizotomy	(rye-**ZOT**-oh-mee)	Section (cutting) of a nerve root
spondylosyndesis	(**spon**-dih-loh-**SIN**-dee-sis)	Surgical fusing of vertebrae
sympathectomy	(**sim**-pah-**THECK**-toh-mee)	Surgical removal of certain pathways of the sympathetic nervous system
trephination	(**tref**-ih-**NAY**-shun)	Removal of a circular piece of tissue or bone, especially a piece of the skull, with a specialized saw called a trephine
vagotomy	(vay-**GOT**-oh-mee)	Sectioning of the vagus nerve, sometimes used in treating peptic ulcer disease; *medical vagotomy* consists of administering of drugs that prevent function of the vagus nerve.

14.1   Review: System

DIRECTIONS: Cover the left column while you complete the statements on the right side.

central nervous system
peripheral nervous system

There are two major structural divisions of the nervous system. The _____ consists of the brain and spinal cord. The _____ includes all the individual nerves, both cranial and spinal.

neuron

The basic structural and functional unit of the nervous system is the _____ .

afferent
toward

The sensory or _____ neurons transmit impulses (toward) (away from) the central nervous system.

efferent **away from**	The motor or _____ neurons transmit impulses (toward) (away from) the central nervous system.
synapse	The point where nerve impulses are communicated between neurons is the _____ .
brain	The largest and most complex part of the nervous system is the _____ .
31 **spinal nerves** **voluntary**	The spinal cord has _____ segments, each giving rise to a pair of _____ . _____ nerves are under conscious control.
autonomic	_____ nerves act without conscious control.

14.2   Review: Building Blocks

DIRECTIONS: Write the meanings of these word endings.

1. –algia _____
2. –asthenia _____
3. –cele _____
4. –esthesia _____
5. –glia _____
6. –ism _____
7. –lysis _____
8. –malacia _____
9. –oma _____
10. –phasia _____
11. –plegia _____
12. –sthenia _____

14.3   Review: Building Blocks

DIRECTIONS: Match the terms in the two columns.

1. _____ agor/a		A.	action
2. _____ astr/o		B.	beside
3. _____ auto		C.	body
4. _____ –cyte		D.	cell
5. _____ erg/o		E.	chamber
6. _____ hypnos		F.	diction
7. _____ kinesis		G.	fear
8. _____ –lexia		H.	large
9. _____ –lepsis		I.	marketplace
10. _____ macro–		J.	motion
11. _____ micro–		K.	root
12. _____ mono–		L.	seizure
13. _____ para–		M.	self
14. _____ phobia		N.	single
15. _____ –praxis		O.	sleep
16. _____ radicle		P.	small
17. _____ soma		Q.	star
18. _____ thalam/o		R.	work

14.4   Review: Building Blocks

DIRECTIONS: Write the meanings of the combining forms below.

1. arachn/o   _____

2. atel/o   _____

3. cephal/o   _____

4. crani/o   _____

5. encephal/o   _____

6. men/o   _____

7. mening/o   _____

8. narc/o   _____

9. neur/o   _____

10. psych/o   _____

11. rhiz/o   _____

12. spondyl/o   _____

14.5   Review: Vocabulary

DIRECTIONS: Match the words in the second column with the definitions by placing the correct letter in the space provided.

1. _____ Inability to interpret written language	A.	akinesia
2. _____ Pain in the head	B.	amentia
3. _____ A fainting spell	C.	apathy
4. _____ Abnormal largeness of the head	D.	ataxia
5. _____ Complete or partial loss of muscle movement	E.	autism
	F.	bradykinesia
6. _____ An emotional disorder related to unresolved conflicts	G.	cephalalgia
	H.	delusion
7. _____ Patient withdraws from reality and displays self-centered activity	I.	dyslexia
	J.	ganglion
8. _____ Congenital mental deficiency	K.	hypnology
9. _____ A false belief held without rational explanation	L.	macrocephalia
	M.	narcolepsy
10. _____ Loss of muscular coordination	N.	neurosis
11. _____ A collection of nerve cells outside the brain or spinal column	O.	paresthesia
	P.	syncope
12. _____ Indifference; lack of emotion		
13. _____ Scientific study of sleep		
14. _____ Sensation of numbness or tingling		
15. _____ Chronic recurrent attacks of drowsiness and sleep		
16. _____ Extreme slowness of all motor activity		

14.6   Review: Word Building

DIRECTIONS: Cover the left column as you complete the items

encephal	A building block for brain is _____
	Build a word meaning
encephal/itis	Inflammation of the brain
	_____ / _____
electro/	A tracing of the electrical activity of the brain
encephalo/gram	_____ / _____ / _____
neur	A root form meaning nerve is _____

neur/algia	Build a word meaning Pain in a nerve _____ / _____
neur/ectomy	Excision of a nerve _____ / _____
mening/o	A combining form for membrane is _____
meningi/oma	Build a word meaning A tumor involving a membrane _____ / _____
mening/itis	Inflammation of a membrane _____ / _____
meningo/cele	A congenital hernia involving protrusion of a membrane through an opening of the spinal column _____ / _____
–plegia	A suffix meaning paralysis is _____
quadri/plegia	Build a word meaning Paralysis of all four extremities _____ / _____
para/plegia	Paralysis of the lower portion of the body and of both legs _____ / _____
hemi/plegia	Paralysis of the lower portion of one-half of the body _____ / _____

Reading Comprehension 14.1

DIRECTIONS: Underline the medical terms as you go through the reading exercise.
Then list and analyze the terms. Some will be completely new to you. Consult a medical
dictionary for their meanings. Then re-read the material for better comprehension.

Neurologic Consultation

October 1, 19—

The patient is a 57-year-old woman who sought further neurologic care. She returns for
neurologic care at this time with the specific concern about increase in seizure difficulties
since a motor vehicle accident in 19—. She states that she was broadsided on that occasion and suffered a basal skull fracture. The seat belt slipped and her head was bumped

over the right frontal region. She had swelling the size of a baseball and black and blue areas over the face and head. She was evaluated at Blank Emergency Room and discharged home. She feels that her seizures have increased since that accident.

She does have a history of seizures, beginning in 19—. She had suffered a motor vehicle accident in 19— and her head struck the steering wheel. She was treated initially for the seizures with Dilantin and had exfoliative dermatitis or Stevens-Johnson's syndrome with leukopenia and that was discontinued and she was begun on phenobarbital and Mysoline. She presently is taking phenobarbital 100 mg tablets 1 1/2 to 2 tablets daily. She increases the dose when the seizures are more frequent.

In recent weeks her seizures have been daily and they seem to be worsened by stress. Her husband describes the seizures. Initially she cannot talk, she flutters her eyes and stutters and then she may cry out. She then proceeds to have a full-blown generalized convulsion with loss of consciousness measured in seconds typically. She feels tired and has a headache afterward. She is occasionally incontinent with these spells. She feels that she was at her best when on Mysoline in very low dosages, namely 25 mg daily many years ago. She complains that doctors have not believed her about this low dose of medication. Her seizures have been better in the past week or two but because of their frequent occurrence before that she decided to return for neurologic care.

Patient has a history of multiple traumatic events. She has been in a wheelchair since 19— after a fracture of the hip which was pinned and she feels was an incorrect management of her hip fracture. She had suffered a fall that led to the fracture of the hip. She suffered a fracture in 19— when she fell out of her wheelchair and believes that was a midthoracic spine fracture. She has had fractures of right wrists and right lower extremity which she believes was not set correctly and led to deformity of a permanent nature.

She tells me of an illness with high fever after the accident of 19— and it is at that point that she apparently first encountered Dr. Blank who has dealt with the febrile illness part. It is not clear what the origin of the liver damage is as she denies an alcohol history.

Social History:
She smokes 2 packs of cigarettes daily, does not use alcohol.

Current Medications:
Zantac, 150 mg. BID; Phosfree, vitamin B-12 orally; Nitro-Bid 6.5 mg BID; Digoxin, 1 tablet daily and Lasix occasionally for leg swelling. She also takes OsCal.

Review of Systems:
She is allergic to Dilantin with severe reaction as described above. Her last phenobarbital level is believed to have been 41 mcg per ml and that was about 3 weeks ago.

Neurologic Examination:
Vital Signs: 140/85, pulse 70, respiration 16.

Head and Neck: There is no sign of major cranial deformity, no palpable depression of skull. Carotid pulses are full, no bruits.

Mental Status: She is minimally dysarthric and somewhat labile in her emotional content. There is no aphasic difficulty.

Cranial Nerves: Visual fields are full by confrontation. The optic fundi are normal. Pupils equal and reactive to light. There is a trace of nystagmus on lateral gaze. There is minimal facial asymmetry without major weakness. Pin perception is equal bilaterally. Hearing is intact to finger rub. The remainder of the cranial nerves seem normal.

Motor Examination: There is a spastic left hemiparesis with contracture at heel cord and the knee is held in partial flexion. On the right, the lower extremity is rigid with bony block and equinovarus posture. The right arm has mildly decreased tone but is functional.

Sensaton: Pin testing is normal on the face and the upper extremities. There is a sensory level to pin at about T4 to T6 and this is barely reproducible on repeated testing. Vibratory sense is suppressed bilaterally.

Tendon Reflexes: Hyperactive in both upper extremities. Plantar responses are mute bilaterally.

Coordination: Finger to nose testing with right hand is intact.

Impression:

1. Post-traumatic encephalopathy with seizure disorder
2. History of multiple fractures and probably thoracic spinal fracture with paraparesis
3. Seizure disorder poorly controlled

Disposition:
Patient will continue on phenobarbital 150 mg daily. I have started her on Mysolin 25 mg BID. I asked that she keep track of seizure frequency. She will sign a release for records of a CT from Hospital A over 10 years ago as she was told of brain damage and also of a recent MRI of head and possibly neck done at Hospital B recently. She will return in about 6 weeks for followup.

Reading Comprehension 14.2

DIRECTIONS: Underline the medical terms as you go through the reading exercise. Then list and analyze the terms. Some will be completely new to you. Consult a medical dictionary for their meanings. Then re-read the material for better comprehension.

History and Physical Examination

Present Illness:
This 44-year-old male was transferred from General Hospital, where he was under the care of Dr. S. H. for status epilepticus, resolved metabolic and respiratory acidosis, hypoglycemia and heavy alcohol abuse. The patient was found on the street, sitting on the curb, and then developed status epilepticus which required heroic measures, including phenobarb, Dilantin, and Valium to finally control the seizures, which have not recurred. The patient has continued to slowly improve, with increased mentation prior to transfer. Workups at that time include EEG which is positive for encephalopathy only, negative CAT scan and slow resolution of all the abnormal lab studies.

Past History:
History taken from the family now. The patient denies any previous medical problems or surgery. He was on no medicines, and had no known allergies. The patient quit smoking about a year ago, but his alcohol intake has been quite excessive, up to several beers and martinis per day or higher. The patient has no previous history of ethanol problems in the past.

Social History:
The patient has six children. He is married and works as an accountant.

Family History:
Positive for early myocardial infarctions, father. Brothers and sisters alive and well. Mother still alive, in her 70's. No family history of diabetes or cancer.

Review of Systems:
HEENT: No history of lightheaded spells, headaches or blackout spells. No eye problems or nose, mouth or throat problems.

Endocrine: No history of thyroid disorders or diabetes. No increased nocturia recently.

Cardiorespiratory: Previous walking pneumonia in early 50's. No other problems. No cough, wheezing, asthma. On health screen at work, patient was found to have slightly decreased lung volumes, and was thought to have early COPD, which prompted his cessation of smoking one year ago. Wife states that patient has chronic cough, which is usually clear and a.m. in character. No history of myocardial infarctions, murmurs or palpitations.

GI: No history of jaundice, hepatitis, gallbladder problems, changes in bowel habits. The patient did have ulcer disease years ago.

GU: No history of burning, infections or prostate problems.

Musculoskeletal: No history of arthritis or serious injuries.

Hematological: No history of bleeding disorders.

Neurological: No prior history of seizures, strokes, epilepsies or palsies.

Clinical Exam:
General: The patient appears as a mature male lying in bed, agitated, pulling at his restraints and only partially oriented.

Skin: Clear, except for marked herpes-like lesions around the nose and upper lip.

Vital Signs: BP 110/80, pulse 80 and regular. Temperature 99, respirations 14.

HEENT:
Head normocephalic.
Eyes—pupils equal, reactive, reactive to light and accommodation. Extraocular movements within normal limits. Sclerae are clear, fundi benign.
Ears—tympanic membranes are clear. No Battle's sign noted.
Nose, mouth, throat—mucous membranes are moist.
No inflammation noted.

Neck: Supple. No neck vein distention noted. Carotids are full without bruits. No masses palpable.

Lungs: Scattered rhonchi and coarse rales throughout, clearing with coughing. The patient appears to have some phlegm in his trachea.

Heart: Regular rhythm without gallops or murmurs.

Abdomen: Nontender. Bowel sounds are active. No hepatomegaly appreciated.

Genitalia: Normal male. Foley catheter in place.

Rectal: Stool brown, occult blood negative. No masses palpable.

Extremities: Distal pulses strong. No clubbing, cyanosis or edema noted.

Neurological: Deep tendon reflexes are decreased but symmetrical. Toes are +/− bilaterally.

Assessment:
   1. Status post status epilepticus with slowly recovering mentation.
   2. COPD with bronchitis
   3. History of alcoholism

Plan:
Continuation of IV fluids while attempting PO feeding. Appropriate cultures of the sputum and urine. Continuation of Erythromycin. Continue patient on thiamine as well as

tapering Decadron doses. Continuation of Dilantin, 300 mg per day, with Dilantin level. Appropriate chest x-ray and lab work.

Reading Comprehension Vocabulary

Use the space below to list the medical terms for analysis and definition.

_____

_____

_____

_____

_____

_____

_____

_____

_____

_____

_____

_____

_____

_____

_____

_____

_____

_____

_____

_____

_____

_____

_____

CHAPTER 15

Special Senses: Sight and Hearing

OBJECTIVES

When you have successfully completed Chapter 15, you should be able to:
— Recall terms relating to the structure and function of the eye and ear.
— Write the meanings of building blocks introduced in this chapter.
— Write medical terms when given the definitions.
— Label the structures of the eye and ear on familiar drawings.
— Write the definitions for terms from this chapter.
— Analyze common medical terms related to the eye and ear.
— Build medical terms using the building blocks introduced in this and previous chapters.

amplified	(AM-plih-FIED)	Enlarged or made stronger. For example, a hearing aid amplifies sound.
articulate	(ar-TICK-you-late)	To unite by a joint or joints; to move a joint. Also means to enunciate clearly
atrophy	(AT-roh-fee)	Waste away from lack of nourishment or from disuse
diminished	(dih-MIN-isht)	Made less or smaller
equilibrium	(ee-kwih-LIH-bree-um)	A state of balance
evaluation	(ee-val-you-AY-shun)	The process of determining the value or amount of something. In medicine, judging a patient's state of health
focus	(FOH-kus)	A central point or center of activity; a convergence
habilitation	(hah-bill-ih-TAY-shun)	To equip for working
intraocular	(in-trah-OCK-you-lar)	Within the eye
labyrinth	(LAH-bih-rinth)	A system of intercommunicating cavities or canals
meatus	(mee-AY-tus)	An opening or passageway in soft tissues of the body
medial	(MEE-dee-al)	Pertaining to the middle
motility	(moh-TILL-ih-tee)	The ability to move spontaneously
opaque	(oh-PAYK)	Impervious to light rays; not transparent or translucent
peripheral	(peh-RIH-fer-al)	Situated away from the center
protrusion	(proh-TROO-zhun)	The state of being thrust forward
receptors	(ree-SEP-torz)	Sensory nerves that respond to various stimuli such as light, sound, or touch
refracted	(ree-FRACK-ted)	Caused to deviate or diffuse; for example, a crystal refracts light
rehabilitation	(ree-hah-bill-ih-TAY-shun)	The process of restoring a patient to former capacity or capabilities
stereoscopic	(steh-ree-oh-SKAHP-ick)	Pertaining to seeing objects in three dimensions; that is, as having depth as well as height and width

transparent	(trans-**PAIR**-ent)	Having the property of transmitting light rays
vascular	(**VAS**-kyou-lar)	Supplied with or containing vessels or ducts
vibrations	(vigh-**BRAY**-shunz)	Quivering or trembling motions

OVERVIEW

The *special senses* include vision, hearing, taste, and smell. This chapter will deal with vision and hearing as extensions of the nervous system.

Ophthalmology is the science concerned with the eye and its diseases. *Otology* is the science concerned with the ear, its functions, and its diseases.

An *ophthalmologist* is a physician who specializes in the diagnosis and treatment of diseases of the eye. An *otolaryngologist*, occasionally called otorhinolaryngologist, specializes in the diagnosis and treatment of diseases of the ear, nose, and throat. Both are usually Board certified medical specialists (see Chapter 16). An *optometrist* is trained and licensed to examine and test the eyes and to treat visual defects by prescribing corrective lenses and by establishing programs of eye exercise. Generally, optometrists are not permitted to prescribe drugs. An *optician* is trained in filling prescriptions for corrective lenses. Opticians grind lenses and dispense eyeglasses. An *audiologist* is a licensed practitioner in the evaluation, habilitation and rehabilitation of persons with hearing disorders. He or she may work with a physician or may have an independent practice. Some states require that the audiologist have a statement from a physician indicating the patient's need for a hearing aid before prescribing.

STRUCTURE AND FUNCTION OF THE EYE

The eyes are paired to provide stereoscopic vision, that is, to allow us to perceive depth or mass as well as height and breadth. If the sight of one eye is lost, depth perception is lost. The eye is an extension of the brain and as such may be considered a part of the nervous system. The eye is set in a bony *orbit*, or socket, for protection. All but about one-sixth of the eye is concealed within the orbit. The eyelid further assists in protecting the eyeball from physical trauma. Figure 15.1 shows the external structures of the eye. The eyeball, or *ocular globe*, is a hollow, fluid filled sphere composed of three layers (Figure 15.2).

Sclera

The outer layer of the eyeball, the *sclera*, consists of tough, fibrous tissue and is contiguous with the transparent cornea at the front of the eyeball. The cornea permits light rays to enter the eye. The sclera has no blood vessels but does have sensory nerve endings that transmit the sense of pain.

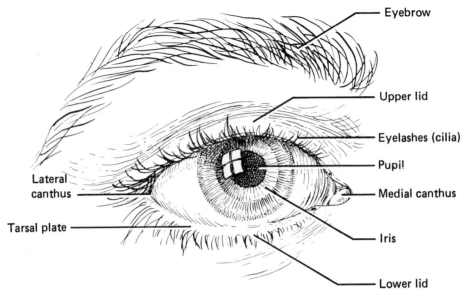

FIGURE 15.1   External view of the eye

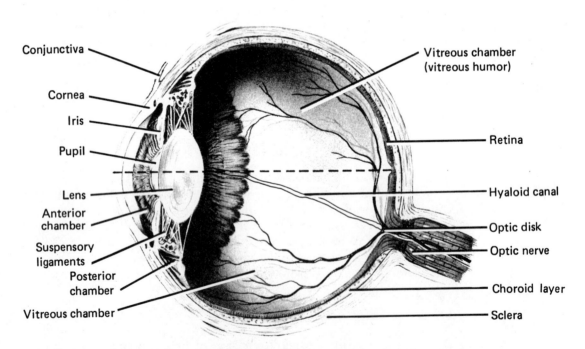

FIGURE 15.2   Internal structures of the eye (From Fong, Ferris, and Skelly, *Body Structures and Functions*, 6th edition, copyright 1984 by Delmar Publishers, Inc.)

Uvea

The middle layer, or *uvea*, contains blood vessels that nourish the eye. It includes:

- The *choroid* layer, which covers a large proportion of the eye globe posteriorly
- The *ciliary* body, which extends anteriorly around the front of the eye
- The *iris* which is under involuntary (autonomic) control and dilates or contracts to allow more or less light, as needed, to enter through the *pupil*, an opening in the center of the iris.

Retina

The inner layer, or *retina*, is open at the front. It contains the light receptors called *rods* and *cones* as well as specialized areas including the macula lutea and the optic disk. The eye's approximately 7 million cones are responsible for daylight vision. Most of the cones are found in a retinal depression called the *fovea centralis*, the area of sharpest vision. The fovea centralis is located within the *macula lutea*, a small yellow spot occupying about one square millimeter in the central region of the retina. The eye's estimated 100 million *rods* are activated only in dim light. They are located in the peripheral areas of the retina. The rods cannot perceive fine details or color, which accounts for our diminished vision at night.

Chambers of the Eye

The hollow part of the eyeball is divided into two distinct cavities, the anterior cavity and the posterior cavity. The iris further divides the anterior cavity into an anterior and a posterior chamber, both of which are filled with a watery fluid called *aqueous humor*. The large cavity behind the lens, the *vitreous chamber*, is filled with a *vitreous humor*, which has about the consistency of raw egg white. The vitreous humor maintains pressure within the eyeball to prevent its collapse. The *aqueous humor*, the lens, and the *vitreous humor* refract light rays and focus them on the retina.

Optic Nerve

In the optic disk, just medial to the fovea centralis, the nerve fibers from the retina leave the eye and become a part of the *optic nerve*, a thick, complex bundle of nerve fibers. Nerve cells (neurons) in the retina receive and transmit visual information via the optic nerve to other areas of the brain where it is processed in such a way as to allow us to see objects. The retina and optic nerve are considered to be extensions of the brain.

VISUAL ACUITY

Most common problems of vision are related either to visual acuity or to disorders of refraction.

Distance vision is tested with the familiar Snellen "E" chart, which has standardized numbers and letters of sizes a person with normal vision should be able to read at stated distances. These letters are sized from large (top) to small (bottom line). The subject is placed 20 feet from the chart. Each eye is tested separately, and the results are recorded as 20/20 (normal) or some other number based on the smallest characters that person can distinguish at a distance of 20 feet. For example, if the smallest characters the subject can distinguish could be read by a normal subject at 40 feet, vision in that eye is recorded as being 20/40. The well-known "E" at the top of the chart can be read by persons with normal visual acuity at 200 feet; a subject who could read only the "E" would have 20/200 vision in that eye.

REFRACTIVE DISORDERS

Refractive disorders generally are caused by problems in ability of the eye to adjust focus at different distances. These problems can be corrected with eyeglasses or contact lenses.

Myopia (nearsightedness), *hyperopia* (farsightedness), and *astigmatism* are common refractive disorders. Astigmatism is a problem in which light rays cannot be sharply focused on the retina.

COMMON OPHTHALMIC DISEASES

The most common ophthalmic disorders include:

- *Strabismus*, a pronounced deviation of one or both eyes ("crossed eyes")
- *Glaucoma*, abnormally increased intraocular pressure
- *Cataract*, in which the lens or its capsule gradually loses its transparency and becomes cloudy and opaque
- *Diabetic retinopathy*, a complication of diabetes that is currently the leading cause of blindness in adults

≡ BUILDING BLOCKS

ROOTS AND COMBINING FORMS

Word Element	Meaning
ambly/o	dull
ametr/o	disproportionate
aqua	water
blephar/o	eyelid
cor/o	pupil
cry/o	cold
cycl/o	ciliary body
cyst	sac
dacry/o	tear
dipl/o	double
goni/o	angle
irid/o	iris
kerat/o	cornea

Word Element	Meaing
lacrim/o	tear
meter	measure
myein	to shut
nyct	night
occul/o	eye
ophthalm/o	eye
phac/o	lens
photo	light
ptosis	falling
scler/o	hard
trich/o	hair
xer/o	dry
stere/o	three dimensional

SUFFIXES

Word Element	Meaning
–ism	condition
–opia	condition of the eye
–scopy	process of examining
–stigma	point
–tropic	turning

PREFIXES

Word Element	Meaning
aniso–	unequal
eso–	inward
exo–	outside
intra–	within
presby–	old age

VOCABULARY

General

accommodation	(ah-**KOM**-moh-**DAY**-shun)	The ability of the eye to adjust to various distances by changing the shape of the lens

anisocoria	(an-is-so-**KOH**-ree-ah)	Inequality of the size of the two pupils, congenital or acquired
bifocal	(by-**FOH**-kal)	Having two foci, (singular, focus) such as the correction for near and far vision in bifocal eyeglasses
emmetropia	(**em**-eh-**TROH**-pee-ah)	The normal condition of the eye in refraction
intraocular	(in-trah-**OCK**-you-lar)	Within the eyeball
miotic	(my-**AH**-tick)	Causing the pupil to contract; also a drug that contracts the pupil
mydriatic	(mid-ree-**AT**-ick)	Causing pupillary dilatation; also, any drug that dilates the pupil
ophthalmologist	(ahf-thal-**MOL**-oh-jist)	A physician who specializes in the treatment of disorders of the eye
ophthalmology	(ahf-thal-**MOL**--oh-jee)	The science dealing with the eye and its diseases
optician	(op-**TIH**-shan)	One who is a specialist in the making of and dispensing of optical appliances
optometrist	(op-**TOM**-eh-trist)	A person specifically trained and licensed to examine and test the eyes, and to treat visual defects with corrective lenses and eye exercises; a Doctor of Optometry
orthoptics	(or-**THOP**-ticks)	The science of correcting defects in binocular vision through eye exercises
visual acuity	(**VIZH**-you-al ah-**KYOU**-ih-tee)	Acuteness or sharpness of vision, which may be determined by use of the Snellen "E" chart

Terms related to Anatomy and Physiology

aqueous humor	(**AY**-kwee-us)	Transparent liquid contained in the anterior and posterior chambers of the eye between the cornea and the lens
canthus	(**KAN**-thus, **KAN**-thigh)	The angle formed at either end of the eye between the eyelids; corner of the eye. Plural, *canthi*.

choroid	(**KOH**-royd)	Vascular middle layer of the eye between the sclera and the retina
cilia	(**SILL**-ee-ah)	Eyelashes. Singular, cilium.
cones	(kohn)	Cells in the outer layer of the retina that are responsible for daylight vision
conjunctiva	(kon-junk-**TIE**-vah)	Mucous membrane that lines eyelids and covers the eyeball
cornea	(**KOR**-nee-ah)	The clear, transparent anterior portion of the fibrous coat of the eye that admits light and comprises about one-sixth of the eye's surface
fovea centralis	(**FOH**-vee-ah sen-**TRAH**-lis	A depression in the center of macula lutea, the area of clearest vision
iris	(**EYE**-rihs)	The circular colored membrane behind the cornea, that controls the amount of light entering through the pupil. Plural, *irides.*
lacrimal gland	(**LACK**-rih-mal)	Gland that secretes tears
lens	(lenz)	The crystalline lens of the eye that functions with the humors of the eye to refract light rays
optic disk	(**OP**-tick disk)	The area in the retina for entrance of the optic nerve; the blind spot
optic nerve		The nerve that carries impulses from the retina to the brain for the sense of sight; cranial nerve II
orbit	(**OR**-bit)	The bony socket in the skull that contains and protects the eyeball.
pupil	(**PYOU**-pil)	The contractile opening at the center of the iris
retina	(**RET**-ih-nah)	Innermost or third layer of the eye, where the rods and cones are located and which receives light rays focused by the lens

rods		Specialized cells in the retina, which respond to dim light
sclera	(SKLEE-rah)	The outer layer of the eyeball. It extends from the optic nerve to the cornea.
uvea	(YOU-vee-ah)	The entire middle layer of the eye which lies immediately beneath the sclera. It encompasses the iris, ciliary body, and choroid.
vitreous humor	(VIT-ree-us)	The gelatinous fluid that fills the vitreous chamber between the lens and the retina and prevents its collapse

Terms Related to Pathology

amaurosis	(am-aw-ROH-sis)	Complete loss of sight; blindness
amblyopia	(am-blee-OH-pee-ah)	Reduction or dimness of vision
ametropia	(am-eh-TROH-pee-ah)	Inability of the eye to focus directly on the retina
anophthalmia	(an-off-THAL-mee-ah)	The absence of one or both eyes
aphakia	(ah-FAY-kee-ah)	Absence of the lens of an eye as might exist after cataract surgery
astigmatism	(ah-STIG-mah-tizm)	Condition in which an irregular curvature of the cornea prevents clear focusing
blepharitis	(blef-ah-RYE-tis)	Inflammation of the edges of the eyelids
blepharoptosis	(blef-ah-roh-TOH-sis)	Drooping of the upper eyelid
cataract	(KAT-ah-rackt)	Condition in which the lens or its capsule gradually loses its transparency and becomes cloudy and opaque
chalazion	(kah-LAY-zee-on)	A cystlike tumor on the eyelid caused by inflammation of a meibomian gland; meibomian cyst
conjunctivitis	(kon-junk-tih-VIGH-tis)	Inflammation of conjunctiva

cycloplegia	(**sigh**-kloh-**PLEE**-jee-ah)	Paralysis of the ciliary muscle which results in a loss of accommodation
dacryocystitis	(**dack**-ree-oh-sis-**TIE**-tis)	Inflammation of a tear sac
dacryoma	(**dack**-ree-**OH**-mah)	A tumorlike swelling caused by obstruction of a tear duct
diabetic retinopathy	(die-ah-**BEH**-tick **ret**-ih-**NOP**-ah-thee)	Disorder of the retina occurring in diabetes and leading to blindness if not treated
diplopia	(dih-**PLOH**-pee-ah)	Double vision; may affect only one eye
ectropion	(eck-**TROH**-pee-on)	A turning outward of the edge of an eyelid
epiphora	(eh-**PIF**-oh-rah)	Abnormal overflow of tears which may be caused by an excess secretion of tears or to obstruction of a lacrimal duct
esotropia	(es-oh-**TROH**-pee-ah)	The turning inward of an eye, crossed eyes
exophthalmos, exophthalmus	(**eck**-sof-**THAL**-mos)	Abnormal protrusion of eyeball
exotropia	(**eck**-soh-**TROH**-pee-ah)	The turning outward of an eye
glaucoma	(glaw-**KOH**-mah)	An incurable disease of the eye characterized by abnormally increased intraocular pressure, which results in blindness unless treated
hemianopia	(**hem**-ee-ah-**NO**-pee-ah)	Blindness in one-half of the field of vision in one or both eyes
hordeolum	(hor-**DEE**-oh-lum)	A stye
hyperopia	(**high**-per-**OH**-pee-ah)	Farsightedness
iridocyclitis	(**ir**-ih-doh-sigh-**KLIGH**-tis)	Inflammation of the iris and ciliary body
iridomalacia	(**ir**-ih-doh-mah-**LAY**-she-ah)	Softening of the iris
iritis	(eye-**RYE**-tis)	Inflammation of the iris
keratitis	(ker-ah-**TIE**-tis)	Inflammation of the cornea

miosis	(my-**OH**-sis)	Abnormal contraction of the pupils
myopia	(my-**OH**-pee-ah)	Nearsightedness
nyctalopia	(**nick**-tah-**LOH**-pee-ah)	Inability to see well in a dim light or at night; night blindness
nystagmus	(nis-**TAG**-mus)	A repeating, involuntary, cyclical movement of the eyeball
phacosclerosis	(**fack**-oh-skleh-**ROH**-sis)	Hardening of the lens of the eye
photophobia	(**foh**-toh-**FOH**-bee-ah)	An abnormal intolerance of light; occurs in disease conditions such as measles, rubella, meningitis, and inflammation of the eye and as a side effect of some medications
pinkeye		Epidemic form of acute conjunctivitis
presbyopia	(**pres**-bee-**OH**-pee-ah)	An impairment of vision in advancing age that involves loss of accommodation or the power of the eye to focus
pterygium	(teh-**RIJ**-ee-um)	A wingshaped, abnormally thickened patch of conjunctiva that extends over part of the cornea
retinitis pigmentosa	(ret-ih-**NIGH**-tis pig-men-**TOH**-sah)	A degenerative disease which may be hereditary, affecting the retinal epithelium, the rod and cone layer, and which causes night blindness
retinoblastoma	(**ret**-ih-noh-blass-**TOH**-mah)	A malignant tumor of the retina composed of neuroglia cells
retinopathy	(**ret**-ih-**NOP**-ah-thee)	Any disease of the retina
scleritis	(sklee-**RYE**-tis)	Inflammation of the sclera
strabismus	(strah-**BIZ**-mus)	Disorder of the eyes in which there is a lack of visual coordination; squint; crossed eyes
sty(e)	(stie)	An inflammatory swelling of one or more sebaceous glands of the eyelid
trachoma	(trah-**KOH**-mah)	A chronic contagious form of conjunctivitis in which the conjunctivae become enlarged,

		follicles form, and other changes ensue
trichiasis	(trick-**EYE**-ah-sis)	Inversion of eyelashes (ingrown hairs) that cause an irritation of the eyeball
uveitis	(**you**-vee-**EYE**-tis)	Inflammation of the uvea
xerophthalmia	(**zee**-roff-**THAL**-mee-ah)	A dryness of the conjunctiva and cornea that is associated with deficiency of vitamin A

Terms Associated with Diagnostic Devices and Procedures

gonioscope	(**GOH**-nee-oh-**skohp**)	An instrument for examining the anterior chamber of the eye
keratometer	(ker-ah-**TOM**-eh-ter)	An instrument for measuring the curves of the cornea
laser	(**LAY**-zer)	Acronym for *l*ight *a*mplification by *s*timulated *e*mission of *r*adiation, a device that emits intense heat and power at close range, and in precise focus. Used in surgery and in diagnostic procedures
Snellen's chart	(**SNEH**-lenz)	The familiar "E" chart imprinted with standardized lines of black letters graduating in size from large at the top to small at the bottom, used for testing visual acuity. Named for Dutch ophthalmologist Herman Snellen, 1834–1908
tonography	(toh-**NOG**-rah-fee)	The recording of changes in pressure; for example, intraocular pressure
tonometry	(toh-**NOM**-eh-tree)	The measurement of pressure or tension of a part, as intraocular tension. Used to detect glaucoma

Terms Related to Surgery and Treatment

enucleation	(ee-**new**-klee-**AY**-shun)	Surgical removal of an entire mass or part; generally used to refer to removal of a tumor or of the eyeball

iridectomy	(ir-ih-**DECK**-toh-mee)	Surgical removal of a portion of the iris
iridesis, iridodesis	(eye-**RID**-eh-sis, ir-ih-**DOD**-eh-sis)	Artificial creation of an iris
keratoplasty	(**KER**-ah-toh-**Plass**-tee)	Plastic operation on the cornea
phacolysis	(fah-**KOL**-ih-sis)	Surgical removal or disintegration of the lens of the eye

STRUCTURE AND FUNCTION OF THE EAR

The *ear* is the organ of hearing and balance and it, like the eye, can be considered a part of the nervous system. It consists of three main subdivisions; the outer ear, the middle ear, and the inner ear. Working in unison, the two ears localize sound.

Outer or External Ear

The part of the ear that projects from the side of the head (Figure 15.3) is the *auricle*

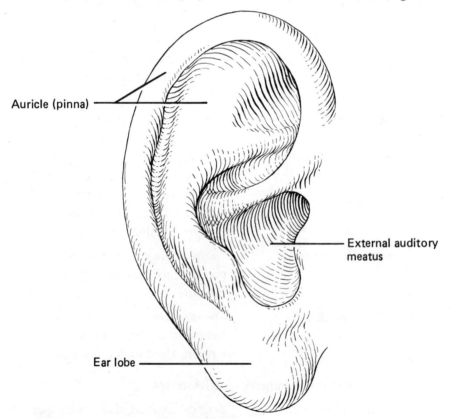

Auricle (pinna)

External auditory meatus

Ear lobe

FIGURE 15.3   External view of the ear

or *pinna*. It is formed mostly of cartilage. Its function is to catch sound waves and direct them inward. The *external auditory meatus*, or *acoustic* meatus, is a canal that conducts sound waves inward to the *tympanic membrane* (eardrum). The canal is lined with glands that secrete a waxy substance called *cerumen*, which helps protect the tympanum from damage by foreign objects.

Middle Ear

The *middle ear* (Figures 15.4 and 15.5) consists of the tympanic membrane (eardrum) and the ossicles. The tympanum is a thin membrane covered on the outside with skin and on the inside with mucous membrane. The membrane vibrates and transmits sound waves to the *malleus* or hammer, the *incus* or anvil, and the *stapes* or stirrup. These three small bones, or ossicles, amplify the sound waves that reach them and transmit this amplified signal to the inner ear.

Eustachian Tube

The *eustachian tube* connects the middle ear with the pharynx. Its function is to equalize air pressure during changes in altitude. As altitude rises above sea level, atmospheric pressure decreases and air trapped inside the middle ear expands, as you may

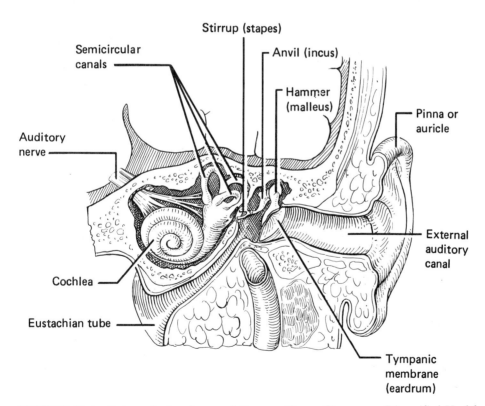

FIGURE 15.4 Internal structures of the ear (From Simmers, *Diversified Health Occupations*, 2nd edition copyright 1988 by Delmar Publishers, Inc.)

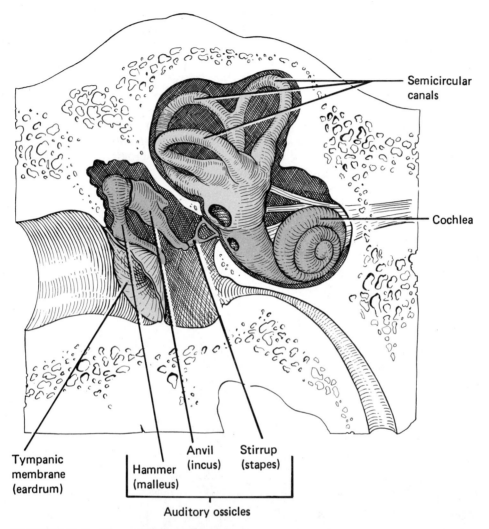

Semicircular canals

Cochlea

Tympanic membrane (eardrum)

Hammer (malleus)

Anvil (incus)

Stirrup (stapes)

Auditory ossicles

FIGURE 15.5 The middle and inner ear

have discovered in airplanes or even elevators. This expansion may cause pain and could damage the ear's internal structures if it could not escape through the eustachian tubes. Swallowing or yawning helps open the tubes and allow the air to escape.

Inner Ear

The *inner ear* is a complex system of tubes and chambers called a *labyrinth*. A membranous labyrinth is contained within a bony labyrinth. The structures within the labyrinth are the cochlea, the semicircular canals, and the vestibule.

COCHLEA The *cochlea* is a spiral, snail-shaped, fluid-filled body that contains the organ of Corti, the final organ of hearing. The vibrations it receives from the middle ear stimulate sensors to emit nerve impulses that are then transmitted from the organ of Corti to the brain by the auditory nerve (cranial nerve VIII).

SEMICIRCULAR CANALS The three *semicircular canals* of the inner ear function in maintaining equilibrium (balance). These canals lie at right angles to each other and are filled with a fluid called *endolymph*. Any movement of the head sets this fluid in motion, stimulating nerve endings of the *vestibulocochlear nerve* (cranial nerve VIII), which transmits impulses to the brain so that it can correct equilibrium as necessary. Patients who have undergone certain operations on the ear experience some disturbance of equilibrium for a brief time after surgery. Viral infections of the ear and other disorders may also interfere with equilibrium.

VESTIBULE The *vestibule* is a chamber that connects the cochlea and the semicircular canals.

COMMON DISORDERS OF THE EAR

Some common disorders affecting the ear are:

- *Otitis media*, or infection of the middle ear
- *Otalgia*, or earache, which may have a number of causes
- *Otosclerosis*, a hardening of the bony tissue of the labyrinth that leads to hearing loss
- *Tinnitus*, a ringing sound in the ears.

BUILDING BLOCKS

ROOTS AND COMBINING FORMS

Word Element	Meaning
audi/o	hearing
aur/i, aur/o	ear
cera	wax
incus	anvil
laryng/o	larynx
lymph	clear fluid
malleus	hammer
myc/o	fungus
myring/o	eardrum
ot/o	ear
pharyng/o	pharynx
staped/o	stirrup; stapes
tympan/o	eardrum

Word Element	Meaning
–cusis	hearing
–dynia	pain
–meter	measure
–phonia	sound
–sclerosis	hardening

PREFIXES

Word Element	Meaning
endo	within
presby–	old age

VOCABULARY

General Terms

acoustic	(ah-**KOO**-stick)	Relating to sound or to the sense of hearing
audiologist	(**au**-dee-**OL**-oh-jist)	A specialist in the evaluation, diagnosis, and rehabilitation of persons with hearing impairment
aural	(**AW**-ral)	Pertaining to the ear
deaf-mute		A person who is unable to hear and unable to speak
deafness	(**DEHF**-ness)	Inability to hear
hearing acuity	(ah-**KYOU**-ih-tee)	The distance at which a person can hear a certain sound
hearing impairment		Diminution of hearing acuity
otolaryngologist	(**oh**-toh-**lar**-in-**GOL**-oh-jist)	Physician who specializes in diagnosis and treatment of the ear, nose, and throat; formerly called otorhinolaryngologist. The root rhino (nose) has been dropped but is still implied.
otology	(oh-**TAHL**-oh-jee)	The science or study of the ear, its function, and its pathology

otopharyngeal	(oh-toh-fah-**RIN**-jee-al)	Relating to the ear and the pharynx

Terms Related to Anatomy and Physiology

auricle, auricula	(**AW**-rih-kal, aw-**RICK**-you-lah)	The portion of the external ear outside the skull; the pinna
cerumen	(see-**ROO**-men)	The waxy, soft, brownish secretion found in the ear canal; earwax
cochlea	(**KOCK**-lee-ah)	A spiral, snail-shaped, fluid-filled body that contains the organ of Corti, the receptor for hearing
endolymph	(**EN**-doh-limf)	Pale, translucent fluid within the semicircular canals of the inner ear
eustachian tubes	(you-**STAY**-kee-an tewbz)	The paired auditory tubes, about 1 to 1½ inches long that connect the middle ear with the nasopharynx
external auditory meatus	(**AW**-dih-**toh**-ree mee-**AY**-tus)	The canal leading from the pinna to the tympanic membrane (eardrum)
incus	(**ING**-kus)	The second of the three ossicles in the middle-ear; the anvil
labyrinth	(**LAB**-ih-rinth)	The internal ear consisting of bony and membranous labyrinths; essential to maintaining physical equilibrium of the body
malleus	(**MAL**-ee-us)	The first and largest of the three ossicles in the middle ear; it articulates with the incus
ossicle	(**AHS**-ih-kal)	Any small bone. *Auditory ossicles* are the three small bones of the middle ear: the malleus, incus, and stapes.
oval window		Oval opening in the wall of the tympanic cavity (middle ear) that holds the base of the stapes
perilymph	(**PER**-ih-limf)	The pale, transparent fluid secreted by cells in the bony labyrinth that circulates in the space between the membranous labyrinth and the bony labyrinth of the internal ear

pinna	(**PIN**-nah)	The auricle or projected part of the external ear.
semicircular canals		The passages forming part of inner ear that are involved with balance and equilibrium
stapes	(**STAY**-peez)	The third ossicle in the middle ear commonly called the stirrup because of its shape
tympanic membrane	(tim-**PAN**-ick)	The membrane that separates the tympanic cavity from the external auditory meatus; the eardrum

Terms Related to Pathology

labyrinthitis	(lab-ih-rin-**THIGH**-tis)	Inflammation of the labyrinth; *otitis externa*
Meniere's disease	(men-ee-**AYRZ**)	A disease of the labyrinth that includes such symptoms as tinnitus, dizziness, a sensation of fullness or pressure in the ears, and progressive loss of hearing
otalgia	(oh-**TAHL**-jee-ah)	Pain in the ear
otitis media	(oh-**TIE**-tis **MEE**-dee-ah)	Inflammation of the middle ear
otodynia	(**oh**-toh-**DIN**-ee-ah)	Pain in the ear; earache
otomycosis	(**oh**-toh-my-**KOH**-sis)	A fungal infection of the external auditory meatus of the ear
otosclerosis	(**OH**-toh-sklee-**ROH**-sis)	A condition in which the formation of spongy bone in the inner ear causes the stapes to become fixed to the oval window, leading to impairment of hearing, especially for low tones
presbycusis	(pres-beh-**KOO**-sis)	Progressive impairment of hearing with advancing age
tinnitus	(tin-**NIGH**-tus)	Ringing or tingling in the ear
vertigo	(**VER**-tih-go)	A type of dizziness that sometimes is caused by disturbances of the semicircular canals

Terms Related to Diagnostic Devices and Procedures

audiogram	(**AW**-dee-oh-gram)	The recording created when hearing is tested by audiometer
audiometer	(aw-dee-**OM**-eh-ter)	An instrument for testing hearing
audiometry	(aw-dee-**OM**-eh-tree)	The testing of the hearing sense
otoscope	(**OH**-toh-skohp)	An instrument for internal examination of the ear

Terms Related to Surgery or Treatment

fenestration	(**fen**-es-**TRAY**-shun)	Surgical creation of an artificial opening into the labyrinth of the ear
labyrinthectomy	(**lab**-ih-rin-**THECK**-toh-mee)	Excision of the labyrinth
myringodectomy	(mih-**ring**-go-**DECK**-toh-mee)	Excision of a part or all of the tympanic membrane; myringectomy
myringoplasty	(mih-**RING**-go-**plas**-tee)	Plastic surgery for repair of the tympanic membrane
otoplasty	(**OH**-toh-**plas**-tee)	Plastic surgery for correction of defects and deformities of the ear
stapedectomy	(**stay**-peh-**DECK**-toh-mee)	Excision of the stapes and replacement by a prosthesis (artificial device) to improve hearing
tympanoplasty	(**tim**-pah-no-**PLAS**-tee)	Any one of several surgical procedures for correction of chronic inflammation or restoration of sound transmission in the middle ear

15.1 Review: Visual System

DIRECTIONS: Cover the left column while you complete the statements on the right side.

orbit

The eye is set in a bony _____ for protection.

sclera	The outer fibrous layer of the eyeball is the
cornea	_____ , the anterior part of which
	is the _____ .
uvea	The middle vascular layer is the _____ .
iris	It contains a pigmented area called the
pupil	_____ , which has a hole in the
	center, the _____ , for the
	passage of light.
retina	The inner layer, the _____ , has
	no anterior portion. This inner layer contains the light
cones	receptors: _____ , which are
	responsible for daylight vision, and
rods	_____ which are activated only in
	dim light. Nerve cells of the eye receive and transmit
	visual information via the _____
optic nerve	_____ to other areas of the brain.
	Light rays are refracted and focused on the inner
aqueous	retina by the anterior _____
lens	humor, the _____ , and the
vitreous	posterior _____ humor. Normal
20/20	vision is usually written as _____ .

15.2   Review: Visual Building Blocks

DIRECTIONS: Write the meanings of the following building blocks.

1. ambly/o _____
2. blephar/o _____
3. cor/o _____
4. cycl/o _____
5. dacry/o _____
6. dipl/o _____
7. irid/o _____
8. kerat/o _____
9. ophthalm/o _____
10. –opia _____
11. phot/o _____
12. plac/o _____
13. trich– _____
14. tropia _____
15. xer/o _____

15.3 Review: Building Visual Terms

DIRECTIONS: Fill in the blanks with the appropriate building block or medical term.

1. The combining form for *eyelid* is _____ .
   _____ means *falling* or *drooping*.
   Write the word for *drooping of the upper eyelid* _____ .

2. The combining form _____ means *tear*.
   _____ is the medical term for *sac* or *bladder*.
   The suffix _____ indicates *inflammation*.
   The term for inflammation of the tear sac is _____ .

3. A suffix for *turning* is _____ .
   The prefix _____ means inward.
   The term _____ means a *turning inward of the eye*.

4. A combining form for *eye* is _____ .
   The prefix _____ means *within*.
   Write the term for *within the eyeball* _____ .

5. The combining form for *cornea* is _____ .
   _____ is the suffix meaning *inflammation*.
   _____ is *inflammation of the cornea*.
   The suffix meaning *surgical repair* is _____ .
   _____ is *surgical repair of the cornea*.

6. The suffix that indicates a *condition of the eye* is _____ .
   The combining form for *dull* or *dim* is _____ .
   Write the word for *dimness of vision* _____ .
   _____ is nearsightedness.
   _____ is farsightedness.

7. A suffix meaning *disease condition* is _____ .
   Write the word for *any disease of the retina.* _____

8. _____ is a combining form meaning *eye*.
   The suffix _____ means the *science or study of*.
   _____ is the *science or study of the eye*.

9. A suffix indicating a *condition of the eye* is _____ .
   The combining form for *dry* is _____ .
   A dryness of the conjunctiva and cornea due to Vitamin A deficiency is called

   _____ .

10. The combining form for *lens* is _____ .
    The suffix _____ means a *hardening*.
    _____ is a hardening of the crystalline lens of the eye.

15.4   Review: Vocabulary

DIRECTIONS: Match the terms in the first column with the definitions in the second column.

_____ 1. accommodation
_____ 2. amaurosis
_____ 3. anisocoria
_____ 4. cataract
_____ 5. conjunctiva
_____ 6. diplopia
_____ 7. glaucoma
_____ 8. miotic
_____ 9. mydriatic
_____ 10. nyctalopia
_____ 11. photophobia
_____ 12. presbyopia
_____ 13. strabismus
_____ 14. trichiasis
_____ 15. visual acuity

A. Squint, or crosseye
B. Agent that causes the pupil to dilate
C. Acuteness or sharpness of vision
D. Defect of vision in advancing age involving loss of accommodation or recession of near point
E. Complete loss of sight
F. Agent that causes the pupil to contract
G. Inversion of eyelashes so that they rub against the cornea
H. Inequality of the size of the pupils
I. Mucous membrane lining the eyelids
J. Double vision
K. The adjustment of the eye for various distances in order to focus an image
L. Lack of transparency of the lens
M. Unusual intolerance to light
N. Disease of the eye characterized by increase in intraocular pressure
O. Night blindness

15.5   Review: Analyzing Visual Terms

Analyze the following terms:

EXAMPLE:	anisocoria		
	aniso	/cor	/ia
	unequal	pupil	condition
1.	amblyopia		
2.	blepharoptosis		
3.	esotropia		
4.	phacosclerosis		
5.	xerophthalmia		

15.6   Review: Visual Anatomy

DIRECTIONS: Label the structures of the eye.

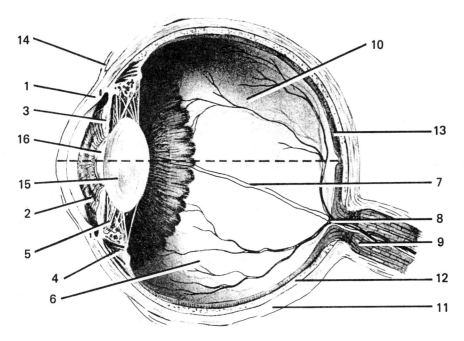

(From Fong, Ferris, and Skelly, *Body Structures and Functions*, 6th edition, copyright 1984 by Delmar Publishers, Inc.)

1. _____   6. _____   11. _____
2. _____   7. _____   12. _____
3. _____   8. _____   13. _____
4. _____   9. _____   14. _____
5. _____   10. _____   15. _____

15.7   Review: Hearing System

DIRECTIONS: Cover the column on the left while you complete the sentences on the right.

outer ear

inner, outer ear

The ear consists of three main subdivisions, which are: (a) _____
(b) _____ , and
(c) _____ .

auricle or pinna

The part of the ear that projects from the side of the head is the _____ .

external auditory meatus	A canal called the _____
tympanum	conducts sound waves to the eardrum, known medically as the _____ .
cerumen	Glands lining the canal secrete a waxy substance
ossicles	called _____ . The eardrum transmits sound waves to three small bones referred to as _____ .
malleus	The names of these bones are the _____ ,
incus	which resembles a hammer; the _____ ,
stapes	which resembles an anvil; and the _____ , the Latin word for *stirrup*.
cochlea	The inner ear contains a spiral, snail-shaped,
Corti	fluid-filled body called the _____ , which contains the organ of _____ and is the end organ of hearing. Also within the inner
semicircular	ear are three _____ canals which function in maintaining equilibrium. The
eustachian tube	_____ connecting with the pharynx equalizes air pressure.

15.8   Review: Aural Building Blocks

DIRECTIONS: Match the meanings in the second column with the building blocks in the first column. Some answers may be used more than once.

_____	1. audi/o	A.	anvil
_____	2. aur/i	B.	clear fluid
_____	3. cer/a	C.	ear
_____	4. –cusis	D.	eardrum
_____	5. –dynia	E.	fungus
_____	6. incus	F.	hammer
_____	7. laryng/o	G.	hardening
_____	8. lymph/o	H.	hearing
_____	9. malleus	I.	larynx
_____	10. myc/o	J.	pain
_____	11. myring/o	K.	stirrup
_____	12. oto–	L.	wax
_____	13. –sclerosis		
_____	14. stapes		
_____	15. tympan/o		

15.9   Review: Building Aural Terms

DIRECTIONS: Fill in the blanks with the appropriate building block or term.

1. The combining form for *hearing* is _____ .
   The word ending _____ means *one who specializes.*
   _____ means one who is a specialist in hearing disorders.
   The suffix _____ means *measure.*
   _____ is the *process of measuring the hearing sense.*

2. The combining form _____ signifies the *eardrum.*
   _____ is the excision of all or part of the eardrum.
   _____ is a surgical repair of the eardrum.

3. _____ is the combining form for *nerve.*
   Severe pain along the course of a nerve is _____ .
   The combining form for *ear* is _____ .
   Severe pain occurring in the ear is _____ .

4. The combining form for *fungus* is _____ .
   _____ is a fungal infection of the external auditory meatus.
   The suffix _____ means *an instrument for viewing.*
   An instrument for viewing the ear is called_____ .

5. The prefix for *old age* is _____ .
   The suffix for *hearing* is _____ .
   _____ means impairment of hearing in old age.

15.10   Review: Aural Vocabulary

DIRECTION: Match the terms in the first column with the definitions in the second column.

_____ 1. acoustic
_____ 2. auditory ossicles
_____ 3. aural

_____ 4. cerumen
_____ 5. endolymph
_____ 6. fenestration
_____ 7. otitis media
_____ 8. otoscope
_____ 9. pinna
_____ 10. tinnitus
_____ 11. tympanic membrane
_____ 12. vertigo

A. Instrument for examining the ear
B. Inflammation of the middle ear
C. Surgical creation of an opening into the labyrinth of the ear
D. Sensation of dizziness
E. The projected part of the exterior ear
F. Eardrum
G. Three bones of the middle ear
H. Ringing or tingling in the ear
I. Pale, translucent fluid within the semicircular canals
J. Relating to sound or to the sense of hearing
K. Pertaining to the ear
L. Secretion found in the external canal of the ear

15.11 Review: Aural Structures

DIRECTIONS: Label the structures of the ear.

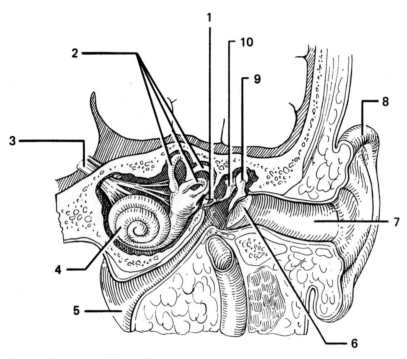

(From Simmers, *Diversified Health Occupations*, 2nd edition copyright 1988 by Delmar Publishers, Inc.)

1. _____   6. _____
2. _____   7. _____
3. _____   8. _____
4. _____   9. _____
5. _____   10. _____

Reading Comprehension 15.1

DIRECTIONS: Underline the medical terms as you go through the reading exercise. Then list and analyze the terms. Some will be completely new to you. Consult a medical dictionary for their meanings. Then re-read the material for better comprehension.

Laser Surgery

Preoperative Diagnosis: Open angle glaucoma

Postoperative Diagnosis: Same

Procedure: Argon laser trabeculoplasty

Surgeon: Dr. A. Blank

Assistant: Dr. B. Blank

Anesthesia: Topical Proparacaine drops

Complications: None

Procedure:
After instillation of Proparacaine drops to the eye in question, the gonio lens was brought onto the surface of the eye and using the Argon laser, a total of 100 spots were applied, 360 degrees in the trabecular meshwork, spot size of 50 microns, duration 0.1 second, power setting of 900 to 1200 milliwatts.

The patient tolerated the procedure well and was taken to the recovery room in satisfactory condition.

Reading Comprehension 15.2

DIRECTIONS: Underline the medical terms as you go through the reading exercise. Then list and analyze the terms. Some will be completely new to you. Consult a medical dictionary for their meanings. Then re-read the material for better comprehension.

Surgical Report

Preoperative Diagnosis: Ectropion

Postoperative Diagnosis: Same

Name of Operation: Ectropion repair

Surgeon: Dr. A. Blank

Anesthetic: 1 cc Xylocaine 2% with epinephrine

Procedure:
After adequate prep and drape and with the patient on cardiac monitor, anesthesia was administered in a slow injection with a 30-gauge needle. After anesthetic was administered a #15 Bard-Parker blade was used to make an incision through skin and tarsal plate but allowing conjunctiva to remain intact. Next the overlying skin was undermined to expose tarsus for approximately one cm. A wedge of tarsus was then excised preserving skin tissue and underlying conjunctiva. The orbicularis oculi was then approached; removed a wedge of muscular tissue of approximately one cm in size from the orbicularis muscle. The tarsus was then approximated and sutured closed using three #6–0 silk sutures through the margin of the tarsus taking care to incorporate a good bite of tarsus into the underlying tissues. These sutures were left long and later used for bridle sutures. The muscle layer was then closed along with the overlying skin by taking deep bites through the skin surface with #6–0 nylon suture in an interrupted fashion. The conjunctiva was then approached and was undermined so that the overlying muscular tissue and tarsus could be closed without creating a defect in either the fornix or the palpebral conjuctiva. Then the bridle sutures which had been used to close tarsus were pulled taut and attached to the brow in a suspension to allow traction upon the tarsal closure and thereby prevent a later defect in scar formation. At the conclusion of the procedure, the patient had done well and was given erythromycin ointment onto the margins of the tarsus, lid margin, globe and overlying skin incision.

Reading Comprehension 15.3

DIRECTIONS: Underline the medical terms as you go through the reading exercise. Then list and analyze the terms. Some will be completely new to you. Consult a medical dictionary for their meanings. Then re-read the material for better comprehension.

Surgical Report

Preoperative Diagnosis: Retinal detachment, right eye

Postoperative Diagnosis: Same

Procedure: Scleral buckle, right eye

Complications: None

Procedure:
After the patient received satisfactory endotracheal anesthesia, the patient's right eye was prepped and draped in the usual fashion. A lid speculum was placed in the lid

fissure and a 360-degree limbal peritomy was made approximately 1 mm posterior to the limbus. Two relaxing incisions were made at 8 o'clock and 4 o'clock and the four rectus sutures were then isolated with #2–0 silk sutures. The sclera was seen to be in good condition in all four quadrants. The indirect ophthalmoscope was then used with cryopexy and the detachment was seen to extend from approximately 12 o'clock to 6 o'clock nasally on the right eye going clockwise, and there appeared to be two small peripheral holes at approximately 12:30. There was some latticing at approximately 1 o'clock with no holes as well as lattice down at 5 o'clock with no holes. The inferior vitreous had old blood remnants. The detachment was carefully examined for any additional holes and none were found. Cryopexy was applied in and around the holes as well as throughout the detachment. The 276 tire was then used with a #40 band and placed into position to extend from 11:30 to 6:30. The band was tied with a clove-hitch knot at 10 o'clock. #4–0 Mersilene sutures were used, two mattress sutures in the superior nasal quadrant and inferior nasal quadrant. They were tied in slip knots. Examination of the fundus was done with the indirect ophthalmoscope at this time to determine the best site of drainage. It was elected to drain at approximately 2:30. Using a #57 Beaver blade, a sclerostomy site was prepared and using diathermy, the lips of the sclera were opened. A needle from a #6–0 chromic suture was rinsed thoroughly and used to perforate the choroid, and clear subretinal fluid was seen to emanate from the drainage. The sutures were then tied up and examination of the fundus revealed good settling of the retina on the buckle. The hole was covered adequately. The Mersilene sutures were then tied permanently, and two anchoring sutures were applied in the superior temporal and inferior temporal quadrants. The anterior chamber was tapped with a paracentesis wound to release some aqueous fluid as the pressure of the eye increased for a very short period of time with the tying of the buckle. The conjunctiva was then closed using #6–0 chromic sutures. A previously made lateral canthotomy was then closed with two #5–0 sutures, interrupted fashion. Subconjunctival Solu-Medrol was injected in addition to irrigation with 20 mg of gentamicin solution. The eye was then patched and shielded and the patient was extubated and taken back to the Recovery Room in satisfactory condition.

Reading Comprehension 15.4

DIRECTIONS: Underline the medical terms as you go through the reading exercise. Then list and analyze the terms. Some will be completely new to you. Consult a medical dictionary for their meanings. Then re-read the material for better comprehension.

Surgical Report

Preoperative Diagnosis: Chronic tonsillitis and serous otitis media, bilaterally

Postoperative Diagnosis: Same

Operation: T & A
Bilateral myringotomy with tubes

Procedure:

Under endotrachael anesthesia, the patient was prepped and draped in the usual fashion for tonsillectomy. Myringotomies were accomplished bilaterally removing thick tenacious fluid from behind both tympanic membranes. #160 polyethylene tubing was placed through the myringotomy incisions without difficulty. The tonsils were then removed with the Sauer tonsillectome using a snare at the inferior pole. Adenoids were removed with LaForce adenotome and curet. Hemostasis was secured with plain #0 ties and electrocautery. The patient tolerated the procedure well and left the operating room in apparent good condition.

Reading Comprehension 15.5

DIRECTIONS: Underline the medical terms as you go through the reading exercise. Then list and analyze the terms. Some will be completely new to you. Consult a medical dictionary for their meanings. Then re-read the material for better comprehension.

Referral Letter

FAMILY HEARING AND SPEECH . . . .

June 1, 19—

Dear Doctor Smith:

I saw your patient, Bob Jones, on 5–15— for an audiological evaluation as per your referral.

Mr. Jones states that he is suffering from a recent onset of vertigo and a high-frequency tinnitus. He denies hearing loss. The external and auditory meati were quite normal. No cerumen was present and the tympanic membranes were clear, with the malleus quite visible.

Pure tone thresholds were normal in the right ear from 250 to 3000 Hz with a severe sensory neural dip at 4000 and 8000 Hz. The left ear was normal from 250 to 8000 Hz. The speech-reception thresholds were in good agreement with the pure tone averages, SRT = 10dB and PIA = 10dB. Speech discrimination was measured at NCL, normal conversational level, of 50 dB HC and 85 dB. The results showed no high-intensity rollover; 100% in all modes tested. Tone decay was negative at 500 Hz and 2000 Hz bilaterally. An ABLB, Alternate Binaural Loudness Balance, test was performed at 4000 Hz. Total recruitment was noted.

Impedance testing shows type A tympanograms with acoustic reflexes present ipsilaterally and contralaterally. Reflex decay was negative at 500 Hz bilaterally.

Results of today's test show that Mr. Jones has normal hearing for the left ear and a high-frequency sensorineural hearing loss for the right ear. The audiological results suggest an absence of middle ear pathology. Site of lesion testing suggests the loss is cochlear in nature.

The patient has been scheduled for electronystagmography and brain stem testing to rule out retrocochlear involvement.

Sincerely yours,

Audiologist

Reading Comprehension 15.6

DIRECTIONS: Underline the medical terms as you go through the reading exercise. Then list and analyze the terms. Some will be completely new to you. Consult a medical dictionary for their meanings. Then re-read the material for better comprehension.

Surgical Report

Preoperative Diagnosis: Tympanic membrane Perforation, right ear

Postoperative Diagnosis: Same with possible early cholesteatoma

Operation: Tympanoplasty

Findings:
Marginal perforation of the posterior superior quadrant overlying the long process of the incus and squamous infiltration extending to the medial surface of the tympanic membrane.

Procedure:
The patient was placed on the operating table in the supine position and general anesthesia was induced via an endotracheal tube. The outer ear was prepped sterilely. The four quadrants of the external canal and postauricular sulcus and temporalis region were injected with 1% lidocaine with epinephrine 1:20,000 fresh mixed. The ear was draped sterilely. Ten minutes were allowed to elapse for hemostatic effect of epinephrine. The operating microscope was then used to visualize the external canal through an operating speculum. The perforation was noted to be larger than it appeared preoperatively because it was obscured by desquamated plates of epithelium which were removed and the perforation was noted to be approximately 10% of the ear drum. In addition there appeared to be some squamous material extending medially from the edges of the perforation.

The edges were freshened using a Rosen needle and cup forceps. Tympanomeatal flap incisions were then made with sickle and round knives; tympanomeatal flap was elevated to the annulus. The annulus was elevated with an annulus elevator and attention was then turned to the postauricular area.

An incision was made in the superior aspect of the postauricular area. An incision was made in the superior aspect of the postauricular sulcus with a scalpel and this was carried down to the temporalis fascia. The temporalis fascia was quite difficult to locate in this patient. There were many layers of adipose-mixed connective tissue. When the temporalis fascia was located a graft was taken approximately 50% larger than the perforation. The postauricular sulcus was then closed in layers using #4–0 chromic catgut for the deep layer and #3–0 nylon for the skin. The graft was placed on gauze and into a graft crusher.

Attention was returned to the external canal. The medial surface of the tympanic membrane was scraped with the round knife and fine suction to remove any squamous epithelial remnants. The middle ear was then filled with crushed Gelfoam squares up to the level of the tympanic membrane in the region of the perforation. The graft was then removed from the gauze and held with an alligator forceps. It was lowered into place on top of the bed of Gelfoam squares with a 7 mm operating speculum and the edges were carefully positioned so as to underlie and contact all edges of the perforation. The tympanomeatal flap was returned to the posterior canal wall and the remaining perforation edges were brought into contact with the graft with careful technique with a Rosen needle.

At this point a Xeroform gauze was applied to the postauricular incision and the patient was awakened and extubated. She was returned to the recovery room in satisfactory condition. A cotton ball with antibiotic ointment was placed in the external canal.

Reading Comprehension Vocabulary

Use the space below to list the medical terms for analysis and definition.

_____
_____
_____
_____
_____
_____
_____
_____
_____
_____
_____

CHAPTER 16

Health Professions

OBJECTIVES

When you have successfully completed Chapter 16, you should be able to:
— Distinguish between medicine, nursing, and allied health.
— Identify the medical specialties as established by the American Board of Medical Specialties.
— Briefly describe the nature of care rendered by the various medical specialties.
— Describe the levels of educational preparation in nursing and name nursing specialties.
— List the principal fields of specialization in allied health occupations.

OVERVIEW

The many professions involved in health care can generally be classified as belonging to one of five major categories:

- Medicine, which includes surgery
- Nursing
- Allied health
- Dentistry, which includes oral and maxillofacial surgery
- Pharmacology

Dentistry and pharmacology, the science dealing with the nature and properties of drugs, will not be discussed here. Medicine, which is practiced by physicians, and nursing, which is practiced by licensed nurses, both involve direct care of patients as well as management of different aspects of patient care. Allied health includes a broad spectrum of support services, many of which are associated with diagnostic procedures, research, or clinical care, and some of which are at least partly clerical.

MEDICINE

Medicine is practiced by physicians, who may be Doctors of Medicine (M.D.s) or Doctors of Osteopathy (D.O.s). This chapter focuses on M.D.s.

Physician assistants (P.A.s) must practice under the supervision of a physician. Educational and licensure requirements for physician assistants, as well as their areas of responsibility, vary.

General Practice

Physicians who do not specialize, or limit their practice, are said to be in *general practice*. General practitioners treat all age groups and usually perform some minor surgery. They refer complicated cases to an appropriately qualified specialist. The old-time "family doctor" was a general practitioner, and many physicians still practice in this way.

Specialty Practice

Physicians who decide to concentrate on a special field of medicine generally seek certification by one of the 23 *specialty boards* under the general supervision of the American Board of Medical Specialties. Approved Specialty Boards of the United States include:

- American Board of Allergy and Immunology
- American Board of Anesthesiology
- American Board of Colon and Rectal Surgery
- American Board of Dermatology
- American Board of Emergency Medicine
- American Board of Family Practice
- American Board of Internal Medicine
- American Board of Neurological Surgery
- American Board of Nuclear Medicine

- American Board of Obstetrics and Gynecology
- American Board of Ophthalmology
- American Board of Orthopaedic Surgery
- American Board of Otolaryngology
- American Board of Pathology
- American Board of Pediatrics
- American Board of Physical Medicine and Rehabilitation
- American Board of Plastic Surgery
- American Board of Preventive Medicine
- American Board of Psychiatry and Neurology
- American Board of Radiology
- American Board of Surgery
- American Board of Thoracic Surgery
- American Board of Urology

Not all specialty areas in medicine are recognized to the extent of having a specialty board. Some are subspecialties within the province of a broader Board category such as Internal Medicine.

AEROSPACE MEDICINE The specialty known as aerospace medicine is concerned with the physiologic, pathologic, and psychologic problems encountered by humans in space. At present, practice of aerospace medicine occurs almost entirely within the space agencies of the federal government.

ALLERGY AND IMMUNOLOGY The *allergist* is specially trained to diagnose and treat problems related to abnormal reactions of the immune system to substances that are ordinarily harmless. Many kinds of medicines and treatments are available to relieve allergic symptoms, but it is essential first to identify the cause. The American Board of Allergy and Immunology is a Conjoint Board of the American Board of Internal Medicine and the American Board of Pediatrics. To become an allergist, a physician already certified in pediatrics or internal medicine must take several years of additional specialty training and must pass a certifying examination in allergy and immunology.

ANESTHESIOLOGY An *anesthesiologist* is a physician who administers local and general anesthesia, usually before and during surgery, but occasionally for relief of pain. An anesthesiologist is also responsible for maintaining respirations while the patient is under general anesthesia, which depresses the respiratory center and other vital functions. The anesthesiologist monitors the patient's blood pressure and heart rate and informs the surgeon of any hazardous changes, both during surgery and until after surgery. An *anesthetist* is a nonphysician trained to administer anesthesia under a physician's supervision.

DERMATOLOGY A *dermatologist* is a physician who has specialized training in the medical and surgical treatment of disorders of the skin, hair, and nails. The treatment may involve the use of medicines, both internal and external, or may involve skin surgery.

EMERGENCY MEDICINE The *emergency medicine physician* specializes in the immediate recognition and treatment of acute illnesses and injuries. Specialists in emergency medicine have traditionally provided around-the-clock coverage in emergency departments of acute care hospitals and may also operate freestanding facilities for treatment of minor emergencies. They also provide the authority and license under which paramedic prehospital care is provided.

FAMILY PRACTICE The *family practice specialist* renders care to the family as a whole and to individual family members regardless of age or sex. These physicians cover a vast range of medical problems. The concept permits continuity of care through the lifespan for the individual and integration of care for the family as a whole.

INTERNAL MEDICINE *Internal medicine* is the specialty concerned with all aspects of caring for adults that do not involve surgery. Physicians who practice this specialty are called *internists*. They not only provide diagnosis and treatment of adult medical disorders but are concerned with health maintenance and wellness. A considerable percentage of the internist's patients are well persons who rely upon the physician to monitor their health through regular physical checkups.

Within the broad specialty of internal medicine are many subspecialties; including cardiology (heart diseases), endocrinology (metabolic diseases), gastroenterology (diseases of the digestive organs), gerontology (disorders of the aged), hematology (diseases of the blood and blood-forming organs), infectious disease, nephrology (kidney diseases), oncology (cancer), pulmonary (lung) diseases, and rheumatology.

NEUROLOGY *Neurologists* are concerned with the nonsurgical management of diseases affecting the nervous system. Generally, the neurologist will manage infectious, metabolic, degenerative, and systemic involvement of the nervous system. Disorders requiring surgery are the province of the *neurosurgeon*.

NUCLEAR MEDICINE In this specialty field, radioactive substances are used for the diagnosis and treatment of disease. For example, many scanning techniques require that solutions containing radioactive isotopes be given orally or parenterally before the test to enhance visibility of an organ.

OBSTETRICS AND GYNECOLOGY The specialty involved in the care and management of women during and immediately after pregnancy, labor, and delivery is known as *obstetrics*. *Gynecology* is the specialty devoted to the medical and surgical treatment of diseases of women, especially those affecting the breasts and reproductive organs, and menstruation and menopause. These two specialties are commonly referred to as OB/GYN.

OPHTHALMOLOGY The diagnosis and treatment of eye and vision disorders using surgery and other corrective techniques is the specialty called ophthalmology.

OTOLARYNGOLOGY Otolaryngology is generally referred to as head and neck surgery in current practice. The specialty encompasses medical and surgical treatment of ear, nose and throat disorders; allergy therapy; cosmetic and reconstructive surgery of the face; and tumors in the head and neck.

Pathology

The science that deals with the causes, mechanism of development, and effects of disease is called pathology. The practice of pathology is divided into two major areas, anatomic pathology and clinical pathology, and further subdivided into numerous subspecialties. The function of the *anatomic pathologist* is to render a diagnosis on the basis of examination of a tissue specimen, and to determine as precisely as possible the extent of disease. The *clinical pathologist* is in charge of the medical laboratory in which a wide variety of diagnostic studies are performed.

Forensic pathology is a subspecialty dealing with various aspects of medicine and the law. The television character "Quincy" was a forensic pathologist.

PEDIATRICS The specialist in *pediatrics* cares for the health of children from birth to adolescence. Pediatric practice encompasses both prevention and treatment of all aspects of childhood diseases, from the problems of acutely ill children to providing guidance to parents regarding the development and preventive care of children who are well. The *neonatologist* deals with the diseases and abnormalities of the newborn. There are also physicians who specialize in *adolescent medicine.*

PHYSICAL MEDICINE AND REHABILITATION The specialist in physical medicine and rehabilitation, called a *physiatrist* is concerned with the diagnosis and treatment of disorders and disabilities of the neuromuscular system. Physiatrists use and prescribe treatments in which heat, cold, water, electricity, weightbearing, and exercise are employed to restore physical function and the capacity for independent living.

PREVENTIVE MEDICINE *Preventive medicine* is concerned with both mental and physical aspects of health and the prevention of illness and disability. Specialists in preventive medicine help patients analyze their health histories, including family histories; present illnesses if any; and lifestyles to plan for health and wellness needs. The fields of occupational medicine and public health also encompass preventive medicine.

PSYCHIATRY A *psychiatrist* is a physician who specializes in the diagnosis and treatment of persons with mental, emotional, or behavioral disorders. Psychiatrists are qualified to conduct psychotherapy and to prescribe medications when necessary. A *clinical psychologist* also treats patients with mental and emotional disorders but is not a doctor of medicine (M.D.) and therefore cannot legally prescribe medications. Some psychologists have Ph. D. (doctor of philosophy) degrees and use the title "doctor" for this reason.

RADIOLOGY Radiology is a specialty in which x-rays (roentgen rays) are used to diagnose and treat a wide variety of disorders. A *diagnostic radiologist* specializes in using such techniques as x-rays, ultrasound, nuclear medicine, computed axial tomography (CAT), and magnetic resonance imaging (MRI) to detect abnormalities throughout the body. *Therapeutic radiology* involves the use of ionizing radiation in the treatment of cancer and other tumors.

SURGERY Surgeons correct deformities, defects, diseases, and injury (trauma) by operative techniques or by manipulation. For example, they may make an incision into body tissue and then remove, rearrange, connect, or dissect diseased or injured tissue. They may replace an organ or a part of an organ, as in a kidney transplant or a skin graft. Surgeons also perform treatments involving manipulation of an injured part, as in reducing ("setting") a fracture. Because surgery can be performed on all body systems and body areas, the broad field of surgery includes not only general surgery but such areas as neurosurgery, oral surgery and dentistry, plastic and reconstructive surgery, cardiovascular surgery, colon and rectal surgery, thoracic surgery, urologic surgery and others.

Colon and rectal surgeons concentrate on surgical treatment of the lower intestinal tract which includes the colon and rectum.

Neurosurgeons specialize in the diagnosis and surgical treatment of the nervous system (the brain, spinal cord, and nerves) and the surrounding bony structures such as the skull and the intervertebral disks.

Orthopedic surgeons treat the musculoskeletal system including injuries and congenital and acquired deformities. Some orthopedic surgeons specialize in treating sports injuries. Also, many musculoskeletal conditions are treated by nonsurgical means, for example, most fractures and many muscle and tendon disorders. The work of orthopedic surgeons may involve surgeons from other specialties, especially neurosurgery.

Plastic and reconstructive surgeons repair injuries or inherited defects of soft tissue. This may be done surgically by graft, tissue transfer, implants, or cosmetic alteration of tissue. Reconstructive plastic surgery is often required by victims of burns or automobile and industrial accidents and by people born with inherited disfigurements. Aesthetic surgery of the face and body contouring for cosmetic reasons is a subspecialty of this surgical discipline. Plastic surgeons often work with orthopedic surgeons and with oral surgeons.

Thoracic surgeons are concerned with the operative treatment of the chest and chest wall, the lungs, and the respiratory passages. Also in this group are specialists involved with heart surgery, including valvular heart surgery, and coronary artery surgery.

Urologic surgeons are concerned with treating urinary diseases and disorders of both sexes as well as problems affecting the male genital tract. (Problems of the female genitalia and reproductive and lactating organs are treated by gynecologists.)

NURSING

Like physicians, nurses are directly involved in patient care. From its traditional role of providing "handmaidens to the physician," nursing has evolved into a distinct profession with roles ranging from day-to-day care of the ill in hospital settings through preventive care and health education in the community to highly technical specialty nursing such as critical care nursing.

Registered Nurses (R.N.) are licensed by the state after completing a course of study and passing qualifying examinations. Today, the trend is toward four-year college programs leading to a B.S.N. (Bachelor of Science in Nursing), although three-year (diploma school) and two-year (associate degree, or A.D.N.) programs also prepare nurses. The R.N. examination must be passed regardless of the type of educational program. Certain nursing functions such as the dispensing of medications are legally restricted to registered nurses.

Licensed Practical Nurses (L.P.N.), also called *Licensed Vocational Nurses*, as the name of their profession implies, are licensed in all fifty states. Their areas of responsibillity are somewhat more limited than those of registered nurses.

Nurse practitioners are registered nurses in independent practice who have had additional preparation and have passed additional qualifying examinations. *Nurse-midwives* specialize in obstetric nursing. Other areas in which nurses may earn special certification include critical care nursing (C.C.N.), urologic nursing, and respiratory care.

Nursing assistants perform many routine patient care functions under the supervision of graduate nurses (R.N.s).

ALLIED HEALTH

The field of allied health encompasses a broad array of supportive services in which there are many subspecialties. Some of these fields overlap. The following discussion describes some of the best known.

Specialty Areas in Allied Health

ELECTROCARDIOGRAPHY In the procedure known as electrocardiography, sensors are attached to specified areas of the body surface so that the electrical activity of the heart may be monitored. The heart's activity is translated into a graph inscribed by a pen on a moving strip of paper. The result is a series of tracings that are collectively referred to as the patient's electrocardiogram (EKG or ECG). This very basic valuable test may be performed by a physician or nurse, but is often performed by medical assistants.

ELECTROENCEPHALOGRAPHY The recording and studying of the electrical activity of the brain is called electroencephalography (EEG). The tracing produced by this technique is called an electroencephalogram (EEG). It is used mainly in the specialty of neurology. The test may be performed by EEG technicians and technologists. The EEG is now being supplemented with computer-aided techniques.

EMERGENCY MEDICAL TECHNICIANS (EMT) AND PARAMEDICS These professionals are usually employed by emergency care centers, fire departments, and independent and hospital-operated ambulance services. They work under the supervision of physicians, often through radio communication. Paramedics have a longer training period than EMTs.

HISTOLOGIC TECHNICIAN Histologists study body tissue at the microscopic level. The histologic technician prepares sections of body tissue by special slicing and staining (dyeing) so that the physician/pathologist can examine their cellular structure. *Histotechnologists* may perform more complex procedures than technicians and may be involved in technician training.

LABORATORY TECHNICIAN In medical laboratories, *technicians* perform routine, less complex procedures such as blood cell counts in hematology, some serum studies, blood banking, urinalyses, microbiologic studies, and clinical chemistry. They may also draw blood samples from patients. A *medical technologist* has a higher level of education and can perform more complex laboratory analyses.

MEDICAL ASSISTANT Medical assistants are employed by physicians to perform both administrative and clinical duties. They may be certified by the American Association of Medical Assistants (CMA) or by the Registered Medical Assistant/AMT Program (RMA). Medical assistants may work in specialized areas. For example, an ophthalmic medical assistant renders supportive services to the ophthalmologist and is qualified by academic and clinical training to carry out diagnostic and therapeutic procedures under the direction and responsibility of the physician.

MEDICAL TRANSCRIPTIONIST *Medical transcriptionists* transcribe medical dictation detailing a patient's health care during an episode of illness, after an injury, or during an operation. Reports like those in the Reading Comprehension exercises in this book are examples of their work. These professionals may be certified by the American Association for Medical Transcription (CMT).

OCCUPATIONAL THERAPIST Occupational therapists (OTs) work in hospitals, in schools, in mental health facilities, and in public agencies. They provide services to individuals whose abilities to cope with the tasks of living are threatened or impaired often by psychologic or emotional conditions.

PHYSICAL THERAPIST Physical therapists (PTs) work in hospitals or nursing homes, in rehabilitation centers, or in schools for the disabled. They work to restore physical function and to prevent disability following disease or injury. For example, a physical therapist might teach a patient how to walk with a leg prosthesis (artificial leg) or help a skier to restore function in a knee after an operation.

RADIOLOGIC TECHNOLOGIST A *radiographer* works under the direct supervision of a physician and is involved in a number of techniques for producing visual images of body parts or body processes. The *radiation therapy technologist* has more advanced training. These allied health professionals assist oncologists (cancer specialists) in administering radiation to treat tumors and other forms of cancer.

RENAL DIALYSIS TECHNICIAN Renal dialysis is a procedure in which toxins (poisons) that build up in the bloodstream of a person whose kidneys have failed are artificially removed, most often by circulating the blood through a filtration device called a hemodialysis machine (artificial kidney). The machine is connected to the patient's blood vessels by an intravenous (actually, intraarterial) line, usually once a week for several hours for life, unless the patient receives a kidney transplant. *Dialysis technicians* assist with this procedure and also instruct patients in home dialysis care.

RESPIRATORY THERAPY The work of respiratory therapists and respiratory therapy technicians is somewhat similar, but technicians have more advanced training. Both perform procedures that help patients maintain or restore normal respiration (oxygen/carbon dioxide exchange). They are most often involved in the care of patients with heart and lung disorders.

SURGICAL TECHNOLOGIST *Certified Surgical Technologists* assist surgeons in hospital operating rooms and in private practice.

VASCULAR TECHNOLOGIST The relatively new field of vascular technology involves study of the blood vessels by use of ultrasound techniques instead of by radiologic means. *Registered Vascular Technologists* are trained to give these tests such as, for example, Doppler imaging.

16.1   Review: Medical Specialties

DIRECTIONS: Write the name of the specialty on the blank line following each of the descriptions:

1. A subspecialty that is concerned with various aspects of medicine and the law

   _____

2. The science of diagnosing and treating disorders of the skin, hair, and nails

   _____

3. The specialty concerned with the physiologic, pathologic, and psychologic problems of humans in space _____

4. The diagnosis and nonsurgical treatment of diseases of the brain, spinal cord, and the nerves _____

5. The specialty involved in the care of the family as a whole regardless of age or sex

   _____

6. The diagnosis and treatment of abnormal reactions of the immune system resulting from unusual sensitivity to foods, pollens, dusts, medicine, or other substances

   _____

7. The use of radioactive substances in the diagnosis and treatment of disease

   _____

8. The specialty concerned with diagnosis and nonsurgical treatment of adult illnesses and with health maintenance of adults _____

9. The science of administering various forms of anesthetics before and during surgery and diagnostic procedures, and for the relief of pain _____

10. Surgical specialty that concentrates on the diagnosis and surgical treatment of the brain, spinal cord and nerves, and the surrounding bony structure

    _____

11. Specialty of immediate recognition and treatment of acute illnesses and injuries

    _____

12. Surgical subspecialty that treats the lower intestinal tract _____

13. Diagnosis and treatment of diseases of the ear, nose, and throat

    _____

14. Specialty concerned with the diagnosis and treatment of diseases or disorders of the kidneys, bladder, ureters, and urethra, and of the male reproductive organs

    _____

15. Surgical subspecialty involving the operative repair of tissues by graft, tissue transfer, or cosmetic alteration of tissue _____

16. Diagnosis and treatment of diseases of the female reproductive organs and the care of women during pregnancy, childbirth, and the interval immediately following

_____

17. Diagnosis and treatment of injuries and deformities of the musculoskeletal systems

_____

18. That branch of medicine concerned with both mental and physical aspects of health and the prevention of illness and disability

_____

19. Science that deals with the causes, mechanism of development, and effects of disease _____

20. The specialty of diagnosing and treating ocular and visual disorders

_____

21. Surgical subspecialty concerned with the operative treatment of the chest and chest wall, the lungs, and the respiratory passages _____

22. Specialty that uses heat, cold, water, electricity, and exercise to help restore physical function and independence _____

23. Specialty concerned with diagnosis and treatment of mental, emotional, or behavioral disorders _____

24. The specialty that cares for the health of children from birth to adolescence

_____

25. The specialty that uses x-rays, ultrasound, nuclear medicine, CAT scanning and MRI scanning in the diagnosis and treatment of disease _____

16.2   Review: Nursing and Allied Health

DIRECTIONS: Complete the following statements by filling in the blanks.

1. The five major categories of professionals involved in health care are:
   a. _____
   b. _____
   c. _____
   d. _____
   e. _____

2. Registered nurses who have had advanced training and who have passed additional examinations qualifying them to engage in independent practice are known as

_____

3. The licensed practical nurse (LPN) has _____ (greater)   or   (lesser) _____ responsibilities than an R.N.

   (cross out the incorrect term)

4. The various career professionals who provide supportive services to physicians are collectively described as _____

5. The _____ _____ is trained to perform both administrative and clinical duties for the physician

6. Both _____ _____ and _____ _____ _____ perform procedures that help patients maintain or restore normal respiration

7. The procedure called _____ involves the attaching of sensors to specified areas of the body surface so that the electrical activity of the heart may be monitored

8. The function of the _____ _____ is to restore physical function and to prevent disability following disease or injury

9. The registered _____ _____ uses ultrasound techniques in studying the blood vessels

10. The technician who prepares sections of body tissue for examination by a pathologist is a _____ _____

11. _____ is the recording and studying of the electrical activity of the brain

12. The _____ _____ technician assists in procedures whereby toxins that have built up in the patient's bloodstream are removed through a filtration device (artificial kidney)

13. The providing of corrective services to individuals whose ability to cope with the tasks of living are threatened is called _____ _____

14. The certified _____ _____ assists surgeons in the hospital operating room and in private practice

15. The technician who performs procedures such as blood cell counts and urinalyses is a _____ _____

APPENDIX I

Additional Medical and Surgical Terms

Chapters 4 through 15 dealt with terms as they related to specific body systems. In practical usage, though, much of our medical vocabulary is not specific to any body system. Also, there is considerable overlapping of application. The terms in this appendix apply to medicine in general and to many of the body systems. Even within the major divisions of this appendix, not everyone will agree about which terms should be chosen and the categories in which they belong. Categories are provided for convenience only and are not intended to suggest that the terms listed under them belong exclusively in any single area.

SELECTED TERMS RELATING TO SIGNS AND SYMPTOMS

afebrile	(ay-FEB-ril)	Without fever; *febrio* = fever
anaphylaxis	(an-ah-fih-LACK-sis)	Violent response of the immune system to a substance, usually after one or more previous exposures to it. Anaphylaxis is an antigen-antibody reaction (*phylaxis* = protection).
asthenia	(as-THEE-nee-ah)	A lack or loss of strength; weakness (*stheno* = strength)
atypical	(ay-TIP-ih-kal)	Not typical; varying from the usual
autogenous	(aw-TAH-jeh-nus)	Taken from or produced by the patient's own body; for example, an autogenous skin graft (*auto* = self + *genesis* = origin)
bacteria	(back-TEE-ree-ah)	A class of microorganism. Singular, *bacterium*.
bilateral	(by-LAH-ter-al)	Two-sided, or relating to both sides of the body (*bi* = two + *latus* = side)
cachexia	(kah-KECK-see-ah)	Severe ill health, usually related to malnutrition (*cac(o)* = bad or ill + *hexis* = habit + *ia* = condition)
clinical	(KLIH-nih-kal)	Having to do with actual symptoms occurring in illness or injury as compared with theoretical or laboratory situations (*klinikos* = pertaining to a bed)

coma	(**KOH**-mah)	A state of unconsciousness from which the patient cannot be aroused
comatose	(**KOH**-mah-tohs)	Being in coma or related to coma
congenital	(kon-**JEN**-ih-tal)	Existing at birth (*congenitus* = born together)
congestion	(kon-**JEST**-yun)	Buildup of blood, lymph, or other body fluid in a local area; for example, nasal congestion
contralateral	(**KON**-trah-**LAH**-ter-al)	At or about the opposite side (*contra* = against + *latus* = side)
contusion	(kon-**TOO**-zhun)	An injury not involving a break in the skin; a bruise
convulsion	(kon-**VUL**-shun)	Violent, uncontrollable, spasmodic contractions of the voluntary muscles
debility	(deh-**BILL**-ih-tee)	Lack or loss of strength
diaphoresis	(**die**-ah-foh-**REE**-sis)	Profuse perspiration
dilatation	(dill-ah-**TAY**-shun)	Stretching or expansion of an organ; the act of dilating or stretching
discrete	(dih-**SKREET**)	Separate, distinct, not blending or merging
diurnal	(die-**ER**-nal)	Occurring during the day (*dies* = day)
dormant	(**DOR**-mant)	Sleeping, inactive (*dormire* = to sleep)
ecchymosis	(eck-ih-**MOH**-sis)	A blood-filled, flat, bluish or purple discoloration in or beneath the skin; bruising
edema	(eh-**DEE**-mah)	Excessive accumulation of fluid in the body tissues; swelling
effusion	(ee-**FEW**-zhun)	An abnormal escape or release of fluid; abnormal fluid within a joint or cavity. (*effusio* = a pouring out)
emaciation	(ee-**may**-see-**AY**-shun)	Extreme thinness; wasting away
exudate	(**ECKS**-you-dayt)	Fluid, for example, blood or plasma, secreted by body tissues in response to irritation, physical injury, or inflammation (*exsudare* = to sweat out)
fatigue	(fah-**TEEG**)	Tiredness; discomfort and reduced efficiency related to prolonged or excessive exertion

febrile	(**FEB**-ril)	Related to fever; having fever
flaccid	(**FLACK**-sid)	Relaxed, not contracted or engorged; for example, a flaccid penis
flatulence	(**FLAT**-you-lens)	Accumulation of air or gas in the gastrointestinal tract
functional	(**FUNK**-shun-al)	In medicine, used to refer to disturbances of physiologic function that have no apparent organic cause
hemorrhage	(**HEM**-or-idj)	Bleeding; usually refers to extensive bleeding from a vein or artery (*hemo* = blood + *rhage* = to burst forth)
hereditary	(heh-**RED**--ih-ter-ee)	Genetically transmitted
homogeneous	(hoh-moh-**JEE**-nee-us)	Having the same composition throughout (*homo* = same + *genos* = kind)
hyperpyrexia	(**high**-per-pie-**RECK**-see-ah)	Extreme fever
idiopathic	(id-ee-oh-**PAH**-thick)	Originating spontaneously; having no known cause (*idio* = self + *pathos* = disease)
idiosyncracy	(**id**-ee-oh-**SING**-krah-see)	A habit or trait peculiar to one individual (*synkrasis* = mixture)
indurated	(**IN**-dyou-ray-ted)	Hardened in such a way that soft tissues become firm but less hard than bone
induration	(**IN**-dyou-**RAY**-shun)	An abnormal hardening of tissue
infiltration	(in-fill-**TRAY**-shun)	Firmness of tissue related to trauma; the presence of a foreign substance, or a growth such as a tumor; *or* instilling fluid into tissue under pressure (for example, with a hypodermic syringe)
inflammation	(in-flah-**MAY**-shun)	An immune response of tissue to infection or injury involving redness and swelling
invagination	(**IN**-vah-jih-**NAY**-shun)	Ensheathing of one part within another; see intussusception
ipsilateral	(ip-sih-**LAH**-ter-al)	At or affecting the same side (*ipsi* = same or self)
lassitude	(**LAH**-sih-tewd)	Weakness or exhaustion

lesion	(LEE-zhun)	A term commonly used to denote any abnormality of tissue, loss of function, or injury
lethargy	(LETH-ar-jee)	Drowsiness, torpor, indifference
malnutrition	(mal-new-TRISH-un)	Any disorder of nutrition, whether associated with insufficient or excessive food, inappropriately selected food, or defects in the body's utilization of food
metastasis	(meh-TASS-tah-sis)	Usually used to refer to cancer; the transfer of disease from one organ or part to another location not adjacent to the original site (*meta* = after, beyond, over + *stasis* = stand)
morbid	(MOR-bid)	Diseased
moribund	(MOR-ih-bund)	Dying
narcosis	(nar-KOH-sis)	Reversible stupor or unconsciousness, naturally or artifically induced (*narco* = numbness)
nausea	(NAW-see-ah)	Abdominal uneasiness or discomfort often leading to vomiting
nocturnal	(nock-TUR al)	Occurring during the night or related to night (*noct* = night)
obesity	(oh-BEE-sih-tee)	Abnormally high proportion of body fat; extreme overweight
optimum	(OP-tih-mum)	The condition that is most favorable to a function
pallor	(PAL-or)	Unnatural lack of skin color
palpitation	(pal-pih-TAY-shun)	Unusually rapid, noticeable action of the heart whether regular or irregular in rhythm
paroxysm	(PAR-ock-sizm)	An uncontrollable seizure, usually spastic
prolapse	(proh-LAPS)	Abnormal descent of an organ from its usual position, particularly the uterus, kidney, or stomach (*pro* = before + *labi* = to fall)
prostration	(pros-TRAY-shun)	Extreme or absolute exhaustion
psychogenic	(sigh-koh-JEN-ick)	Having an emotional or mental rather than a physiologic or

anatomic origin (*psycho* = mind + *gen* = produce)

ptosis	(**TOH**-sis)	Descent or drooping of an organ such as an eyelid, kidney, or stomach (*ptosis* = fall)
purulent	(**PYOU**-roo-lent)	Consisting of or containing pus; for example, purulent discharge.
relapse	(re-**LAPS**)	Return of a disease after it had apparently ended
seizure	(**SEE**-zhur)	The sudden onset or recurrence of a disease. Often used to indicate a convulsion
senility	(seh-**NILL**-ih-tee)	A general term for a variety of physical and mental conditions thought to be associated with old age
sign	(sighn)	Any objective evidence of an abnormal state or disease
suppuration	(**sup**-you-**RAY**-shun)	The formation of pus (*sub*[p] = under + *puris* = pus)
symptom	(**SIMP**-tum)	Any subjective experiential evidence of disease or of a patient's condition
syncope	(**SIN**-koh-pee)	A temporary loss of consciousness related to insufficient flow of blood to the brain; fainting
unilateral	(you-neh-**LAH**-ter-al)	Affecting only one side (*uni* = one + *latus* = side)
vertigo	(**VER**-tih-go)	An illusion of movement; often associated with diseases of the inner ear
viscous	(**VIS**-kus)	Sticky or gummy
void	(voyd)	to pass wastes from the body, particularly urine, but also feces

SELECTED TERMS RELATING TO EXAMINATION AND TREATMENT

abrasion	(ah-**BRAY**-zhun)	A scraping off of tissue due to trauma or by mechanical means; also, the resulting scraped skin surface

abscess	(**AB**-ses)	A localized collection of pus in a cavity formed by the disintegration of tissues (*ab* = away + *cedere* = to go)
adhesion	(ad-**HEE**-zhun)	An abnormal uniting of tissues that often occurs during the healing process; also, the resultant sticking together of tissues
administer		To instill a drug or effect a treatment
ampule	(**AM**-pewl)	A small glass container that can be sealed to preserve sterility of its contents
analgesia	(**an**-al-**JEE**-zee-ah)	The absence or loss of the normal sense of pain; the relief of pain without loss of consciousness (*an* = not + *algos* = pain)
anesthesia	(an-es-**THEE**-zee-ah)	Natural or artificially induced absence or loss of sensation or feeling (*esthes* = feeling)
antibiotic	(**an**-tih-by-**OTT**-ick)	A drug that employs chemicals produced by molds or bacteria to destroy other bacteria or suppress their activity. Used mainly in treating infectious diseases (*anti* = against + *bio* = life)
antidote	(**AN**-tih-doht)	A substance that counteracts a particular poison or a group of poisons
antigen	(**AN**-tih-jen)	A substance in the blood that stimulates a specific immune response and promotes the formation of antibodies (*anti* = against + *gennan* = to produce)
antisepsis	(**an**-tih-**SEP**-sis)	Prevention of infection (*sepsis* = decay)
antiseptic	(**an**-tih-**SEP**-tick)	An agent used to prevent or treat infection
antispasmodic	(**an**-tih-spaz-**MOD**-ick)	An agent that relieves spasm
antitoxin	(**an**-tih-**TOCK**-sin)	An antibody produced in the bloodstream of animals in response to the injection of certain toxins; for example, tetanus antitoxin (*tox* = poison)

asepsis	(ah-**SEP**-sis)	The absence of infection; sterility
auscultation	(aws-kul-**TAY**-shun)	The act of listening for sounds within the body, especially in examining the lungs, heart, pleura, abdomen, and other organs (*auscultare* = to listen to)
chemotherapy	(**kee**-moh-**THER**-ah-pee)	Generally, the treatment or prevention of disease by the use of chemical compounds; now usually used only to refer to treatment of cancer
convalescence	(kon-vah-**LESS**-ens)	The period of recovery from illness, injury, or surgery
diagnose	(**DIE**-ag-nos)	To identify the nature of a disease (*dia* = through, complete + *gnosis* = knowledge)
diagnostic	(die-ag-**NOS**-tick)	Related to diagnosis; also has a special meaning referring to a sign or symptom that definitely identifies a disease or condition; for example, the presence of a certain substance in the blood may be "diagnostic of" a specific disease
diluent	(**DILL**-you-ent)	An agent used for thinning (diluting) the medication to which it is added
disinfectant	(dis-in-**FECK**-tant)	An agent used to destroy pathogenic bacteria
dissection	(die-**SECK**-shun)	The process of cutting apart or separating tissues for anatomical study
emesis	(**EM**-eh-sis)	The act of vomiting
emetic	(eh-**MET**-ick)	A substance that induces vomiting
enema	(**EN**-eh-mah)	Introduction of liquid into the rectum to promote defecation or to administer a drug
eradicated	(eh-**RAD**-ih-kay-ted)	Removed, exterminated, literally to pluck out by the roots (*e–* = out, away + *radix* = root)
generic	(jeh-**NER**-ick)	In medicine, used to refer to the name of a drug that describes or indicates its composition as opposed to trade or brand names.

		Generic names are not capitalized. For example, acetophenophen is the generic name of the drug sold as Tylenol.
geriatrics	(jeh-ree-**AH**-tricks)	The study and treatment of old age and aging (*geras* = old age)
germicide	(**JER**-mih-sighd)	Any agent applied externally to kill pathogenic microorganisms
Hippocrates	(hih-**POCK**-rih-teez)	Greek physician, living in the fifth century B.C., who is considered to be the Father of Medicine
homologue	(**HOM**-oh-log)	A biologic term referring to a body part or structure that has the same evolutionary origin as a corresponding part in another species, whether or not the parts appear similar; for example, a horse's leg and a whale's flipper
incision	(in-**SIH**-zhun)	A cut. Also a wound produced by cutting with a sharp instrument; for example, a surgical incision (*ciso* = cut)
inhalation	(**in**-hah-**LAY**-shun)	Voluntarily drawing air or gas into the lungs. Inspiration is automatic inhalation.
ligation	(lie-**GAY**-shun)	Tying up something to close it, usually a blood vessel during surgery. The ties are called *ligatures*.
lumen	(**LOO**-men)	The hollow channel within a tube or tubular organ, especially a blood vessel; or the diameter of the channel; for example, the lumen of a catheter
malaise	(may-**LAYZ**)	Vague generalized fatigue or discomfort
manipulation	(mah-**nip**-you-**LAY**-shun)	In medicine, procedure or treatment in which the hands are used to move the body or a body part
outpatient		Patient who is diagnosed or treated at a hospital without being admitted or staying overnight; opposite of *inpatient*
palliative	(**PAL**-ee-**ah**-tiv)	Treatment or drug that relieves but does not cure a condition

parenteral	(pah-**REN**-ter-al)	Introduced into the body by some way other than by mouth; for example, by injection or infusion
patent	(**PAT**-ent)	In medicine, open or unobstructed; used most often to refer to a tube or duct; for example, a patent airway
percussion	(per-**KUSH**-un)	Diagnostic procedure involving striking a part with short, sharp blows to evaluate its condition according to the sound produced
pharmacology	(**far**-mah-**KOL**-oh-jee)	The science that deals with the study of the nature of drugs and their effect on living systems
placebo	(plah-**SEE**-boh)	A drug or treatment considered to have no organic effect on the body given to satisfy psychologic needs; in clinical tests, used to evaluate the effect of an active substance on paired subjects with similar or identical conditions with neither group of subjects knowing whether the treatment they are receiving is an active or inactive one (*controlled blind study*). If those giving the drug do not know either, the study is a *double-blind study.*
prescribe	(pree-**SKRYB**)	To designate a remedy and direct how it should be used
prognosis	(prog-**NO**-sis)	The physician's considered prediction about the course of a disease and its probable outcome
prophylactic	(**pro**-fih-**LACK**-tick)	Preventive of disease or condition; a preventive agent
prophylaxis	(**pro**-fih-**LACK**-sis)	Preventive treatment
proprietary	(pro-**PRY**-eh-tah-ree)	In regard to drugs, a patented formulation marketed under a registered trade name by its originator or a licensee. A proprietary drug name must be capitalized. See *generic.*
prosthesis	(pros-**THEE**-sis)	An artificial part; for example, dentures or an artificial leg
regimen	(**REJ**-ih-men)	A prescribed, systematic course of action; for example, a drug

		regimen, a dietary regimen (a "diet"). Often confused with *regime*, which is incorrect in this meaning.
resuscitation	(ree-sus-ih-**TAY**-shun)	Restoration of life or consciousness to an apparently dead person; for example, cardiopulmonary resuscitation (CPR)
sedative	(**SED**-ah-tiv)	Soothing or calming
soporific	(sop-oh-**RIFF**-ick)	Sleep-inducing (*sopor* = sleep)
suture	(**SUE**-chur)	Closing a wound by bringing its edges together or the thread, wire, or other material used in suturing. Also, the interlocking of two bones at their edges, as in the skull
syndrome	(**SIN**-drohm)	A set of symptoms that occur together. Many symptoms are diagnostic.
tactile	(**TACK**-till)	Having to do with touching; discernible through touch
therapeutic	(ther-ah-**PEW**-tick)	Having to do with the treatment of disease
therapy	(**THER**-ah-pee)	The treatment of disease or disorder
vestigial	(ves-**TIJ**-ee-al)	In anatomy, a body part persisting from an earlier evolutionary stage or from embryonic development and having no function; for example, the vermiform appendix
vital signs		Temperature, respiration, and pulse (TPRs)

SELECTED TERMS RELATING TO DIAGNOSTIC PROCEDURES

aspiration	(as-pih-**RAY**-shun)	Inhaling; or removing fluids or gases from a cavity by suction
autopsy	(**AW**-top-see)	Examination by dissection of a cadaver (dead body) to determine the cause or causes of death
biopsy	(**BY**-op-see)	The surgical removal of a small portion of tissue for examination and diagnosis. The removed tissue is properly called the *biopsy specimen*.

cadaver	(kah-**DAH**-ver)	Any dead human body, but especially one used for dissection in the teaching of anatomy
catheter	(**KATH**-eh-ter)	A tube used to withdraw liquids from a body cavity (for example, a urinary catheter) or to introduce liquids
catheterization	(**kath**-eh-ter-ih-**ZAY**-shun)	Using or inserting a catheter
cautery	(**KAW**-ter-ee)	Therapeutically destroying tissue using heat produced by electricity or chemical reaction. Use of cold for this purpose is called *cryocautery*.
clysis	(**KLIE**-sis)	Instilling fluids into the body other than by mouth, often to wash out a body cavity
diagnosis	(**die**-ag-**NOH**-sis)	Identifying the nature of a disease or disorder
dilation	(die-**LAY**-shun)	The act of stretching or expanding an opening or tubular structure of the body
infusion	(in-**FEW**-zhun)	Introducing fluid into the body by gravity flow; for example, an intravenous infusion
instillation	(**in**-stih-**LAY**-shun)	Introducing liquid into a cavity, or wound, usually by drops
insufflation	(in-suh-**FLAY**-shun)	Introducing air, gas, or an airborne substance into a body cavity or tubular body structure by blowing
lavage	(lah-**VAHZH**)	Irrigating an organ or a body cavity to cleanse it; for example, gastric lavage
palpation	(pal-**PAY**-shun)	Diagnostic technique of pressing the hands or fingers against the external surface of the body to feel the underlying structures
pathogen	(**PATH**-oh-jen)	Any microorganism or material that produces disease
pathology	(pah-**THOL**-oh-jee)	The branch of medical science concerned with the originating cause of disease and the study of tissues and organs to determine changes in structure and function associated with disease. A *pathologic condition* is the disease itself.

specimen	(**SPEH**-sih-men)	A sample or part taken for diagnostic purposes; for example, a urine specimen
speculum	(**SPECK**-you-lum)	A tubular instrument that is inserted into a hollow organ or part, often expanding it, so that it can be examined or treated; for example, a vaginal speculum
STAT report		An immediate report (*statim* = at once)
stethoscope	(**STETH**-oh-skohp)	An instrument used for listening to sounds within the body

SELECTED TERMS RELATING TO A DISEASE OR CONDITION

acidosis	(ass-ih-**DOH**-sis)	An acid-base disturbance in which the ratio of acids to alkalis (bases) in the blood is too high. The reverse is *alkalosis*.
acute	(ah-**KYOUT**)	Having a sudden onset and a relatively short, severe course
addiction	(ah-**DICK**-shun)	A physiologic or psychologic dependence on the use of a substance, for example, alcohol addiction; may be of genetic origin
adenopathy	(add-eh-**NOP**-ah-thee)	Disease or enlargement of the lymphatic glands, or of any gland
adventitious	(add-ven-**TISH**-us)	Unnaturally produced or located; for example, adventitious heart sounds
allergy	(**AL**-er-jee)	Abnormal sensitivity of the immune system to a natural substance
amorphous	(ah-**MOR**-fus)	Having no definite form; shapeless
anomaly	(ah-**NOM**-ah-lee)	A severe deviation from the normal standard. A *congenital anomaly* is an anomaly present at birth, often but not necessarily inherited.
aplasia	(ah-**PLAY**-zee-ah)	The congenital absence or extreme underdevelopment of an organ or body part
asphyxia	(as-**FICK**-see-ah)	Condition caused by insufficient intake of oxygen

atopic	(ah-**TOP**-ick)	Out of its normal or ordinary position
atrophy	(**AH**-troh-fee)	The wasting away of a previously normal part or an entire organ, sometimes through disuse; for example, muscular atrophy
benign	(bee-**NINE**)	Not malignant (cancerous) or not recurrent or life-threatening; for example, a benign tumor
carcinogenic	(**kar**-sih-noh-**JEN**-ick)	Producing, or capable of producing cancer
chronic	(**KRON**-ick)	Having a slow onset and long duration; compare with *acute*
cicatrix	(sick-**AY**-tricks)	A scar; the new tissue formed in the healing of a wound. Plural, *cicatrices* (sick-**AY**-trih-seez).
coma	(**KOH**-mah)	A state of unconsciousness from which the patient cannot be aroused. Properly referred to as being in coma (not in *a* coma).
contagious	(kon-**TAY**-jus)	Capable of being transmitted from one person to another. Compare with *infectious*.
degeneration	(dee-**jen**-er-**AY**-shun)	Deterioration in cells or tissue, usually leading to loss of function
dysfunction	(dis-**FUNK**-shun)	Disturbance, impairment, or abnormality of the functioning of an organ or system
ectopia	(eck-**TOH**-pee-ah)	Being out of a normal location; abnormally located; for example, ectopic pregnancy
endemic	(en-**DEM**-ick)	Continually present in a specific community or continually present at low levels in the human community
epidemic	(ep-ih-**DEM**-ick)	A situation in which an infectious disease simultaneously attacks large numbers of people. Compare *endemic* and *pandemic*.
etiology	(**eh**-tee-**OL**-oh-jee)	Properly used to refer to the study of the origins of a disease or of an abnormal condition; often used as a synonym for cause or origin

exacerbation	(egg-**zass**-er-**BAY**-shun)	Worsening of a disease or any of its symptoms. See *remission*.
gangrene	(**GANG**-green)	Death (necrosis) of tissue, with or without infection, usually due to deficient blood supply
imperforate	(im-**PER**-foh-rayt)	Not open; abnormally closed, as imperforate anus
incidence	(**IN**-sih-dens)	The rate of occurrence of a disease or disorder within a specified time
infection	(in-**FECK**-shun)	The invasion and multiplication of microorganisms in body tissues; also, the resulting condition
in situ	(in **SIGH**-too)	Restricted to the site of origin without invasion of neighboring tissues; for example, carcinoma in situ
labile	(**LAY**-beyel)	Gliding or fluctuating between conditons; for example, emotionally labile
laceration	(lass-er-**AY**-shun)	A wound made by tearing or cutting and having rough edges
latent	(**LAY**-tent)	Used in medicine to describe a disease process that is concealed or hidden
malignant	(mah-**LIG**-nant)	Tending to grow worse and to result in death; most often used to mean cancerous. Compare with *benign*.
mortality	(mohr-**TAL**-it-ee)	Death. Also, the rate of occurrence of death in a given population or from a given disease in a specified time
neoplasm	(**NEE**-oh-plasm)	Any new and abnormal growth; most often a tumor
nodule	(**NOD**-youl)	A small, solid swelling detectable by touch
nonviable	(non-**VIE**-ah-bul)	Unable to sustain life
pandemic	(pan-**DEM**-ick)	Occurring over a wide geographic area and affecting a large proportion of the population
remission	(ree-**MISH**-un)	A reduction in or cessation of the symptoms of a disease. (See *exacerbation*.)

residual effect	(ree-**ZID**-you-al)	The effect that remains or is left behind
sequela	(see-**KWEE**-lah)	A lesion or systemic effect that follows or is caused by an injury or disease. Plural, sequelae.
shock		A reduction in the basic, automatic functions of the body, including slowing of circulation and respiration, that follows any sudden assault on the body by injury, toxins, or microorganisms. Life-threatening and progressive if not reversed
slough	(sluf)	Casting off of dead tissue, or the substance being shed
stenosis	(steh-**NOH**-sis)	Any narrowing or constriction of a canal, duct, or vessel
stricture	(**STRICK**-chur)	Narrowing in a canal, duct, or vessel caused by scarring or the presence of abnormal tissue
systemic	(sis-**TEM**-ick)	Pertaining to, or affecting, the body as a whole
toxic	(**TOCK**-sick)	Poisonous
trauma	(**TRAW**-mah)	A wound or injury; often used to refer to severe or life-threatening injury
viability	(vie-ah-**BILL**-ih-tee)	The ability to sustain life
virulence	(**VIR**-you-lens)	The degree of disease-producing power possessed by microorganism

APPENDIX II

Commonly Used Abbreviations

Be careful about using abbreviations. Even frequently used abbreviations may have additional meanings that you are not aware of. Notice that even within medicine, similarities and overlaps exist. Be sure to use abbreviations *in context*, and use the context of abbreviations you encounter to help determine which meaning is intended. Note that some abbreviations may be used with or without periods according to local custom; consult a current medical dictionary.

a.c.	before meals (ante cibum)
A&P	auscultation and percussion
A&W	alive and well
abd	abdomen
ABG	arterial blood gas
ACTH	adrenocorticotropic hormone
AD	right ear (auris dexter)
ad lib	at pleasure (ad libitum)
ADH	antidiuretic hormone
ADLs	activities of daily living
AE	above elbow
AFP	alphafetoprotein
Ag	antigen
agit	shake, stir
AgNO$_3$	silver nitrate
AHD	arteriosclerotic heart disease
AID	automatic implantable defibrillator
	acute infectious disease
AIDS	acquired immune deficiency syndrome
AKamp	above knee amputation
alt dieb	alternate days
alt hor	alternate hours
alt noct	alternate nights
AMI	acute myocardial infarction
amp	ampule *or* ampere
amt	amount
Anesth	anesthetic
ANS	autonomic nervous system
AP	anteroposterior
aq	water
ARC	AIDS-related complex
ARD	acute respiratory disease
AS	aortic stenosis *or* left ear (auris sinister)
ASCVD	arteriosclerotic cardiovascular disease
ASHD	arteriosclerotic heart disease
AU	both ears (aures unitas)
AV	atrioventricular

Ba	barium
BAC	blood alcohol concentration
BBT	basal body temperature
BE	below elbow *or* barium enema
BHA	butylated hydroxyanisole
bid	twice a day (bis in die)
bil	bilateral
BIN, bin	twice a night (bis in noctus)
BK	below knee
BKAmp	below knee amputation
BM	bowel movement *or* basal metabolism
BMR	basal metabolic rate
BOM	bilateral otitis media
BP	blood pressure
BPH	benign prostatic hypertrophy
BR	bed rest
BRP	bathroom privileges
BS	blood sugar *or* bowel sounds *or* breath sounds
BUN	blood urea nitrogen
BV	blood volume
B_x	biopsy
C	Celsius; centigrade
c̄	with (cum)
C/S	Cesarean section
C&S	culture and sensitivity
Ca	calcium *or* cancer
CA	carcinoma
CAB	coronary artery bypass
CAD	coronary artery disease
cal	calorie; see *kcal*
cap	capsule
CAPD	continuous ambulatory peritoneal dialysis
CAT	computerized axial tomography; also CT
cath	catheter, catheterize
CBC	complete blood count
CBR	complete bed rest
CC	chief complaint *or* cardiac cycle
cc	cubic centimeter (same as a *ML*)
CCPD	continuous cycle peritoneal dialysis
CCT	cranial computed tomography
CCU	coronary care unit
CEA	carcinoembryonic antigen
CF	cystic fibrosis
¢ gl	with correction, with glasses
Ch; Chol	cholesterol
CHD	coronary heart disease *or* childhood disease

CHF	congestive heart failure
CHO	carbohydrate
CI	coronary insufficiency
cib	food (cibus)
CIS	carcinoma in situ
ck	check
CL	critical list
cm	centimeter
CMA	Certified Medical Assistant
CNS	central nervous system
CO	carbon monoxide
CO_2	carbon dioxide
comp	compound
contra	against
COPD	chronic obstructive pulmonary disease
CP	cerebral palsy
CPR	cardiopulmonary resuscitation
CRD	chronic respiratory disease
CS	central supply
CSF	cerebrospinal fluid
CT	computed tomography
CV	cardiovascular
CVA	cerebrovascular accident (stroke)
CVD	cardiovascular disease
cysto	cystoscopy, cystoscopic examination
D/C, DC	discontinue
D&C	dilatation and curettage
DCC	direct current cardioversion
DDS	Doctor of Dental Surgery
DEA	Drug Enforcement Administration
DES	diethylstilbestrol
diag	diagnosis
diff	differential
dil	dilute
disch	discharge
disp	dispense
DJD	degenerative joint disease
DM	diabetes mellitus
DNA	deoxyribonucleic acid
DNR	do not resuscitate
D.O.	Doctor of Osteopathy
DOA	dead on arrival
DOB	date of birth
DOE	dyspnea on exertion
DPT	diphtheria, pertussis, tetanus
Dr	doctor

DR	delivery room *or* digital radiography
DRG	diagnosis-related group
DSA	digital subtraction angiography
DTs	delirium tremens
DVA	distance visual acuity
D_x	diagnosis
E. coli	*Escherichia coli*
EBL	estimated blood loss
EC/IC	extracranial-intracranial (bypass operation)
ECG	electrocardiogram; also EKG
ECHO	echocardiogram
EDC	estimated date of confinement
EDD	estimated date of delivery
EEG	electroencephalogram
EENT	eye, ear, nose and throat
Ej	elbow jerk
EKG	electrocardiogram; also ECG
elix	elixir
EM	electron microscope *or* emmetropia
EMG	electromyogram
ENT	ear, nose, and throat
EOMs	extraocular movements
EP	ectopic pregnancy *or* evoked potential
ER	emergency room
ERG	electroretinogram
EST	electric shock therapy
et	and
ET	esotropia
etiol	etiology
EUA	examination under anesthetic
exp	expiration
expl lap	exploratory laparotomy
ext	external *or* extract
f or F	female
F.	Fahrenheit
F.A.C.P.	Fellow of the American College of Physicians
F.A.C.S.	Fellow of the American College of Surgeons
FB	foreign body
FBS	fasting blood sugar
FDG	fluorodeoxyglucose
Fe	iron
FECG	fetal electrocardiogram
FH	family history
FHS	fetal heart sounds
FHT	fetal heart tones

fl	fluid
FME	full mouth extraction
FP	family practice
FRC	functional residual capacity
FROM	full range of motion
FS	frozen section
FSH	follicle-stimulating hormone
FTG	full thickness graft
FTND	full term normal delivery
FU	followup
FUO	fever of unknown origin
F_x	fracture
g	gram
GA	gastric analysis *or* general anesthesia
GB	gallbladder
GC	gonorrhea
GE	gastroenterology
GG	gamma globulin
GH	growth hormone
GI	gastrointestinal
GLTT	glucose tolerance test
gm	gram
GP	general practice
gr	grain
grav I	first pregnancy, primigravida
GS	general surgery
GTT	glucose tolerance test
gtt	drops (guttae)
GU	genitourinary
GYN	gynecology
H	hydrogen *or* hypodermic
h	hour
H&P	history and physical (examination)
H_2O	water
HASHD	hypertensive arteriosclerotic heart disease
HB	heart block
HBP	high blood pressure
HCG	human chorionic gonadotropin
HCl	hydrochloric acid
hct	hematocrit
HCVD	hypertensive cardiovascular disease
HD	hearing distance
HDL	high-density lipoprotein
HEENT	head, ears, eyes, nose, throat
Hg	mercury

hgb	hemoglobin
HIV	human immunodeficiency virus
HLA	human leukocyte antigen
HLAC	human lymphocyte antigen complex
HPN	hypertension
hr	hour
hs	at bedtime (hora somni)
HSV	herpes simplex virus
ht	hematocrit *or* height
HV	hospital visit
H$_x$	history
hypo	hypodermic
I&D	incision and drainage
I&O	intake and output
ICCU	intensive coronary care unit
ICS	intercostal space
ICU	intensive care unit
ID	infectious disease
IDS	immunity deficiency state
IGT	impaired glucose tolerance
IH	infectious hepatitis
IHD	ischemic heart disease
IM	intramuscular *or* infectious mononucleosis
inc	increase
inf	inferior *or* infusion
inj	injection
int & ext	internal and external
IO	intraocular
IP	inpatient
IPPB	intermittent positive pressure breathing
IQ	intelligence quotient
IS	intercostal space
ISG	immune serum globulin
IT	inhalation therapy
ITP	idiopathic thrombocytopenic purpura
IU	international unit
IUD	intrauterine device
IV	intravenous *or* intervertebral
IVC	inferior vena cava
IVF	in vitro fertilization
IVP	intravenous pyelogram
JOD	juvenile-onset diabetes (type I)
JRA	juvenile rheumatoid arthritis
jt	joint
JVP	jugular venous pulse

K	potassium (kalium)
KB	ketone bodies
Kcal	kilocalorie
kg	kilogram
KJ	knee jerk
KS	Kaposi's sarcoma
KUB	kidney, ureter, and bladder
KVO	keep vein open
L	left *or* liter
l	liter
L&A	light and accommodation
L&D	labor and delivery
lab	laboratory
lac	laceration
lap	laparotomy
LASER	Light Amplification by Stimulated Emission of Radiation
lat	lateral
LBBB	left bundle branch block
LD	lethal dose
LDL	low-density lipoprotein
LE	lupus erythematosus *or* left eye
lg	large
LH	luteinizing hormone
liq	liquid
LK&S	liver, kidney, and spleen
LLE	left lower extremity
LLQ	left lower quadrant
LMP	last menstrual period
LOM	limitation of motion
LP	lumbar puncture *or* light perception
LPN	Licensed Practical Nurse
LSD	lysergic acid diethylamide
lt	left
LUE	left upper extremity
LUQ	left upper quadrant
LVN	Licensed Vocational Nurse
m	male *or* meter
MBC	maximal breathing capacity
MBD	minimal brain damage
mcg	microgram
MCHC	mean corpuscular hemoglobin concentration
MCT	mean circulation time
MCV	mean corpuscular volume
M.D.	Doctor of Medicine
MD	muscular dystrophy

MED	minimum effective dose
mEq	milliequivalent
MFT	muscle function text
mg	milligram
mg %	milligrams per cent (mg per l00 ml)
MH	marital history
MI	myocardial infarction
ml or mL	milliliter
mm	millimeter
mm Hg	millimeters of mercury (used for blood pressure)
MR	metabolic rate *or* mental retardation
MRFIT	multiple risk factor intervention trial
MRI	magnetic resonance imaging
MS	multiple sclerosis
MSL	midsternal line
My	myopia
myel	myelogram
n.b.	note well (nota bene)
N/C	no complaints
N&V	nausea and vomiting
NA	not applicable
Na	sodium (natrium)
NAD	no acute disease *or* no apparent distress
NB	newborn
NED	no evidence of disease
neg	negative
neuro	neurology
NG	nasogastric
NICU	neurologic intensive care unit
NMR	nuclear magnetic resonance
noct	night
NP	neuropsychiatric
NPN	nonprotein nitrogen
NPO	nothing by mouth (non per os)
NR	no response
NREM	no rapid eye movements (a sleep phase)
NS	not sufficient *or* normal saline
NSR	normal sinus rhythm
NTG	nitroglycerin
NYD	not yet diagnosed
O.R.	operating room
O&C	onset and course (of a disease)
OB	obstetrics
OB-GYN	obstetrics and gynecology
OC	office call *or* oral contraceptive

od	every day (omni die)
OD	overdose *or* right eye (oculus dexter)
OGTT	oral glucose tolerance test
oint	ointment
OM	otitis media
OP	outpatient
OPD	outpatient department
Ophth	ophthalmic
Orth	orthopedics
OS	left eye (oculus sinister)
os	mouth
OT	occupational therapy
OTC	over the counter (drugs)
OU	both eyes (oculi unitas)
oz	ounce
p	pulse
P	after
P&A	percussion and auscultation
PAC	premature atrial contraction
Pap	Papanicolaou
paren	parenterally
Path	pathology
PBI	protein-bound iodine
PBO	placebo
PBZ	pyribenzamine
pc	after meals (post cibum)
PCCU	post coronary care unit
PCU	progressive care unit
PCV	packed cell volume
PDR	*Physician's Desk Reference*
PE	physical examination
Peds	pediatrics
PEG	pneumoencephalogram
PERRLA	pupils equal, round, regular, react to light & accommodation
PET	positron emission tomography *or* preeclamptic toxemia
PFT	pulmonary function test
PG	pregnant *or* prostaglandin
PGH	pituitary growth hormone
pH	acidity, hydrogen ion concentration
PH	past history
PI	present illness
PID	pelvic inflammatory disease
PKU	phenylketonuria
PLA	polylactic acid
PM	after death (post mortem) *or* physical medicine *or* afternoon (post meridian)

PMH	past medical history
PMN	polymorphonuclear neutrophils
PMP	previous menstrual period
PMR	paramedic run *or* physical medicine and rehabilitation
PMS	premenstrual syndrome
PND	paroxysmal nocturnal dyspnea *or* postnasal drip
PNS	peripheral nervous system
PO	postoperative
po	by mouth (per os)
pos	positive
post-op	postoperatively
PP	postprandial (after a meal)
PPBS	postprandial blood sugar
PR	pulse rate *or* peer review
PRBC	packed red blood cells
preg	pregnant
preop	preoperative
prep	prepare
prn	when needed (pro re nata)
pro time	prothrombin time
prog	prognosis
PROM	premature rupture of membranes
PSRO	Professional Standards Review Organization
Psych	psychiatry
pt	patient
PT	physical therapy *or* paroxysmal tachycardia
PTH	parathyroid hormone
PU	peptic ulcer
PV	polycythemia vera
PVC	premature ventricular contraction
PVD	peripheral vascular disease
pvt	private
PX	physical examination
P_x	prognosis
q	every (quaque)
qd	every day (quaque die)
qh	every hour (quaque hora)
qid	four times a day (quater in die)
qm	every morning (quaque mane)
qn	once every night (quaque nocte)
qns	quantity not sufficient
qod	every other day
qoh	every other hour
qs	sufficient quantity (quantum satis)
qt	quiet
quad	quadrant

R	right *or* respiration
R/O	rule out
R&R	rate and rhythm (of pulse)
RA	rheumatoid arthritis *or* right arm *or* right atrium
Ra	radium
rad	radiation absorbed dose
RAI	radioactive iodine
RAT	radiation therapy
RBBB	right bundle branch block
RBC	red blood corpuscle (cell) *or* red blood count
RBCV	red blood cell volume
RCA	right coronary artery
RD	respiratory distress
RDA	recommended dietary allowance or recommended daily allowance
reg	regular
rehab	rehabilitation
REM	rapid eye movement (a phase of sleep)
resp	respirations
RF	rheumatic fever *or* rheumatoid factor
RFS	renal function study
Rh neg	Rhesus factor negative
Rh pos	Rhesus factor positive
RHD	rheumatic heart disease
RLC	residual lung capacity
RLE	right lower extremity
RMA	Registered Medical Assistant
RN	Registered Nurse
RNA	ribonucleic acid
ROM	range of motion *or* rupture of membrane
ROS	review of systems
RP	retrograde pyelogram
rpm	revolutions per minute
RR	recovery room
RSR	regular sinus rhythm
RT	radiation therapy
R_x	prescription *or* therapy
S	single
s	without
S-A	sinoatrial
SC	subcutaneous
SCD	sudden cardiac death
SD	septal defect *or* sudden death
SDS	sudden death syndrome
sec	second
sed rate	sedimentation rate
SEM	scanning electron microscopy

seq	sequela
SF	spinal fluid *or* scarlet fever
SG	serum globulin *or* skin graft
SGOT	serum glutamic oxalacetic transaminase
SGPT	serum glutamic pyruvic transaminase
SH	social history *or* serum hepatitis *or* sex hormone
SICU	surgical intensive care unit
SIDS	sudden infant death syndrome
sig	label; write (signa)
SLE	systemic lupus erythematosus
SM	simple mastectomy
sm	small
SMR	submucous resection
SNS	sympathetic nervous system
SO	salpingo-oophorectomy
SOB	shortness of breath
SOP	standard operating procedure
sp gr	specific gravity
SPBI	serum protein-bound iodine
SR	sedimentation rate *or* system review
SS	signs and symptoms
ss	half
staph	staphylococcus
stat	immediately (statim)
STD	sexually transmitted disease *or* skin test dose
STG	split thickness graft
STH	somatotropic hormone
strep	streptococcus
STSG	split thickness skin graft
subq	subcutaneous
SUI	stress urinary incontinence
supp	suppository
surg	surgery
SVC	superior vena cava
SWD	short wave diathermy
S_x	symptoms
T	temperature
T&A	tonsillectomy and adenoidectomy
TA	therapeutic abortion
tab	tablet
TB	tuberculosis
TBW	total body weight
TD	total disability
TES	treadmill exercise score
TFS	thyroid function studies
THR	total hip replacement

TIA	transient ischemia attack
TIA—IR	transient ischemia attack—incomplete recovery
tid	three times a day (ter in die)
tinct	tincture
TKO	to keep open
TKR	total knee replacement
TLC	tender loving care *or* total lung capacity
TND	term normal delivery
top	topically
TPR	temperature, pulse, respiration
TPUR	transperineal urethral resection
tr	tincture
trach	tracheostomy
TSH	thyroid stimulating hormone
TSS	toxic shock syndrome
TUR	transurethral resection (of prostate)
TV	tidal volume
T_x	traction
U	unit
U&C	usual and customary
UA	urinalysis
UCHD	usual childhood diseases
UCR	unconditioned reflex
UE	upper extremity
UG	upper gastrointestinal *or* urogenital
UHF	ultra high frequency
UK	unknown
ung	ointment
ur	urine
UR	utilization review
URD	upper respiratory disease
URI	upper respiratory infection
urol	urology
URQ	upper right quadrant
USP	United States Pharmacopeia
ut dict	as directed (ut dictum)
UTI	urinary tract infection
UV	ultraviolet
VA	visual acuity
vag	vaginal
VB	viable birth
VC	vital capacity
VD	veneral disease
VDRL	Venereal Disease Research Laboratory
VDS	venereal disease—syphilis

VHD	valvular heart disease *or* ventricular heart disease
VI	volume index
vit cap	vital capacity
VLDL	very-low-density lipoprotein
VO	verbal order
vol. %	volume per cent
VPB	ventricular premature beat
VPC	ventricular premature contraction
VS	vital sign
VSD	ventricular septal defect
W	water
w/f	white female
w/m	white male
w/o	without
Wass	Wasserman test
WBC	white blood cell *or* while blood count
wd	wound
WDWN	well developed, well nourished
WNL	within normal limits
wt	weight
X	times, sign of multiplication
XM	cross-match
XR	x-ray
XT	exotropia
YOB	year of birth
yr	year
Z	atomic number (symbol for) *or* zero *or* standard score (for statistics)

APPENDIX III

Glossary of Building Blocks

PREFIXES

Word Element	Meaning
a–, an–	not, without
ab–	away from
acro–	extremity
ad–	to, toward, near; also, increase
ambi–	both
an–	absence of, without, not
ana–	without
aniso–	unequal
ante–	before
anti–	against
apo–	separation; also, derived from
atel–	incomplete, imperfect
auto–	self
bi–	two, both, double
brady–	slow
circum–	around, surrounding
co–, con–	together, with
contra–	against, opposite
de–	from, down, not, lack of
di–	double, two
dia–	across, apart, through, complete
dis–	separate from, apart
dys–	bad, painful, difficult
e–, ec–	out, away
ecto–	outer, outside
em–, en–	in, within
endo–	within, in
epi–	upon, at, in addition to, above
eso–	inward
eu–	good, normal, healthy
ex–	out, away from, over
exo–	outside, away from
extra–	outside
hemi–	half
homeo–	similar, same
hyper–	above, beyond, excessive
hypo–	below, beneath, deficient
inter–	between
intra–	within, inside

Word Element	Meaning
intro–	into, within
iso–	equal
leio–	smooth
macro–	large
meso–	middle
meta–	change, beyond
metr–	measure
micro–	small
mito–	thread
mono–	single
neo–	new
nulli–	none
pan–	all
para–	beside, around; also, abnormal, accessory
peri–	around, about, surrounding
post–	after, behind (in time or place)
pre–	before, in front of
presby–	old age
primi–	first
pro–	before, forward, in front of
proto–	first
pyo–	pus
quadri–	four
re–	again, back
retro–	behind, backward
sanguin–	bloody
semi–	half
sub–	under, below
super–, supra–	above, beyond; also, extreme
sym–, syn–	with, together, beside
tachy–	fast, rapid
trans–	across, over, beyond, through
tri–	three, third
ultra–	excessive, beyond
uni–	one

ROOTS AND COMBINING FORMS

MEDICAL: ENGLISH

Word Element	Meaning
acanth/o	thorny, spiny
actin/o	ray
aden/o	gland
adren/o	adrenal gland
agor/a	open area
alb/o, albin/o	white

Word Element	Meaning
aliment/o	food, nutritive material
ambly/o	dull
ametr/o	disproportionate
amni/o	amnion
an/o	anus
andr/o	male
angi/o	vessel
ankyl/o	crooked, bent, stiff
append/o	appendix
aqua	water
arteri/o	artery
arthr/o	joint
astr/o	star
atel/o	imperfect
ather/o	fatty substance
atri/o	atrium
audi/o	hearing
aur/i	ear
balan/o	glans penis
bil/i	bile, gall
blephar/o	eyelid
brachi/o	arm
bronch/o	bronchus
bucc/o	inner cheek
cac/o	bad, ill
calcane/o	calcaneous, heelbone
card/i, cardi/o	heart
carp/o	carpus, wristbone
caud/o	lower part of body, tail
caus/o	burn
cec/o	cecum
cephal/o	head
cer/a	wax
cerebr/o	brain
cervic/o	neck, cervix
cheil/o	lip
chol/e	bile, gall
cholecyst/o	gallbladder
choledoch/o	common bile duct
chondr/o	cartilage
chrom/o	color
chym/o	pour
cleid/o	clavicle, collarbone
clon/o	turmoil
col/o	colon, large intestine
colp/o	vagina

Word Element	Meaning
coni/o	dust
cor/o	pupil
corpus	body
cortex	outer layer, bark
cost/o	rib
crani/o	skull
crine	secrete
cry/o	cold
crypt/o	hidden
culd/o	cul de sac
cutane/o	skin
cyan/o	blue
cycl/o	ciliary body
cyst/o	sac, cyst; also, urinary bladder
cyt/o	cell
dacry/o	tear
dactyl/o	finger, toe
derm/o, dermat/o	skin
diaphor/o	sweat
dipl/o	double
dips/o	thirst
duct	carry
duoden/o	duodenum
edemat/o	swelling
encephal/o	brain
endocrin/o	internal secretion
enter/o	small intestine
episi/o	vulva
epitheli/o	outer skin
erg/o	work
erythem/o	redness, flushing
erythr/o	red
esophag/o	esophagus
esthesi/o	sensation, perception
fasci/o	fascia
flex	bend
flux	flow
galact/o	milk
gastr/o	stomach
gen/o	producing
genit/o	genital
ger/o, geront/o	old age
gingiv/o	gums
gloss/o	tongue
gluc/o, glyc/o	sweet, sugar, glucose
gon/o	seed

Word Element	Meaning
goni/o	angle
graph/o	write
gravid/o	pregnancy
gynec/o	woman, female
hem/o, hemat/o	blood
hepat/o	liver
heter/o	other
hidr/o	sweat
histi/o	tissue
hom/o	same
home/o	same, similar
hydr/o	water
hyster/o	uterus, womb, hysteria
ile/o	ileum
ili/o	ilium
immun/o	protection, safe
irid/o	iris
ischi/o	ischium
kal	potassium
kerat/o	horny tissue; also, cornea
keton	ketone, acetone
kinesis	motion
kym/o	wave, quiver
labi/o	lip
lacrim/o	tear
lact/o	milk
laryng/o	larynx
leuk/o	white
lien/o	spleen
lingu/o	tongue
lip/o	fat, lipid
lith/o	stone
loc/o	place
lumb/o	lower back, loin
lymph, lymph/o	lymph, clear fluid
lytos	soluble
mamm/o, mast/o	breast
meat/o	meatus
melan/o	black
men/o	month; also, mind
mening/o	membrane
mes/o	middle
meter	measure
metr/o	uterus, womb
muc/o	mucus
my/o	muscle

Word Element	Meaning
myc/o	fungus
myein	to shut
myel/o	spinal cord; also, marrow
myring/o	eardrum
myx/o	mucus
narc/o	numbness, sleep
nas/o	nose
nat/i	birth
necr/o	death
nephr/o	kidney
neur/o	nerve
noct/i	night
nucle/o	nucleus, kernel
nyct/o	night
obstetrix	midwife (Latin)
ocul/o	eye
olig/o	little, scanty
onc/o	tumor
onych/o	nail
oo/	ovum, egg
oophor/o	ovary
ophthalm/o	eye
or/o	mouth
orchi/o	testis
orth/o	straight
osm/o	odor
oste/o	bone
ot/o	ear
ov/o	ovum, egg
pachy/o	heavy, thick
palat/o	palate
pancreat/o	pancreas
paresis	slight paralysis, weakness
path/o	disease
ped, ped/o	child; also, foot
perine/o	perineum
phac/o	lens
phag/o	eat, swallow
pharyng/o	pharynx
phas/o	speech
phleb/o	vein
phobia	fear
phot/o	light
phren/o	diaphragm; also, mind
phyt/o	plant
pil/o	hair

Word Element	Meaning
pin/o	to drink
plastic	building up or restoring
pleur/o	pleura
pnea	breath, breathe
pneum/o, pneumon/o, pulmon/o	lung, air
pod/o	foot
praxis	action
proct/o	rectum, anus
prostat/o	prostate
pseud/o	false
psych/o	mind, soul, related to mind
ptosis	falling, downward displacement
ptyal/o	saliva
pulmon/o	lung
py/o	pus
pyel/o	renal pelvis
pylor/o	pylorus, pyloric sphincter
radicle	little root
rect/o	rectum, anus
ren/o	kidney
renal, ren/o	pertaining to kidney
rhin/o	nose
rhiz/o	root
salping/o	uterine tube
sarc/o	flesh
scapul/o	scapula, shoulder blade
scler/o	hard, sclera (white of eye)
scoli/o	crooked, bent
seb/o	sebum
ser/o	serum
sial/o	saliva
sin/o	sinus
soma	body
spermat/o	spermatozoa
sphygm/o	pulse
spir/o	breathe
splen/o	spleen
spondyl/o	vertebra
squam/o	scale
steat/o	fat, lipid; also, sebum
sten/o	narrow, contracted
stere/o	three-dimensional, having depth
steth/o	chest
sthen/o	strength
stom/o; stomat/o	mouth
sudor	sweat

Word Element	Meaning
thalam/o	chamber
therm/o	heat
thorac/o	chest
thromb/o	clot, thrombus
thym/o	thymus gland
thyroid/o	thyroid gland
tom/o	incision, cut
ton/o	tension
tort/i	twisted
toxic/o	poison
trache/o	trachea
trachel/o	neck
trich/o	hair
tympan/o	eardrum
ungu/o	nail
ur/o	urine, urinary tract
ureter/o	ureter
urethr/o	urethra
uter/o	uterus, womb
vagin/o	vagina
vas/o	vessel, duct
ven/i, ven/o	vein
ventr/o	belly, cavity
ventricul/o	ventricle
version	turning
vertebr/o	vertebra
vesicul/o	seminal vesicle
viscer/o	internal body organs
xanth/o	yellow
xer/o	dry
zoster	girdle, encircling

SUFFIXES

MEDICAL: ENGLISH

Word Element	Meaning
–ac, –al, –ar, –ary	pertaining to
–algia	pain, painful condition
–arche	beginning
–asthenia	weakness
–blast	immature stage
–capnia	carbon dioxide
–cele	hernia, pouching
–centesis	surgical puncture (for aspiration)
–cide	to kill
–clasis	break

Word Element	Meaning
–cusis	hearing
–cyesis	pregnancy
–cyte	cell
–dermic	pertaining to skin
–desis	binding, fixation
–diastasis	separation
–dynia	pain
–eal	pertaining to
–ectasia, –ectasis	dilatation, expansion, distention
–ectomy	excision
–emesis	vomiting
–emia	blood condition
–esthesia	sensation
–genesis	production, development, formation
–genic	originating
–glia	glue
–gram	a record
–graphy	process of recording
–hexia	condition, habit
–iac, –ic, –id	pertaining to, affected by
–iasis, –ism	condition
–itis	inflammation
–lepsis	seizure
–lexia	diction
–logy	study or science of
–lysis	dissolution, breaking down, loosening, destruction
–malacia	softening
–mastia	breast condition
–megaly	enlargement
–meter	measure
–oid	resembling, like
–oma	tumor, swelling
–opia	sight condition
–ose, –ous	pertaining to
–osis	abnormal condition or increase
–osmia	smell
–ostomy	surgically formed artificial opening
–otomy	process of cutting, incision
–pathy	disease
–penia	abnormal reduction, deficiency
–pexy	to fix or put in place
–phagia, phagy	eating, swallowing
–phasia	speaking
–philia	attraction for, love
–phobia	exaggerated fear, dislike
–phonia	voice, sound

Word Element	Meaning
–phragm	fence, wall off
–physis	to grow
–plasia	to form, development
–plasm	mold, shape
–plasty	surgical repair, mold, to shape
–plegia	paralysis, stroke
–pnea	breathe
–poiesis	formation, making
–porosis	passage
–ptosis	downward displacement, prolapse
–ptysis	spitting
–rhage, rhagia	excessive flow, hemorrhage
–rhaphy	process of suturing, sewing
–rhea	discharge, flow
–rhexis	rupture
–salpinx	uterine tube
–sclerosis	hardening
–scope	examining instrument
–scopy	process of examining
–spasm	sudden contraction of muscles
–spermia	spermatozoa
–sphyxia	pulse
–stalsis	contraction
–stasis	standing, not flowing
–staxis	hemorrhage
–stenosis	narrowing
–sthenia	strength
–stigma	point
–stomy	creation of an opening
–tasis	stretching
–tic	pertaining to
–tocia	labor, birth
–tomy	incision
–tripsy	crushing, friction
–trophy	nourishment
–tropia	turning
–uria	urine, urination
–version	a turning

PREFIXES

ENGLISH: MEDICAL

English Meaning	Medical Prefix
abnormal	para–
above	epi–
	super–

English Meaning	Medical Prefix
	supra–
above, beyond, excessive	hyper–
absence of	a–, an–
accessory	para–
across	trans–
	dia–
after, behind (in time or place)	post–
again, back	re–
against	anti–
	contra–
all	pan–
apart	dis–
around, surrounding	peri–
	circum–
away from	ab–
bad, painful	dys–
before, in front of	pre–
before	ante–
behind, backward	retro–
below	hypo–
beneath	hypo–
beside	para–
between	inter–
beyond	meta–
	trans–
	ultra–
bloody	sanguin–
both	ambi–
	bi–
change	meta–
complete	dia–
deficient	hypo–
difficult	dys–
double, two	di–
equal	iso–
excessive	ultra–
extremity	acro–
fast, rapid	tachy–
first	primi–
	proto–
forward, in front of, before	pro–
four	quadri–
from, down, not, lack of	de–
good	eu–
half	hemi–
	semi–

English Meaning	Medical Prefix
healthy	eu–
imperfect	atel–
in, within	em– en–
incomplete, imperfect	atel–
increase	ad–
into, within	intro–
inward	eso–
large	macro–
measure	metr–
middle	meso–
near	ad–
new	neo–
none	nulli–
normal	eu–
not	an–
not, without	a–
	an–
old age	presby–
one	uni–
out, away	e–
	ec–
	ex–
outer, outside	ecto–
outside, away from	exo–
outside	extra–
painful, bad	dys–
pus	pyo–
self	auto–
separate from, apart	dis–
separation, derived from	apo–
similar, same	homeo–
single	mono–
slow	brady–
small	micro–
smooth	leio–
surrounding, around	circum–
	peri–
thread	mito–
three	tri–
through	trans–
to, toward	ad–
together, with	co–
	con–
two, both, double	bi–
under, below	sub–
unequal	aniso–

English Meaning	Medical Prefix
upon, at, in addition to	epi–
with, together, beside	sym–
	syn–
within, in, inside	endo–
	intra–
without	an
	ana–

ROOTS AND COMBINING FORMS

ENGLISH: MEDICAL

English Meaning	Medical Root/Combining Form
acetone, ketone	keton
action	praxis
adrenal gland	adren/o
air	pneum/o, pneumon/o, pulmon/o
amnion	amni/o
angle	goni/o
anus	an/o
	proct/o
	rect/o
appendix	append/o
arm	brachi/o
artery	arteri/o
atrium	atri/o
bad, ill	cac/o
bark, outer layer	cortex
belly	ventr/o
bend	flex
bent	ankyl/o
	scoli/o
bile	bil/i
	chol/e
birth	nat/i
black	melan/o
blood	hem/o, hemat/o
blue	cyan/o
body	corpus
	soma
bone	oste/o
brain	cerebr/o
	encephal/o
breast	mamm/o, mast/o
breath, breathe	pnea
	spir/o
bronchus	bronch/o

English Meaning	Medical Root/Combining Form
build up	plastic
burn	caus/o
calcaneous	calcane/o
carry	duct
cartilage	chondr/o
cavity	ventr/o
cecum	cec/o
cell	cyt/o
chamber	thalam/o
cheek (inner)	bucc/o
chest	steth/o
	thorac/o
child	ped/, ped/o
ciliary body	cycl/o
clot, thrombus	thromb/o
cold	cry/o
collarbone (clavicle)	cleid/o
colon, large intestine	col/o
color	chrom/o
common bile duct	choledoch/o
contracted	sten/o
cornea	kerat/o
crooked	ankyl/o
	scoli/o
cul de sac	culd/o
death	necr/o
diaphragm	phren/o
disease	path/o
disproportionate	ametr/o
double	dipl/o
downward displacement	ptosis
drink	pin/o
dry	xer/o
dull	ambly/o
duodenum	duoden/o
dust	coni/o
ear	aur/i
	ot/o
eardrum	myring/o
	tympan/o
eat, swallow	phag/o
egg	oo
	ov/o
esophagus	esophag/o
eye	ocul/o
	ophthalm/o

English Meaning	Medical Root/Combining Form
eyelid	blephar/o
falling	ptosis
false	pseud/o
fascia	fasci/o
fat	steat/o
fat, lipid	lip/o
fatty substance	ather/o
fear	phobia
female	gynec/o
finger	dactyl/o
flesh	sarc/o
flow	flux
flushed	erythem/o
food	aliment/o
foot	ped/o
	pod/o
fungus	myc/o
gall	bil/i
	chol/e
gallbladder	cholecyst/o
genital	genit/o
girdle, encircling	zoster
gland	aden/o
glans penis	balan/o
glucose	gluc/o, glyc/o
gums	gingiv/o
hair	pil/o
	trich/o
hard	scler/o
head	cephal/o
hearing	audi/o
heart	card/i, cardi/o
heat	therm/o
heavy, thick	pachy/o
heelbone	calcane/o
hidden	crypt/o
horny tissue	kerat/o
hysteria	hyster/o
ileum	ile/o
ilium	ili/o
imperfect	atel/o
incision, cut	tom/o
internal secretion	endocrin/o
iris	irid/o
ischium	ischi/o
joint	arthr/o

English Meaning	Medical Root/Combining Form
kernel, nucleus	nucle/o
kidney	nephr/o
	ren/o
larynx	laryng/o
lens	phac/o
light	phot/o
lip	cheil/o
	labi/o
lipid, sebum	steat/o
liver	hepat/o
loin, lower back	lumb/o
lung	pneum/o
	pneumon/o
	pulmon/o
lymph, clear fluid	lymph, lymph/o
male	andr/o
marketplace	agor/a
marrow	myel/o
measure	meter
meatus	meat/o
membrane	mening/o
middle	mes/o
midwife	obstetrix (Latin)
milk	galact/o
	lact/o
mind	men/o
	phren/o
	psych/o
month	men/o
motion	kinesis
mouth	or/o
	stom/a, stomat/o
mucus	muc/o
	myx/o
muscle	my/o
nail	onych/o
	ungu/o
narrow	sten/o
neck, cervix	cervic/o
	trachel/o
nerve	neur/o
night	noct/i
	nyct/o
nose	nas/o
	rhin/o
numbness	narc/o

English Meaning	Medical Root/Combining Form
nutritive material	aliment/o
odor	osm/o
old age	geront/o, ger/o
open area	agor/a
organ, internal	viscer/o
other	heter/o
outer skin	epitheli/o
ovary	oophor/o
palate	palat/o
pancreas	pancreat/o
paralysis (slight)	paresis
perception	esthesi/o
perineum	perine/o
pharynx	pharyng/o
place	loc/o
plant	phyt/o
pleura	pleur/o
poison	toxic/o
potassium	kal
pour	chym/o
pregnancy	gravid/o
producing	gen/o
prostate	prostat/o
protection	immun/o
pulse	sphygm/o
pupil (of eye)	cor/o
pus	py/o
pyloric sphincter	pylor'
pylorus	p˙ ˙r/o
quiver	ĸym/o
ray	actin/o
rectum	proct/o
	rect/o
red	erythr/o
redness	erythem/o
renal pelvis	pyel/o
restore	plasty
rib	cost/o
root	radicle
	rhiz/o
sac, cyst	cyst/o
safe	immun/o
saliva	ptyal/o
	sial/o
same	hom/o
scale	squam/o

English Meaning	Medical Root/Combining Form
scanty, little	olig/o
sclera (white of eye)	scler/o
sebum	seb/o
secrete	crine
seed	gon/o
seminal vesicle	vesicul/o
sensation	esthesi/o
serum	ser/o
shoulder blade, scapula	scapul/o
shut	myein
similar, same	home/o
sinus	sin/o
skin	cutane/o
	derm/o
	dermat/o
skull	crani/o
sleep	narc/o
small intestine	enter/o
soluble	lytos
soul, related to the mind	psych/o
speech	phas/o
spermatozoa	spermat/o
spinal cord	myel/o
spiny	acanth/o
spleen	lien/o
	splen/o
star	astr/o
stiff	ankyl/o
stomach	gastr/o
stone	lith/o
straight	orth/o
strength	sthen/o
sugar	gluco/o
	glyc/o
swallow, eat	phag/o
sweat	diaphor/o
	hidr/o
	sudor
sweet	gluc/o
	glyc/o
swelling	edemat/o
tail, lower part of body	caud/o
tear	dacry/o
	lacrim/o
tension	ton/o
testis	orchi/o

English Meaning	Medical Root/Combining Form
thirst	dips/o
thorny	acanth/o
three-dimensional	stere/o
thymus gland	thym/o
thyroid gland	thyroid/o
tissue	histi/o
toe	dactyl/o
tongue	gloss/o
	lingu/o
trachea	trache/o
tumor	onc/o
turmoil	clon/o
turning	version
twisted	tort/i
ureter	ureter/o
urethra	urethr/o
urinary bladder	cyst/o
urine, urinary tract	ur/o
uterine tube	salping/o
uterus, womb	hyster/o
	metr/o
	uter/o
vagina	colp/o
	vagin/o
vein	phleb/o
	ven/i, ven/o
ventricle	ventricul/o
vertebra	spondyl/o
	vertebr/o
vessel, duct	vas/o
vessel	angi/o
vulva	episi/o
water	aqua
	hydr/o
wave	kym/o
wax	cer/a
weakness	paresis
white	alb/o, albin/o
	leuk/o
woman	gynec/o
womb	hyster/o
	metr/o
	uter/o
work	erg/o
wrist, carpus	carp/o
write	graph/o

English Meaning	Medical Root/Combining Form
yellow	xanth/o

SUFFIXES

English Meaning	Medical Suffix
abnormal condition	–osis
attraction for	–philia
beginning	–arche
binding, fixation	–desis
birth	–tocia
blood condition	–emia
breaking down	–lysis
break	–clasis
breast condition	–mastia
breathing	–pnea
carbon dioxide	–capnia
cell	–cyte
condition (adjective)	–iasis, –ism
condition (noun)	–hexia
contraction of muscles	–spasm
contraction	–stalsis
crushing	–tripsy
cutting	–otomy
deficiency	–penia
destruction	–lysis
development	–genesis
diction	–lexia
dilatation	–ectasia, –ectasis
discharge	–rhea
disease	–pathy
displacement downward	–ptosis
dissolution	–lysis
distention	–ectasia, –ectasis
eating	–phagia, phagy
enlargement	–megaly
examining instrument	–scope
examining process	–scopy
excision	–ectomy
fear or dislike (exaggerated)	–phobia
fence	–phragm
fixation	–pexy
flow	–rhea
flow (excessive)	–rhage, rhagia
form, develop	–plasia

English Meaning	Medical Suffix
formation	–genesis
	–poiesis
friction	–tripsy
glue	–glia
grow	–physis
habit	–hexia
hardening	–sclerosis
hearing	–cusis
hemorrhage	–rhage, rhagia
	–staxis
hernia, pouching	–cele
immature stage	–blast
incision	–otomy, –tomy
increase	–osis
inflammation	–itis
kill	–cide
labor	–tocia
like	–oid
loosening	–lysis
love, affinity for	–philia
measure	–meter
mold, shape	–plasm
narrowing	–stenosis
nourishment	–trophy
opening (creation of)	–ostomy, –stomy
origin	–genic
pain, painful condition	–algia
	–dynia
paralysis	–plegia
passage	–porosis
pertaining to, having to do with	–ac, –al, –ar, –ary, –eal, –iac, –ic, –id, –ose,
	–ous, –tic
point	–stigma
pregnancy	–cyesis
production	–genesis
prolapse	–ptosis
pulse	–sphyxia
record	–gram
recording process	–graphy
reduction	–penia
resembling	–oid
rupture	–rhexis
seizure	–lepsis
sensation	–esthesia
separation	–diastasis
sight condition	–opia

English Meaning	Medical Suffix
skin	–dermic
smell	–osmia
softening	–malacia
sound	–phonia
speaking	–phasia
spermatozoa	–spermia
spitting	–ptysis
standing, still	–stasis
strength	–sthenia
stretching	–tasis
stroke	–plegia
study or science of	–logy
surgical puncture	–centesis
surgical repair	–plasty
suturing process	–rhaphy
swallowing	–phagia, phagy
swelling	–oma
tumor	–oma
turning	–tropia
	–version
urine, urination	–uria
uterine tube	–salpinx
voice	–phonia
vomiting	–emesis
walling off	–phragm
weakness	–asthenia

INDEX

abduction, 38
abductor, 117
aboral, 21
absorption, 196
acanthosis, 64
acceleration, 310
accommodation, 367
acetabulum, 94
acetonuria, 206
achalasia, 211
achlorhydria, 211
acne, 64
acoustic, 378
acquired immune deficiency syndrome
   (AIDS), 238
acromegaly, 16, 320
acrophobia, 344
Addison's disease, 320
adduction, 21, 39, 117
adenitis, 211
adenohypophysis, 318
adenoid, 18
adhesion, 211
adipose, 44
adnexa, 262
adolescence, 310
adolescent medicine, 399
adrenal glands, 318
adrenaline, 316
adrenocorticotropic hormone (ACTH), 316
adrenomegaly, 320
aerophagia, 211
afebrile, 411
afferent, 38, 340
agoraphobia, 16, 345
akinesia, 346
albino, 56
albuminuria, 296
aldosterone, 316
alimentary, 196
allergen, 148
allergic rhinitis, 181
allergist, 397
alopecia, 64
alveolus, 179, 262
Alzheimer's disease, 346
amastia, 21
amaurosis, 370
ambidextrous, 21
amblyopia, 370
ambulation, 117
amenorrhea, 267

amentia, 346
ametropia, 370
amnesia, 346
amniocentesis, 269
amnion, 262
amplified, 362
ampulla, 259
amputation, 98
amyotrophic lateral sclerosis, 120
analgia, 15
anaphylaxis, 154
anaplasia, 45
anastomosis, 215
anatomic pathologist, 399
anatomist, 32
anatomy, 14, 32
androgen, 235
androsterone, 316
anemia, 154
anencephaly, 346
anergic, 340
anesthesia, 340
anesthesiologist, 397
aneurysm, 154
angiectasis, 15
angiitis, 64
angina pectoris, 154
angiocardiography, 157
angioedema, 64
angiorrhexis, 17
angiospasm, 148
angiotomy, 18
anisocoria, 368
ankylosis, 97
anophthalmia, 370
anorchism, 237
anorexia, 211
anorexia nervosa, 346
anoscope, 17
anosmia, 178
anovular, 259
anoxia, 178
antagonist, 118, 332
anteflect, 21
anteflexion, 259
antenatal, 259
antepartum, 259
anterior, 38, 310
antibody, 150
antidiuretic, 293
antidiuretic hormone (ADH), 316
antigen, 150

antimycotic, 21
anuria, 296
anus, 208
aorta, 150
apathy, 346
apex, 150
aphagia, 211
aphakia, 370
aphasia, 15, 346
apical, 206
aplasia, 45, 422
apnea, 178
aponeurosis, 110, 118
appendage, 56
appendectomy, 17, 215
appendix, 208
apraxia, 346
aqueous humor, 368
arachnitis, 346
arachnoid, 340
areola, 262
arrhythmia, 154
arteriography, 157
arteriole, 150
arteriosclerosis, 17, 18, 154
artery, 150
arthralgia, 18
arthrectomy, 98
arthritis, 97
arthrocentesis, 98
arthroclasia, 99
arthrodesis, 17, 99
arthroplasty, 99
articulate, 362
articulation, 93
ascend, 228
ascites, 211
aspermatogenesis, 237
aspermia, 237
asphyxia, 178
aspiration, 179
asplenia, 148
asthenia, 120, 346
asthma, 181
asthmatic, 310
astigmatism, 370
astrocyte, 341
asystole, 154
ataxia, 120, 346
atelectasis, 181
atelencephalia, 346
atherosclerosis, 154

atherosclerotic, 134
atopic, 423
atresia, 211
atrioventricular node, 150
atrium, 134, 150
atrophy, 45, 120, 310, 362
audiogram, 381
audiologist, 378
audiometer, 381
audiometry, 381
aural, 378
auricle, auricula, 379
auscultation, 178
autism, 345
autogenesis, 22
autograft, 149
autonomic nervous system (ANS), 341
axilla, 250
axillary, 134
axon, 341
azoospermia, 237
azotemia, 267

bacteria, 56
balanitis, 237
Bartholin's glands, 262
benign prostatic hyperplasia, 237
biceps, 118
bicuspid, 22, 149
bifocal, 368
bile, 208
bipara, 259
blepharitis, 370
blepharoptosis, 16, 370
bolus, 196, 206
Bowman's capsule, 294
brachial, 93
brachialgia, 120
bradycardia, 134, 155
bradykinesia, 346
bradypnea, 181
bradytocia, 267
bronchiectasis, 181
bronchiole, 179
bronchitis, 16, 182
bronchogenic, 178
bronchoscopy, 183
bronchus, 179
buccal, 206
buccal cavity, 196
bulbourethral glands, 235
bulbous, 228
bulimia, 212, 346

bulla, 64

cachexia, 212, 320
calcaneus, 94
calcitonin, 316
calculus, 293
callus, 64
calyx, 294
cancellous bone, 78
canthus, 368
capillary, 150
carbohydrate, 310
carbuncle, 65
carcinogenic, 15
cardia, 208
cardiac arrest, 155
cardiac catheterization, 157
cardiac tamponade, 155
cardioptosis, 18
cardioscope, 18
cardioversion, 149
caries, 93
carpus, 94
cartilage, 44, 95, 170
cataract, 370
catecholamine, 316
catheter, 293
caudal, 38
causalgia, 65
cauterization, 269
cavernous, 228
cavities, 35
cecum, 208
cell body, 341
cellulitis, 65
cementum, 208
central, 38
central nervous system (CNS), 342
cephalad, 18, 38
cephalalgia, 347
cephalocentesis, 17
cerebellum, 342
cerebral hemorrhage, 347
cerebral palsy, 347
cerebromalacia, 347
cerebropathy, 18
cerebrospinal fluid, 342
cerebrum, 342
certified surgical technologist, 402
cerumen, 379
cervical, 93, 134
cervicitis, 267
cervix, 262

cesarean section, 270
chalazion, 370
chancre, 237
cheilitis, 212
cheiloplasty, 215
cheilosis, 18
Cheyne-Stokes respiration, 182
choana, 179
cholecystectomy, 215
cholecystitis, 212
cholelithiasis, 16, 212
chondrocyte, 19
chondroma, 120
chordotomy, cordotomy, 350
chorea, 347
chorion, 262
choroid, 369
chromosome, 235
chyme, 208
cicatrix, 62
cilia, cilium, 369
circulatory system, 149
circumcision, 239
circumduction, 39
circumscribed, 22
cirrhosis, 212
clavicle, 95
cleft palate, 212
clinical, 32
clinical pathologist, 399
clinical psychologist, 399
clitoris, 262
clonic, 117
clonus, 117
coagulation, 150
coccyx, 95, 263
cochlea, 379
coitus, 234, 259
colectomy, 215
colic, 212
colon, 208
colon and rectal surgeon, 400
colostomy, 215
colpocleisis, 270
colpohysterectomy, 270
colporrhaphy, 270
colposcope, 259
colpotomy, 270
coma, 320
comedo, 65
compact bone, 78
concave, 286
conception, 259

concha, 179
condom, 234
condyloma, 267
cones, 369
congenital, 22, 56
congenital malformation, 332
congestive heart failure (CHF), 155
conical, 286
conjunctiva, 369
conjunctivitis, 370
Conn's syndrome, 320
constipation, 212
contraception, 22, 259
contracture, 120
convex, 286
convulsion, 120
copulation, 234, 259
cor pulmonale, 155
corium, 56
cornea, 369
coronary artery, 151
coronary vein, 151
corpus albicans, 263
corpus cavernosum, 235
corpus luteum, 263
corpuscle, 151
cortex, 318
corticosteroid, 316
cortisol, 316
cortisone, 317
costectomy, 19
costochondral,178
Cowper's glands, 235
cranial, 340
craniectomy, 350
craniometer, 19
craniotomy, 350
cranium, 95
cretinism, 315
cryosurgery, 68
cryptorchism, 237
cul de sac, 263
culdocentesis, 270
culdoscopy, 269
curettage, 68, 270
Cushing's syndrome, 321
cuticle, 64
cyanosis, 65
cycloplegia, 371
cystitis, 296
cystocele, 267
cystogram, 298
cystolith, 19

cystoscope, 293
cystoscopy, 17
cytoblast, 19
cytolysis, 16
cytopenia, 16
cytoplasm, 32, 44

dacryocystitis, 371
dacryoma, 371
deaf-mute, 378
deafness, 378
debility, 212
deceleration, 22
decubitus ulcer, 65
deep, 38
defecation, 206
deglutition, 207
dehiscence, 259
deltoid, 117
delusion, 345
dendrite, 342
dentin, 208
deoxyribonucleic acid (DNA), 318
deposition, 250
dermatitis, 65
dermatologist, 56, 397
dermatology, 56
dermatosis, 16
dermis, 56
dermomycosis, 19
desquamation, 62, 65
diabetes insipidus, 296, 321
diabetes mellitus, 296, 321
diabetic retinopathy, 371
diagnostic radiologist, 399
dialysis, 299
dialysis technician, 402
diaphoresis, 62, 65
diaphragm, 44, 118, 179
diaphysis, 95
diarrhea, 212
diarthrosis, 93
diastole, 151
diastolic pressure, 151
diathermy, 22
diencephalon, 342
digestion, 196
dilatation, 270
dilation & curettage (D&C), 270
diminished, 362
dimorphous, 22
diplegia, 347
diplopia, 371

directional terms, 38
diskectomy, 99
dislocation, 97
disorientation, 345
dissect, 22
distal, 38, 117, 196
diuresis, 297
diuretic, 293
diverticulitis, 212
diverticulum, 212
dorsal, 38
ductus deferens, 235
dumping syndrome, 212
duodenum, 209
dura mater, 337, 342
dwarfism, 315
dysentery, 213
dyslexia, 347
dysmenorrhea, 267
dyspareunia, 267
dyspepsia, 213
dysphagia, 15, 213
dysphasia, 22, 347
dysphonia, 182
dyspnea, 182
dysrhythmia, 134
dystocia, 267
dystonia, 120
dysuria, 297

eccentric, 22
ecchymosis, 65, 155
echocardiography, 157
echogram, 157
ectocytic, 22
ectopic pregnancy, 267
ectropion, 371
eczema, 65
edema, 182
efferent, 38, 340
ejaculation, 234
electrocardiogram, 157
electrocardiography, 157
electrodesiccation, 68
electroencephalogram (EEG), 350
electrolyte, 293, 318
electromyography (EMG), 117, 350
embolus, 155
embryo, 44, 263
emergency medical technician, 401
emergency medicine physician, 398
emesis, 213
emmetropia, 368

emphysema, 182
empyema, 22, 182
encapsulated, 22
encephalitis, 347
encephalocele, 19
endarterectomy, 157
endocardial, 22
endocarditis, 134
endocarditis, acute bacterial, 154
endocardium, 151
endocervicitis, 267
endocrine glands, 310, 319
endocrinologist, 315
endocrinology, 315
endolymph, 379
endometriosis, 267
endometritis, 267
endometrium, 263
endosteum, 95
endothelium, 151
enteritis, 213
enterocele, 15
enterospasm, 19
enterostomy, 17
enucleation, 373
enuresis, 297
enzyme, 209
epicardium, 151
epidermis, 56
epidermolysis, 65
epidermophytosis, 65
epididymectomy, 239
epididymis, 235
epididymitis, 237
epidural space, 342
epigastric, 44, 144
epiglottis, 179
epilepsy, 347
epinephrine, 319
epiotic, 22
epiphora, 371
epiphysis, 95
episioplasty, 270
episiotomy, 270
epispadias, 237
epistaxis, 155, 182
epithelial, 56
equilibrium, 362
erectile tissue, 228
eructation, 207
eruption, 62
erythema, 62
erythrocyte, 134, 151

erythrocytosis, 155
erythropoiesis, 93, 151
erythropoietin, 293
esophagitis, 213
esophagus, 209
esotropia, 371
estradiol, 263
estrogen, 263
eucrasia, 23
eunuch, 234
eupnea, 178
eustachian tube, 180, 379
euthyroid, 315
eutocia, 263, 267
evaluation, 362
excoriation, 62
excretory organ, 134, 250
exhalation, 180
exocrine, 315
exocrine glands, 310
exogenous, 23
exophthalmos, exophthalmus, 321, 371
exostosis, 97
exotropia, 371
expectoration, 178
expiration, 180
exploratory laparotomy, 215
extension, 39
external, 38
external auditory meatus, 379
extrabuccal, 23
extremity, 23

fallopian tubes, 263
family practice specialist, 398
fascia, 118
fasciectomy, 122
fasciitis, 120
fascioplasty, 122
fat, 310
feces, 207
femur, 78, 95
fenestration, 381
fertilization, 259
fetus, 264
fibrillation, 120
fibroid, 16
fibroidectomy, 270
fibroma, 267
fibromyitis, 120
fibrosis, 120
fibrositis, 120
fibrous, 56

fibula, 95
filtrate, 286
filtration, 293
fimbria, 264
fissure, 62, 93
fistula, 213
flaccid, 117
flagellum, 235
flatulence, 207
flatus, 207
flexion, 39
flush, 62
focus, 362
follicle, 56, 250, 264
follicle stimulating hormone (FSH), 264
fontanelle, 93
foramen, 93
foramen magnum, 342
forensic pathology, 399
foreskin, 235
fossa, 93
fovea centralis, 369
fracture, 93
fragment, 134
friction, 170
frigidity, 259
frontal bone, 95
frontal lobe, 342
fulguration, 69
function, 32
functional, 332
fundus, 209, 264
furuncle, 66

galactorrhea, 267
gallbladder, 209
gamete, 264
ganglion, 342
ganglionectomy, 350
gangrene, 66
gastrectomy, 19, 215
gastritis, 213
gastrocele, 213
gastrocnemius, 118
gastrodynia, 15
gastroenterology, 196, 207
gastrostomy, 216
general practice, 396
genitalia, 236, 264
gestation, 260
gigantism, 321
gingivae, 209
gingivitis, 213

glans penis, 236
glaucoma, 371
glomerulonephritis, 297
glomerulus, 294
glossitis, 213
glossoplegia, 19
glossorrhaphy, 17
glottis, 180
glucagon, 317
glucocorticoid, 317
glycemia, 16
glycogen, 319
glycogenesis, 319
glyconeogenesis, 319
glycosuria, 297
goiter, 321
gonad, 228, 264
gonadotrophic hormone, 317
gonioscope, 373
gonorrhea, 239
gout, 98, 321
graafian follicle, 264
granular, 286
granulation, 62
gravida, 260
gynecology, 250, 260, 398
gynecomastia, 237, 321

habilitation, 362
halitosis, 207
hallucination, 345
harelip, 213
hearing acuity, 378
hearing impairment, 378
hematemesis, 213
hematologist, 134
hematosalpinx, 268
hematuria, 17, 297
hemianopia, 371
hemifacial, 23
hemiparesis, 347
hemiplegia, 16, 347
hemisphere, 332
hemocyte, 19
hemoglobin, 151
hemophilia, 155
hemoptysis, 149
hemorrhage, 413
hemorrhoidectomy, 216
hemorrhoids, 213
hemothorax, 182
hepatitis, 19, 213
hernia, 213

hernioplasty, 122
herniorrhaphy, 122, 216
herpes, 66
herpes genitalis, 239
herpes simplex, 213
heterosexual, 234
hiatal hernia, 214
hiccup, 207
hidradenitis, 66
hidropoiesis, 15
hilum, 295
hirsutism, 315
histotechnologist, 401
homeostasis, 44, 294, 315
homosexual, 234
hordeolum, 371
hormone, 134, 228, 310, 317
human chorionic gonadotropin (HCG), 264
humerus, 95
Huntington's chorea, 347
hyaline cast, 294
hydration, 196
hydrocele, 237
hydrocephalus, 348
hydrocortisone, 317
hydronephrosis, 297
hydrosalpinx, 268
hymen, 264
hyperactivity, 310
hypercapnia, 182
hyperesthesia, 348
hyperextension, 39
hyperglycemia, 321
hypergonadism, 321
hyperinsulinism, 322
hyperkalemia, 322
hyperkinesis, 348
hypernatremia, 322
hypernephroma, 297
hyperopia, 371
hyperplasia, 45, 66
hyperpnea, 182
hypertension, 23, 155
hyperthyroidism, 310, 322
hypertrophy, 45
hyperventilation, 178
hypnology, 341
hypoactivity, 310
hypocalcemia, 322
hypochondriac, 44
hypodipsia, 23
hypoglycemia, 322
hypoinsulinism, 322

hypophysectomy, 323
hypophysis, 319
hypoplasia, 45
hypospadias, 238
hypotension, 155
hypothalamus, 342
hypoxemia, 182
hypoxia, 178
hysterectomy, 19, 270
hysterosalpingectomy, 271
hysterosalpingo-oophorectomy, 271
hysterotomy, 271

icterus, 66, 214
identification, 32
ileitis, 214
ileum, 209
ileus, 214
iliac crest, 95
iliac fossa, 95
ilium, 95
immunity, 149
immunoglobulin, 149
impetigo, 66
impotence, 233
impulse, 332
incontinence, 214, 297
incus, 379
induration, 207
inertia, 341
infarction, 134
inferior, 38
infiltration, 178
infundibulum, 264
inguinal, 134, 207
inhalation, 180, 418
inherent, 134
inhibit, 250
innervate, 332
insertion of muscle, 110, 119
inspiration, 180
insulin, 209, 317
integument, 64
integumentary, 56
intercostal, 23
interferon, 149
intermediate, 38
internal, 38
internal medicine, 398
interstitial, 134
interventricular, 149
intervertebral, 78
intralobar, 23

intraocular, 362, 368
intrauterine, 260
introflexion, 23
intussusception, 214
inversion, 341
involuntary muscle, 119
iridectomy, 374
iridesis, iridodesis, 374
iridocyclitis, 371
iridomalacia, 371
iris, 369
iritis, 371
ischemia, 66, 134
ischium, 95
islets of Langerhans, 209, 319
isometric, 117
isotonic, 117
isthmus, 260

jaundice, 214
jejunum, 209
junction, 78, 250

keloid, 63
keratin, 56
keratitis, 371
keratometer, 373
keratoplasty, 374
keratosis, 63
ketonuria, 297
kyphosis, 94

labia, 264
labile, 424
laboratory technician, 401
labyrinth, 362, 379
labyrinthectomy, 381
labyrinthitis, 380
laceration, 63
lacrimal gland, 369
lactation, 260
lactiferous, 260
laminectomy, 98, 350
lanugo, 56
laryngectomy, 184
laryngoscopy, 183
laryngostasis, 182
larynx, 180
laser, 373
lateral, 38, 250, 286
leiomyoma, 121
lens, 369
leukemia, 156

leukocyte, 15, 135, 151
leukoderma, 66
leukoplakia, 66
leukorrhea, 268
licensed practical nurse, 401
licensed vocational nurse, 401
ligament, 95, 119, 250
lingua, 209
lingual, 178
lipid, 310, 319
lipoma, 16
lithotripsy, 18, 299
liver, 209
lobe, 180
lobectomy, 184
lobotomy, 350
lochia, 205
locomotion, 110
longitudinal, 250
lordosis, 94
lubricate, 56, 170
lumbar, 94
lumen, 151
lumpectomy, 271
lung scan, 183
lunula, 64
luteinizing hormone (LH), 265
lymph,152
lymph node, 152
lymphadenectomy, 158
lymphadenopathy, 156
lymphadenotomy, 158
lymphatics, 135
lymphocyte, 135, 152
lymphocytopenia, 156
lymphocytosis, 156
lymphoid tissue, 135
lymphoma, 156
lymphosarcoma, 156

macrocephalia, 348
macrophage, 152
macula, 63
malar, 94
malleus, 379
mammary glands, 265
mammography, 269
mammoplasty, 19, 271
mandible, 95
manubrium, 96
marrow, 78
mastectomy, 271
mastication, 196, 207

mastitis, 19, 268
maxilla, 96
meatotomy, 299
meatus, 295, 362
meconium, 265
medial, 38, 286, 362
median, 38
mediastinal, 135
mediastinum, 180
medical assistant, 402
medical technologist, 402
medical transcriptionist, 402
medulla, 94, 295, 319
medulla oblongata, 343
medullary, 78
meiosis, 44
melanin, 56
melanocyte, 56
melanoderma, 67
melanoma, 67
melatonin, 317
melena, 214
membrane, 32, 44
menarche, 260
Meniere's disease, 380
meninges, 343
meningioma, 348
meningitis, 348
meningocele, 348
meniscus, 96
menopause, 260
menorrhagia, 268
menorrhea, 265, 268
menstruation, 265
mesentery, 209
mesial, 38
mesocolon, 210
metabolism, 44, 210
metacarpus, 96
metatarsus, 96
metritis, 268
metrorrhagia, 268
microcephalus, 343
micturition, 294
milia, 63
miosis, 372
miotic, 368
mitosis, 44
mitral valve prolapse, 156
mole, 63
monocyte, 135
monoplegia, 348
mons pubis, 265

motile, 228
motility, 362
motor neuron, 334, 343
mucosa, 170
mucous membrane, 180
multipara, 260
multiple sclerosis, 121, 348
muscle, 119
muscle, voluntary, 120
muscular dystrophy, 121
myalgia, 121
myasthenia gravis, 121, 348
mycosis, 67
mydriatic, 368
myelitis, 348
myelography, 350
myeloma, 98
myitis, 121
myoatrophy, 20
myoblast, 15, 119
myocardial, 135
myocardium, 110, 152
myoclonus, 121
myodiastasis, 121
myoedema, 121
myofibroma, 121
myogenesis, 15
myoid, 117
myokymia, 121
myology, 110, 117
myolysis, 121
myoma, 121
myomalacia, 121
myometritis, 268
myometrium, 265
myopathy, 121
myopia, 372
myoplasty, 123
myorrhaphy, 123
myorrhexis, 121
myosarcoma, 122
myosclerosis, 122
myositis, 122
myospasm, 122
myotasis, 117
myotome, 117
myotomy, 123
myotonia, 122
myotrophy, 118
myringodectomy, 381
myringoplasty, 381
myxedema, 322

narcolepsy, 348
nares, 180
nasogastric tube, 20
nasopharynx, 180
nausea, 214
necrosis, 78
neonatal, 260
neonatologist, 399
nephrectomy, 299
nephritis, 297
nephrolithiasis, 297
nephron, 297
nephropathy, 297
nephropexy, 299
nephroptosis, 20, 297
nephrosclerosis, 297
nephrotomy, 18
nerve tract, 343
neuralgia, 348
neurasthenia, 345
neurectomy, 20, 351
neuritis, 349
neuroglia, 343
neurohypophysis, 319
neurologist, 341, 398
neurology, 338
neurolysis, 351
neuromuscular, 118
neuron, 343
neurosis, 349
neurosurgeon, 398, 400
neurotransmitter, 343
nevus, 63
nitrogenous waste, 294
nocturia, 297
node, 135
nodule, 67
norepinephrine, 317
nostrils, 56
nucleus, 44
nullipara, 260
nurse practitioner, 401
nursing assistant, 401
nutrient, 135
nutrition, 56
nyctalopia, 372
nystagmus, 372

obsession, 345
obstetrics, 250, 260, 398
occipital bone, 96
occipital lobe, 343
occlusion, 156

occupational therapist, 402
oculogyric, 20
oligomenorrhea, 268
oligospermia, 238
oliguria, 297
oncologist, 135
onychia, 67
oocyte, 265
oogenesis, 265
oophorectomy, 271
opaque, 362
ophthalmia, 20
ophthalmologist, 368
ophthalmology, 368, 398
optic disk, 369
optic nerve, 369
optician, 368
optometrist, 368
oral, 178
orbit, 369
orchiectomy, 239
orchiopexy, 17, 239
orchitis, 238
orgasm, 234
orifice, 170, 260
origin of muscle, 110, 119
oronasal, 20
orthopedic surgeon, 400
orthopnea, 182
orthoptics, 368
ossicle, 379
ostectomy, 98
osteectopia, 20
osteoarthritis, 98
osteology, 78
osteoma, 98
osteomalacia, 98
osteoplasty, 98
osteotomy, 98
otalgia, 20, 380
otitis media, 380
otodynia, 380
otolaryngologist, 378
otolaryngology, 398
otology, 378
otomycosis, 380
otopharyngeal, 379
otoplasty, 17, 381
otosclerosis, 380
otoscope, 381
oval window, 379
ovary, 265
oviduct, 265

ovulation, 265
ovum, 265
oxygenation, 135
oxytocin, 317

pacemaker, 152
palate, 180, 210
pallor, 63
palmar, 38
palpation, 152, 207
palpitation, 152
palsy, 349
pancreas, 319
panhysterectomy, 271
Papanicolaou test, 269
papilla, 295
papilledema, 349
papule, 67
paracentesis, 216
paralysis, 122, 349
paramedian, 23
paranasal, 170, 178
paranoia, 345
paraphimosis, 238
paraplasm, 23
paraplegia, 349
parasympathetic, 341
parathormone, 318
parathyroid gland, 319
parathyroidectomy, 323
parenchyma, 295
parenteral, 207
paresis, 349
paresthesia, 349
parietal, 94, 149, 178, 286
parietal lobe, 343
paronychia, 67
parotid, 207
parturient, 260
parturition, 261
passive movement, 118
patella, 96
pathogen, 149
pathology, 14
pectoralis, 119
pediculosis, 67
pemphigus, 67
penis, 236
percussion, 178
pericardial, 32
pericardiectomy, 158
pericarditis, 135, 156
pericardium, 135, 152

perilymph, 379
perimetrium, 266
perineum, 236, 266
periosteum, 96
peripheral, 38, 362
peripheral nervous system (PNS), 344
perisplenic, 23
peristalsis, 110, 196, 210, 286
peritoneum, 286
perpetuate, 228
perspiration, 56
pertussis, 182
petechiae, 67
pH, 294
phacolysis, 374
phacosclerosis, 372
phagocytosis, 45
phalanx, 96
pharyngeal, 20
pharyngitis, 214
pharynx, 181
phenylketonuria, 297
pheochromocytoma, 322
phimosis, 238
phlebitis, 156
phlebosclerosis, 156
phlebostenosis, 20
phlebotomy, 158
phobia, 345
photophobia, 372
physiatrist, 399
physical therapist, 402
physician assistant, 396
physiology, 14, 32
pia mater, 344
pigment, 63, 250
pineal body, 319
pinkeye, 372
pinna, 380
pinocytosis, 45
pituitary gland, 320
placenta, 266
plane, 32
planes, 34
plantar, 38, 64
plasma, 152
plastic and reconstructive surgeon, 400
plethora, 135
plethysmograph, 135
pleura, 181
pleural, 32
pleurisy, 183
pleurodynia, 183

pneumatosis, 20
pneumectomy, 20
pneumocentesis, 184
pneumoconiosis, 183
pneumoencephalography, 350
pneumonectomy, 184
pneumonia, 183
pneumothorax, 183
poliomyelitis, 349
polydipsia, 214, 322
polyemia, 268
polyphagia, 322
polyuria, 298
pons, 344
popliteal, 119
pore, 64
posterior, 38
postpartum, 261
postprandial, 23
posture, 118
potential, 170
precostal, 23
prenatal, 261
prepuce, 236
presbycusis, 380
presbyopia, 372
preventive medicine, 399
prime mover, 119
primipara, 261
procidentia, 268
proctitis, 214
proctocele, 21, 32
progesterone, 266
projection, 78
prolapse, 250, 268
pronation, 39
propagation, 228
propel, 135
prostatalgia, 238
prostate, 236
prostatectomy, 240
prostatitis, 238
prostatomegaly, 238
protein, 310
protoplasm, 45
protrusion, 23, 362
proximal, 38, 118, 196
pruritus, 67, 214
pseudocyesis, 268
psoriasis, 67
psychiatrist, 399
psychiatry, 338
psychosis, 345

psychosomatic, 341, 345
pterygium, 372
puberty, 228, 235, 261
pubic, 45, 94
pudendum, 266
puerpera, 261
puerperium, 261
pulmonary function test, 184
pulse, 152
pulse pressure, 153
pupil, 369
Purkinje fiber, 153
purpura, 67
purulent, 63, 415
pustule, 67
pyelitis, 298
pyelogram, 298
pyelolithotomy, 299
pyelonephritis, 298
pyeloplasty, 299
pyloric stenosis, 214
pylorospasm, 214
pylorus, 210
pyorrhea, 17, 215
pyosalpinx, 269
pyrexia, 215
pyrosis, 215
pyuria, 298

quadriceps, 118
quadriplegia, 349

radiation therapy technologist, 402
radical mastectomy, 271
radiculitis, 349
radiographer, 402
radius, 96
rales, 183
receptor, 64, 362
rectocele, 269
reflect, 135
reflected, 24
reflex, 110, 341
reflux, 294
refracted, 362
region, 32
registered nurse, 400
regurgitation, 207
rehabilitation, 362
relaxation, 118
renal corpuscle, 295
renal cortex, 295
renal pelvis, 295

renal pyramids, 295
renal sinus, 295
renal transplantation, 299
renal tubules, 295
renal veins, 295
renin, 296, 320
reproduction, 228
reservoir, 196, 286
residual urine, 294
resonant, 179
respiration, 170, 181
respiratory, 135
respiratory therapist, 402
respiratory therapy technician, 402
retina, 369
retinitis pigmentosa, 372
retinoblastoma, 372
retinopathy, 372
retrocecal, 24
retroflexion, 261
retroversion, 261
Reye's syndrome, 349
rheumatoid arthritis, 98
rhinitis, 20, 183
rhinoplasty, 184
rhinorrhagia, 16
rhinorrhea, 183
rhizotomy, 351
rhythmic, 135, 196
rigor mortis, 118, 122
rods, 370
rotation, 118
rotation, lateral, 39
rotation, medial, 39
Rubin's test, 269
rugae, 266

sacrum, 96
saliva, 210
salpingectomy, 271
salpingitis, 269
salpingo-oophorectomy, 271
sanguineous, 149
scabies, 67
scapula, 96
sciatic, 341
sciatica, 349
sclera, 370
scleritis, 372
scleroderma, 68
scoliosis, 94
scrotum, 236
sebaceous, 57, 250

seborrhea, 68
sebum, 57
secretory, 250
secundines, 266
segment, 181
sella turcica, 320
semen, 236
semicircular canals, 380
semilunar, 24, 149
seminal vesicle, 236
seminiferous tubules, 236
sensorium, 344
sensory neuron, 334, 344
septectomy, 184
septum, 135, 149, 181
sequestrum, 94
serosanguineous, 149
serum, 153
sheath, 332
shin splints, 122
shock, 332
sigmoid, 210
silicosis, 183
Simmond's disease, 322
singultus, 208
sinoatrial node, 153
sinus, 170, 181
sinus rhythm, 153
Skene's glands, 296
slough, 57
Snellen's chart, 373
somatotropin, 318
spasm, 122
spasticity, 122
spermatocele, 238
spermatogenesis, 236
spermatozoa, 236
spermaturia, 235
spermicide, 235
sphincter, 119
spinal, 341
spinal cord, 344
spiral, 250
spleen, 153
splenectomy, 21, 158
splenitis, 156
splenomalacia, 16
splenomegaly, 156
splenotomy, 158
spondylosis, 98
spondylosyndesis, 351
sprain, 98
stapedectomy, 381

stapes, 380
steatoma, 68
stereoscopic, 362
sterility, 261
sterilization, 240
sternum, 78, 96
steroid hormone, 310, 318
stertor, 179
stimulant, 310
stomach, 210
stomatitis, 20
strabismus, 372
striated, 118
striated muscle, 119
structural, 332
structure, 32
sty(e), 372
subarachnoid space, 344
subclavian, 135
subcostal, 208
subcutaneous, 57, 250
subdural space, 344
subjacent, 24
sublingual, 208
subluxation, 98
submandibular, 208
sudoriferous, 57
sulcus, 94
superficial, 38
superflexion, 24
superior, 38
supination, 39
supraocular, 24
surgery, 14
sympathectomy, 351
sympathetic, 341
symphysis pubis, 97, 266
synapse, 344
syncope, 350
syndactylism, 98
syndactyly, 24
synergist, 118
synovia, 119
syphilis, 239
systole, 153
systolic pressure, 153

tachycardia, 136, 156
tachypnea, 183
talipes, 98
tarsus, 97
temperature, 57
temporal bone, 97

temporal lobe, 344
tendinitis, 122
tendolysis, 123
tendon, 110, 119
tenodesis, 123
tenodynia, 122
tenolysis, 123
tenoplasty, 123
tenosynovitis, 122
testicle, 236
testis, 237
testosterone, 237
tetany, 322
thalamus, 344
therapeutic radiology, 399
thoracentesis, 184
thoracic, 45
thoracic surgeon, 400
thoracotomy, 21, 184
thorax, 83
thrombophlebitis, 156
thrombus, 156
thymectomy, 158, 323
thymitis, 157
thymus gland, 153
thyroidectomy, 323
thyroiditis, 323
thyrotoxicosis, 323
thyroxine, 318
tibia, 97
tinea, 68
tinnitus, 380
tissues, 34
tongue, 211
tonography, 373
tonometry, 373
tonus, 119
torticollis, 122
toxic shock syndrome (TSS), 269
trachea, 181
tracheloplasty, 271
tracheostenosis, 183
tracheostomy, 184
tracheotomy, 184
trachoma, 372
transection, 24
transparent, 363
transurethral resection of the prostate
        (TURP), 240
transverse, 45
trephination, 351
trichiasis, 373
Trichomonas, 261

trichomoniasis, 239
tricuspid, 149
trigone, 296
triiodothyronine, 318
trimester, 262
tripod, 24
trochanter, 97
tunica adventitia, 136, 153
tunica intima, 136, 153
tunica media, 136, 153
tympanic membrane, 380
tympanoplasty, 381

ulcer, 68, 215
ulna, 97
ultraviolet, 24, 57
umbilical, 45
umbilical cord, 266
unipara, 262
urea, 296
uremia, 298
ureter, 296
ureterocele, 298
ureterography, 21
urethra, 237, 296
urethritis, 21, 298
uric acid, 296
urinalysis, 299
urinary bladder, 296
urinary retention, 298
urinary stress incontinence, 298
urologic surgeon, 400
urologist, 294
urology, 294
uropathy, 16, 298
urticaria, 68
uterine tube, 266
uteroplasty, 21
uterus, 266
uvea, 370
uveitis, 373
uvula, 211

vaccine, 150
vagina, 266
vaginitis, 269
vaginoperineotomy, 271
vagotomy, 216, 351
valve, 154
valvotomy, 158
varicocele, 238
varicose vein, 157
vas deferens, 237

vascular, 363
vascular technologist, 403
vasectomy, 240
vasoconstriction, 157
vasodilation, 158
vasopressin, 318
vein, 154
venipuncture, 158
venography, 157
ventral, 38
ventrally, 250
ventricle, 136, 154, 344
venule, 154
vernix caseosa, 266
version, 262
vertebra, 97

vertigo, 380
vesical, 294
vesication, 63
vesicle, 68, 228, 294
vesiculitis, 238
vestibule, 266
vibrations, 363
virilism, 323
viscera, 110
visceral, 118, 150
viscosity, 150
viscus, 211
visual acuity, 368
vitreous humor, 370
void, 294

vomiting, 215
vulva, 267

wart, 68
wheal, 68
Wilms' tumor, 298
wound, 63

xanthoma, 68
xeroderma, 63
xerophthalmia, 373
xerosis, 63
xiphoid, 97

zygote, 267